Critical Factors
in Cancer
Immunology

MIAMI WINTER SYMPOSIA

MIAMI WINTER SYMPOSIA - VOLUME 10

Critical Factors in Cancer Immunology

edited by
J. Schultz
R. C. Leif

PAPANICOLAOU CANCER RESEARCH INSTITUTE
MIAMI, FLORIDA

Proceedings of the Miami Symposia, January 13-17, 1975
Sponsored by The Papanicolaou Cancer Research Institute
Miami, Florida

Academic Press, Inc.   New York   San Francisco   London 1975

A Subsidiary of Harcourt Brace Jovanovich, Publishers

ACADEMIC PRESS, INC.
111 Fifth Avenue, New York, New York 10003

United Kingdom Edition published by
ACADEMIC PRESS, INC. (LONDON) LTD.
24/28 Oval Road, London NW1

Library of Congress Cataloging in Publication Data
Main entry under title:

Critical factors in cancer immunology.

(Miami winter symposia ; v. 9)
Bibliography: p.
Includes index.
1.   Cancer—Immunological aspects—Congresses.
I.   Schultz, Julius, (date)   II.   Leif, R. C.
III.   Papanicolaou Cancer Research Institute.   IV.   Se-
ries.   [DNLM: 1.   Neoplasms.   2.   Immunology—Con-
gresses.   W3 M1202 v. 9 1975 / QZ200 C934 1975]
RC261.A1C74   616.9'94'079   74-27790
ISBN 0−12−632740−8

PRINTED IN THE UNITED STATES OF AMERICA

CONTENTS

Free Communications

CONTENTS

SPEAKERS, CHAIRMEN, AND DISCUSSANTS

P. Alexander (Session Chairman), Chester Beatty Research Institute, Belmont, Sutton, Surrey, England

D. Axler, Battelle Memorial Institute, Columbus, Ohio

F.H. Bach, University of Wisconsin, Madison, Wisconsin

B. Becker, Purdue University, Fort Wayne, Indiana

C. Bell, University of Illinois, Chicago, Illinois

R. Bollinger, Duke University, Durham, North Carolina

Z. Brada, Papanicolaou Cancer Research Institute, Miami, Florida

B. Cameron, Papanicolaou Cancer Research Institute, Miami, Florida

C. Chang, Tufts University School of Medicine, Boston, Massachusetts

R. Citrobaum, University of California, Los Angeles, Los Angeles, California

M. Cohn (Session Chairman), Salk Institute for Biological Studies, San Diego, California

G.M. Edelman (Session Chairman), Rockefeller University, New York, New York

E.G. Elias, State University of New York, Buffalo, New York

E. Farber, Fels Research Institute, Temple University, Philadelphia Pennsylvania

N. Felberg, Wills Eye Hospital and Research Institute, Philadelphia Pennsylvania

H.H. Fudenberg, University of California School of Medicine, San Francisco, California

R.K. Gershon, Yale University, New Haven, Connecticut

A. Ghaffar, University of Edinburgh, Edinburgh, Scotland

A.L. Goldstein, University of Texas, Galveston, Texas

L.J. Greenberg, University of Minnesota Medical School, Minneapolis, Minnesota

E. Harber, Harvard Medical School, Boston, Massachusetts

R. Hard, Medical College of Virginia, Richmond, Virginia

K.E. Hellstrom, University of Washington, Seattle, Washington

L.A. Herzenberg, Stanford University School of Medicine, Stanford, California

R. Hiramoto, University of Alabama, Birmingham, Alabama

V. Janson, College of Medicine and Dentistry of New Jersey, Newark, New Jersey

E.A. Kabat, Columbia University, New York, New York

E. Klein (Session Chairman), Karolinska Institute, Stockholm, Sweden

G.M. Kollmorgen, Oklahoma Medical Research Foundation, Oklahoma City, Oklahoma

E.W. Lamon, University of Alabama, Birmingham, Alabama

H.S. Lawrence, New York University School of Medicine, New York, New York

R.C. Leif, Papanicolaou Cancer Research Institute, Miami, Florida

E.L. Lloyd, Argonne National Laboratory, Argonne, France

D.M. Lopez, University of Miami Medical School, Miami, Florida

P. Maurer, Jefferson Medical College, Philadelphia, Pennsylvania

L. Muschel, American Cancer Society, New York, New York

A. Nisonoff, University of Illinois, College of Medicine, Chicago, Illinois

R.E. Parks, Jr., Brown University, Providence, Rhode Island

T. Pretlow, University of Alabama Medical Center, Alabama

F.W. Putnam, Indiana University, Bloomington, Indiana

E. Revoltella, Central Nationale Research, Rome, Italy

G. Schiffman, State University of New York, Brooklyn, New York

I. Schenkein, New York University, New York, New York

M.R. Schinitsky, Eli Lilly and Company, Indianapolis, Indiana

J. Schultz, Papanicolaou Cancer Research Institute, Miami, Florida

M. Sela, Weizmann Institute of Science, Rehovot, Israel

M.M. Sigel, University of Miami School of Medicine, Miami, Florida

E.L. Springer, University of California, Berkeley, California

M. Teodorescu, University of Illinois, Chicago, Illinois

W.D. Terry, National Cancer Institute, Bethesda, Maryland

J.T. Thornthwaite, Papanicolaou Cancer Research Institute, Miami, Florida

G. Warchalowski, Rutgers—The State University, New Brunswick, New Jersey

A White, Syntex Research, Palo Alto and Stanford School of Medicine, Stanford, California

H. Whitten, University of Alabama, Birmingham, Alabama

PREFACE

This volume devoted to cancer immunology includes a series of reports presented at the Seventh Miami Winter Symposia following the presentation organized by the Biochemistry Department of the University of Miami Medical School. That session opened with an address by Nobel Laureate G. Edelman. One could not help but muse about the happening in Justrus Van Liebig's Laboratory shortly after 1839 when Mulder, who worked there, had just coined the word "protein." It was then that he received a visit from Dr. Bence-Jones. Dr. Bence-Jones hearing of this new class of compounds brought to Mulder for examination a sample of urine from a patient with bone cancer (Multiple Myeloma). The substance found therein was like the albuminous material from blood serum, wheat glutin, and other natural substances of a similar nature. Thus Bence-Jones protein came into being. The finding that this was part of the myeloma protein and thence to the structure of gammaglobulins over 100 years later laid the quantitative organic structural basis that placed immunology on a molecular level. With Drs. Putnam and Milstein and others developing the primary sequences, the genetic relationships of gammaglobulin further tightened up this area of biochemistry in a rapid fashion. Now in these volumes one finds the clinical, biological, physiological, and genetic consequences. As a result of those discoveries, an entirely new level of interrelationships, highly specialized, yet interdisciplinary was reached, so as to establish a new discipline.

Most affected by the burst of new knowledge is progress in the immunological interpretation of the cancer problem. The immune system is probably responsible for both the initial immunosurveillance which eliminates the nascent cancer cells before they can develop into tumors and also is responsible for the final elimination of residual tumor cells after the tumor mass has been greatly reduced by surgery and/or chemotherapy. Conversely the immune response may be, in part, responsible for metastasis by circulating tumor cells via the lymphatics. The underlying immunophilosophical tenet of this Miami Winter Symposia was that the immune response was multifaceted and particularly the duality of T and B cell response was, as are almost all good models in science, an oversimplification. It has been well known that B cells were involved in the production of the various classes of immunoglobulins, usually one at a time; although there were those cells which "would rather switch than fight" (H. Fudenberg, this volume). In the case of T cells, the concept of suppressor cells was one of the major themes so that at least helper and suppressor cells exist to modulate immunoglobulin synthesis and recognition and cytotoxic effector cells exist for cell killing. Evidently the various stages of development of these T cells are controlled by thymosin and specificity can be imparted by transfer factor. In addition to all of this, the macrophage or possibly the macrophages, are doing everything from processing antigen as the efferent end of the immune response to actually killing tumor cells. In short we are finding out that there is more to immunology than was contained in any of our immunophilosophies.

Lastly, it is suggested to the reader that he or she acquire the companion volume to this series since the subject matter of the meeting overlaps in the two books.

J. Schultz
R. C. Leif

ACKNOWLEDGMENTS

Acknowledgment is made here to Abbott Laboratories, Boehringer Mannehim Corporation, Eli Lilly, Hoffmann-La Roche, and The Upjohn Company for their financial contributions. The editors wish also to thank Dr. Karl E. Hellstrom of the University of Washington and Dr. Frank Putnam of the Indiana University for suggesting participants for the Symposia. Special recognition is due to Miss Pat Bell and her girls in the "boiler room" who transcribed the discussions and worked so hard to follow up the edited comments to be included in time for the publication.

STRUCTURE AND FUNCTION OF IMMUNOGLOBULINS

F. W. PUTNAM
Department of Zoology
Indiana University   Bloomington, Ind.

Abstract: Structural study of Bence Jones proteins and myeloma globulins has led the way to molecular immunology
and to many practical applications in clinical and cellular immunology. The principles of immunoglobulin
structure are now established, and the relationship to
antibody specificity is being elucidated. However, many
questions on the genetic control of antibody diversity
and on the mechanism of other biological activities of
immunoglobulins are still unanswered. To solve these
problems continued comparative structural study of immunoglobulins is needed with special emphasis on iso-
types and allotypes and on rare variants, especially
those giving evidence of deletions or other genetic
aberrations.

INTRODUCTION

Few advances have had such a profound impact on the
development of a science as determination of the structure
of Bence Jones proteins and of myeloma globulins has had on
the transformation of classical immunology to the "new
immunology."

The preceding papers bear witness to this. Both at the
molecular level and at the cellular level, knowledge of immunoglobulin structure has destroyed old myths and led to new
concepts, much in the way that the DNA helix led to a revolu-
tion in modern genetics and molecular biology. But unlike
the case of the DNA helix where solution of the structure of
DNA led to the cracking of the genetic code and the under-

standing of the mechanism of protein biosynthesis, the answer to the antibody problem has not yet been found. Nonetheless, we can identify many advances in immunochemistry, immunobiology, immunogenetics, and immunopathology that are directly attributable to the new knowledge of immunoglobulin structure. Examples include the nature of the antibody combining site and antibody variation, theories for the generation of antibody diversity, the nature of cell surface receptors and antigen recognition, evolution and mutation of immunoglobulin genes and the diversity of genes coding for antibodies, structural relationships between antibodies and histocompatibility antigens, and restriction of clonal responses as a model for understanding differentiation. All of these are subjects covered by preceding speakers. None of these advances deal directly with cancer immunology, though some are undoubtedly critical to further understanding of the cancer problem.

So often it is said that to learn more about the abnormal, one must study the normal, but here we have a case in reverse. Study of a special type of tumor, one involving the antibody-forming cells, has taught us more about the normal than about cancer. Table I lists some of the results, research tools, and practical applications that have been derived from basic research on Bence Jones proteins, myeloma globulins, and pathological macroglobulins. The first three listed are directly applicable to study of the myeloma patient and to quantitative evaluation of the aberrations in protein metabolism in this group of lymphomatous diseases. The next four are the basis for our understanding of the relationship between immunoglobulin structure and antibody diversity, and the problems posed for the genetic control of antibody variability and the nature of the combining site. Among the practical applications has been the development of class-specific antisera for the detection and quantitation of immunoglobulins in many diseases and also for cellular localization of antibodies and identification of immunoglobulin surface receptors on lymphocytes. The applications for immunogenetics are just beginning, but the significance of IgE for allergy is now well appreciated. One of the recent advances is the identification of light chains and light chain fragments as the paramyloid protein causing primary amyloidosis. Still to be fully elucidated are the nature of autoimmune reactions and the binding site of complement. The unknown areas include the conformational changes undergone on complement binding, and the question whether conformational changes in one's own immunoglobulins may expose hidden antigenic sites that are

2

TABLE 1

Results, research tools and practical applications derived from basic research on Bence Jones proteins, myeloma globulins and macroglobulins.

1. Clinical test for Bence Jones proteinuria in the diagnosis of multiple myeloma. Modification of the heat test.
2. Elucidation of the aberration of protein synthesis in multiple myeloma, macroglobulinemia and related diseases.
3. Identification of kappa and lambda light chains in normal immunoglobulins. Quantitation in normal immunoglobulins.
4. Classification of normal "gamma globulin" into IgG, IgA, IgM, IgD and IgE. Quantitation of normal abundance.
5. Principles of structure of antibodies.
6. Amino acid sequence diversity of antibodies and immunoglobulins. Theories of genetic control of antibody biosynthesis.
7. Models for X-ray analysis of antibody binding sites.
8. Antisera for detection and quantitation of Ig types in hypergammaglobulinemia in many diseases and in hereditary hypogammaglobulinemia and agammaglobulinemias.
9. Antisera for routine quantitation of Ig types in plasma proteins by automated immunoprecipitation.
10. Antisera for cellular localization of antibodies.
11. Antisera for detection of surface receptors on immunocytes for study of antibody biosynthesis.
12. Immunogenetics--discovery of genetic differences in immunoglobulins of possible value in transfusion reactions and organ transplantation.
13. Immunogenetics--applications to population genetics, forensic medicine and evolution of immunoglobulins.
14. Discovery of normal IgE and its function as the skin-sensitizing antibody. Quantitative RIA and RAST tests.
15. Identification of Bence Jones protein as the paramyloid protein causing primary amyloidosis.
16. Nature of antibody-mediated autoimmune reactions, e.g., rheumatoid factor IgM as the antibody to IgG.
17. Binding site of complement. Conformational changes.
18. Cellular system for study of mutation and clonal variation.
19. Subcellular study of protein biosynthesis and mutation.
20. Animal and cellular models for clonal restriction and cellular differentiation.

erroneously recognized as "foreign," leading to autoimmune responses. The myeloma protein system will prove invaluable in investigation of the etiological basis of both acute and chronic autoimmune diseases. To this list must be added examples of the increasing importance of the myeloma cell system as a tool for genetic research, so well exemplified by earlier papers and discussion in this Symposium.

Although the cellular and subcellular myeloma systems and the induced animal myelomas are now providing us with new experimental tools, it was the myeloma patient, the unfortunate experiment of nature, who provided the first clues to the principles of structure of immunoglobulins and the aberrations of structure in disease. The patient is not just a factory for producing proteins invaluable to the biochemist and immunologist. He is a person dying because of a perversion of his immunological defenses and a shunting of the pathway of antibody biosynthesis to the production of enormous amounts of a protein unique to himself. Often the excess of this protein exacerbates his problems because of its peculiar physicochemical properties, which may cause some of the symptoms of the disease.

Fig. 1 illustrates what I have called the "plasma cell shunt" (1). This is the neoplastic transformation of normal antibody-mediated immunity into a malignant plasmacytoma. We do not know whether the transformation of normal B lymphocytes into a monoclonal plasma cell tumor is induced by a carcinogen or a virus. In the case of susceptible inbred mouse strains the putative transforming agent need not be a unique chemical carcinogen or oncogenic virus; it may be an unusually active immunostimulant acting at the B cell level. However, there is also usually a progressive loss of T cell function in myeloma patients. Everything seems to be telling us that the transformation is occurring at the genetic level, that is, at the DNA level. The individual shunting is one of the most characteristic signs of this disease with respect to the natural history of the tumor development. The cardinal sign is given by the motto: E pluribus unum. One cell of many becomes the founder of the malignant clone-- a clone in which there has been a unique event, the repression of the vast genome for the normal repertoire of immunoglobulins and derepression of just one set of Ig genes specific for a unique amino acid sequence. This suggests that the inducing agent doesn't trigger the cancer by interaction with an antibody-like receptor on the plasma cell analogous to antigen-induced blast formation and antibody production. Else, there would

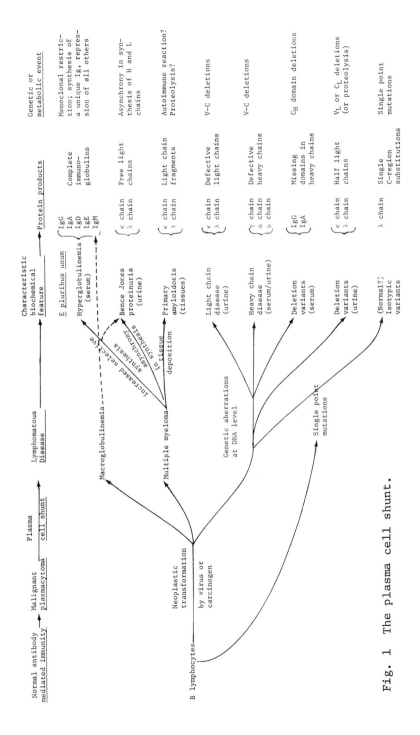

Fig. 1 The plasma cell shunt.

have to be a different carcinogenic agent or a different oncogenic virus for each myeloma patient, for each patient
produces a unique antibody-like protein. The critical event
is the shunt, and the shunt has to be associated with the
integration of a carcinogen or viral product into the genome
of the founder cell.

The three principal protein aberrations in the disease
are hyperglobulinemia, Bence Jones proteinuria (sometimes
called light chain disease), and primary amyloidosis resulting
from the deposition of light chains or light chain fragments
in the tissues(2). A patient may have any one, two or all
three of these errors. There are rarer examples of the
formation of defective proteins that we may call deletion
variants; these are proving very instructive for understanding aberrations at the genetic level of protein biosynthesis.
The protein products may be a complete immunoglobulin of any
one of the five classes, but always one with a sequence
unique for the patient (3,4). The product may be a Bence
Jones protein or free light chain of either the κ or λ type,
but again one of a unique sequence, or a fragment of a light
chain, or a free heavy chain with a large deletion. The
remarkable thing is that each patient produces his own protein. This tells us immediately that although the disease
may have similar clinical symptoms in all or most of the
patients, the transformation of the tumor cell has struck at
a different site-- albeit the site is always at the level of
genetic control of immunoglobulin biosynthesis.

The myeloma proteins were at first thought to be abnormal proteins characteristic of a tumor. The big puzzle was
first the unique physicochemical and antigenic individuality
-- the idiotypy of these proteins, and later the fact that
each myeloma globulin or Bence Jones protein had an amino
acid sequence unique for the patient (3,4). The myeloma
proteins are now regarded as normal members of the immunoglobulin family of antibodies. Each myeloma protein may be
regarded as a random sample of the unending variety of normal
antibodies; a collection of a thousand myeloma globulins
would closely simulate normal pooled gamma globulin. Indeed,
the frequency of the five different classes of immunoglobulins and of the two kinds of light chains closely parallels
the natural abundance of each class in normal pooled immunoglobulins.

In discussing the myeloma proteins as models for study
of antibody structure it is customary to emphasize the homo-

geneity of the pathological globulin and the relative ease of sequencing compared to the normal potpourri of immunoglobulins. I have chosen to emphasize the infinite variety produced, although each is individual for the patient. The genetic and metabolic events involve not only monoclonal restriction of synthesis of a unique Ig and repression of all others, but sometimes an asynchrony of synthesis of heavy and light chains. There are also examples of defective proteins where the defects seem to involve translocation errors in the genes. Isn't it probable that the myeloma cell system is just mirroring the random breakdown of normal processes and that the rate of random breakdown is reflected by the proportion of patients that produce defective proteins? If so, the myeloma system offers a unique opportunity to study degenerative errors in protein biosynthesis. Perhaps some of these errors are a reflection of the aging process because the average onset or at least time of detection of multiple myeloma in man is around age 65. This, too, suggests the need for development of much more sensitive methods to enable earlier detection of the disease at the stage of a solitary myeloma when it can be cured. This is one of the objectives towards which our research at the molecular and cellular level of cancer immunology should be directed.

PRINCIPLES OF IMMUNOGLOBULIN STRUCTURE

With this introduction of the relationship of our studies to cancer immunology, we can next consider the principles of immunoglobulin structure. These will be presented in broad view, rather than in exquisite detail of the latest results of our laboratory. The intention is to identify current problems and future directions of research. Because of the enormous amount of sequence data available, it is most instructive to present the principles with schematic figures rather than in detail.

The essential characteristics of immunoglobulin structure and the general relationship of immunoglobulin structure to antibody specificity are now largely established through complete amino acid sequence analysis of human Bence Jones proteins and myeloma globulins. From partial structural studies on myeloma proteins from the mouse and on purified animal antibodies, the findings have been generalized to give a comprehensive classification of immunoglobulins that is believed to apply throughout the vertebrate world. These principles are summarized in Fig. 2. This shows schematically the basic tetrapolypeptide chain structure of the monomer-

7

Number of Amino Acid Residues

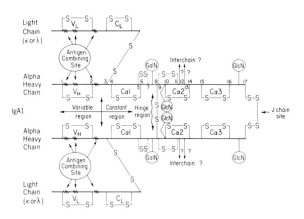

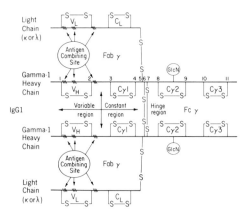

Fig. 2

8

ic units of the three major classes of human immunoglobulins: IgM, IgA, and IgG. The structure for IgM is based upon the complete sequence analysis by Putnam et al. (5), that for IgA is assembled from the tentative unpublished sequence of our laboratory (6,7), and that for IgG from data of other workers (8,9). For each immunoglobulin the tetrachain structure consists of a pair of heavy chains disulfide-bonded to a pair of light chains. The heavy chains are so-called because they have a molecular weight of 50,000 to 70,000, whereas the light chains have a molecular weight of about 23,000. The class of immunoglobulin is determined by the nature of the heavy chain (μ for IgM, α for IgA, and γ for IgG), but a molecule of any class may have a pair of identical light chains of either the κ or the γ type though not a hybrid mixture. There is an overall homology in structure among the heavy chains, of the order of 30-35%, but they differ individually in primary sequence, carbohydrate content, antigenic determinants and even in size.

There are two types of light chains, κ and λ. These are homologous to each other and have about 40% identity in amino acid sequence. Light chains are almost equally homologous to heavy chains with which they share about 30% identity in sequence. As shown by the scale in Fig. 2, all heavy and light chains are divided into homologous units or domains of about 110 amino acids in length, each of which contains an intrachain disulfide loop enclosing some 60 amino acids. It is thus obvious that there is a fundamental structural relationship among heavy and light chains, bespeaking evolutionary development from an ancestral gene coding for about 110 amino acid residues.

Polypeptide chain formulas may be written for each class of immunoglobulin, for example, $\kappa_2\gamma_2$ or $\lambda_2\gamma_2$ for IgG, which is a monomeric unit with a molecular weight of approximately 160,000 or $(\kappa_2\mu_2)_n$ and $(\lambda_2\mu_2)_n$ for IgM, where n is five because IgM is a pentamer of about one million molecular weight. In myeloma globulins, and as far as we know in normal immunoglobulins also, hybrid molecules are not formed in which the pairs of light chains or of heavy chains are non-identical. Except possibly in some antibodies there seems to be no preferential association of one kind of light chain with any kind of heavy chain. However, this needs further investigation. In IgA myeloma globulins our work and that of Capra et al. (10) indicates a high frequency of α chains with an uncommon subgroup of λ chains.

9

The three major classes of immunoglobulins depicted in Fig. 2 as well as the two minor classes IgD and IgE, which are not shown, are all made by healthy individuals. Because there are subclasses and allotypes of some of these, and many idiotypes of each, the number of different immunoglobulin molecules or antibodies that any healthy individual can make ranges in the thousands. Yet, in multiple myeloma or macroglobulinemia, a single one of these is selected for massive synthesis to the virtual exclusion of all others. Bence Jones protein is identical in structure to the light chain of the myeloma globulin or macroglobulin produced by the patient and is representative of normal light chains of either the κ or the λ type. The solution to the structure of immunoglobulins and thus of antibodies began with the complete amino acid sequence analysis of Bence Jones proteins in our laboratory (11,12).

Each chain is divided into a variable or V region comprising the first 110-120 amino acid residues at the amino terminus and into a constant or C region that defines the class of the chain and comprises the remainder of it. Each chain is also made up of a series of homology regions or domains containing about 110 amino acid residues, of which about half are enclosed in an intrachain disulfide loop. There are two such domains in both κ and λ light chains, four in γ and α heavy chains, and five in the μ chain. The variable regions are designated V_L and V_H for the heavy and light chains, respectively. The domains in the C region are numbered with reference to the chains, e.g., $C\mu1$ to $C\mu4$ for the μ chain. The homology of light and heavy chains creates strong interactions which determine the three-dimensional structure. The interaction of the V regions determines the combining site.

Fig. 2 also illustrates that an antibody molecule in its monomeric form has two identical combining sites. The site is largely shaped by interaction of the three hypervariable segments in the V regions of both the light and heavy chains. These are designated by the arrows in Fig. 2-- two near the half-cystine residues and one in the middle of the loop. The IgM molecule may undergo limited cleavage by trypsin or other proteolytic enzymes to form two kinds of fragments with different biological properties, namely an Fab piece that is univalent with respect to antigen and retains specific combining ability and an Fc piece that has other biological properties but no antibody specificity. The Fab fragment consists of the entire light chain disulfide bonded to the first two domains of the heavy chain. X-ray data show that the hypervariable regions of the L and H chains are in close proximity (13). Most of the X-ray crystallographic studies have been made on such Fab fragments of IgG myeloma globulins. The Fc fragment of IgM is a cyclic pentamer with a molecular weight of about 340,000. Attempts to crystallize this in a form suitable for X-ray analysis are now underway.

An enormous amount of amino acid sequence data on light chains and an increasing amount on heavy chains has validated the concept that all immunoglobulin chains are divided into a V region and a C region. This unique structural principle is both the basis of antibody specificity and the paradox that still defies explanation by genetic theory. The V region is the amino-terminal portion of any immunoglobulin chain which has multiple substitutions-- from 10 to 60 in the first 110 residues-- when chains of the same class and species are compared. The C region is the carboxyl-terminal portion of any immunoglobulin chain and has a unique invariant sequence characteristic of the class and animal species --invariant, that is, except for minor allotypic changes.

Although antibody specificity is determined by the V regions of the light and heavy chains, various other biological properties of immunoglobulins as well as some of the cooperative interactions affecting antibody-antigen combination are governed by the constant regions of the heavy chains. These properties include complement fixation, placental transfer, turnover time, and susceptibility to limited proteolytic cleavage to yield Fab and Fc fragments. Comparative study of the μ, α, and γ heavy chains will aid in elucidating the structural basis of these important properties, and this is one of the principal objectives of our current work.

CLASS-SPECIFIC STRUCTURE OF HEAVY CHAINS

Although all five classes of human immunoglobulins have the same basic four-chain structure in the monomeric form, they differ characteristically in the amino acid sequence of their class-specific heavy chains. This difference is restricted to the constant region sequences which are homologous but unique to each class of heavy chain. Furthermore, as illustrated in Fig. 2 and summarized in Table 2, the C region sequences determine other characteristic differences in immunoglobulin class structure such as: 1) the length of the chain, 2) the number of domains, 3) the number and location

of the interchain and intrachain disulfide bridges, 4) the
position, number and kind of oligosaccharides attached to the
heavy chain, and 5) the degree of polymerization of the immunoglobulin molecules. Nonetheless, the symmetrical models
shown in Fig. 2 suggest a great deal about the evolutionary
development and structural relationships of antibodies of all
classes and species. First, that immunoglobulins developed
through tandem duplication of a primordial gene coding for
about 110 amino acids, and thus that we must anticipate much
structural homology among all the light and heavy chains and
even within the chains. Second, that two genes, a V gene and
a C gene, may code for a single antibody chain. Third, that
many of the properties of antibodies are governed by interactions of these homologous subunits and domains, and fourth,
that we should be able to make some deductions about the
evolutionary development and genetic control of immunoglobulins by means of comparative study of IgM, IgA, and IgG.

TABLE 2

Structural characteristics of human
μ, α, γ, and ε heavy chains

Chain	Approximate Number of Residues	Half-Cystines	Constant Region Characteristics			
			Inter-Chain Bridges	Position of H-L Bridge	Oligosaccharides GlcN	GalN
μ	576	14	4	≈ 140	5	0
$\alpha 1$	470	≈ 17	(5)	≈ 130	2	1
$\alpha 2$ (Am$_2$+)	460	<17	(5)	missing	(3)	0
$\alpha 2$ (Am$_2$−)	460	<17	(5)	130?	(2)	0
$\gamma 1$	446	11	3	220	1	0
ε	550	15	3	127	6	0

HYPERVARIABLE REGIONS AND THE SWITCH POINT IN HEAVY AND
LIGHT CHAINS

In preceding work we and others have emphasized the existence of at least three hypervariable regions in both heavy
and light chains. Supporting evidence for the involvement of
these hypervariable regions has come from 1) X-ray diffraction analysis of hapten-binding myeloma proteins (13); 2)
hapten-binding studies of myeloma globulins and antibodies
by the affinity labeling method (14), and 3) amino acid sequence analysis of animal antibodies of defined specificity
and restricted heterogeneity (14).

Fig. 3 shows schematically by the vertical shaded lines the location of the hypervariable regions in a series of μ heavy chains that have been sequenced in our laboratory (15, 16). Although we have emphasized three hypervariable regions, the figure shows four shaded segments where the sequence of these μ chains differs characteristically. Other evidence for four hypervariable regions based on comparative sequence analysis has been given by Capra et al. (17). However, to date X-ray diffraction analysis and affinity labeling have not implicated one of these segments as being involved in the combining site, i.e., that around position 80. As a result, we have not given emphasis to this hypervariable region.

Fig. 4 summarizes the structural features common to μ, γ, and α heavy chains. The V region (114-124 residues) consists of a subgroup-specific region (90 residues) followed by a conservative region (positions 91-99) and a hypervariable deletion region. The subgroup-specific region consists of three segments that are comprised of what are called "framework residues" that are intercalated among the three principal hypervariable regions. The latter are indicated by by the zig-zag lines after Cys-22, around position 60, and after position 99. The framework residues do vary somewhat from one chain to another even among chains of the same class and subgroup. However, the framework residues are highly conserved not only in human heavy chains of different classes but also throughout the animal kingdom. These portions of the V region form a fairly rigid framework that supports the combining site, which is largely composed of the three hypervariable regions. Because of the variation in length of the hypervariable region and also because of the subgroup-specific gaps in the first 90 residues, the V region varies in length. The segment immediately following the first disulfide bridge we call the hypervariable deletion region because it is the locus of the greatest variation in sequence as well as in length. The hypervariable deletion region plays a very important role in shaping the combining site and in determining antibody specificity and affinity.

Three heavy chain subgroups in human immunoglobulins (V_{HI}, V_{HII}, and V_{III}) have previously been defined largely by reference to the complete V_H sequences of a series of μ, γ, and α chains determined by our laboratory and others. Although each heavy chain class has a unique C region sequence characteristic for the class, the three V_H subgroups are shared by all classes of heavy chains. The switchover from a variable sequence to a constant sequence characteristic of

13

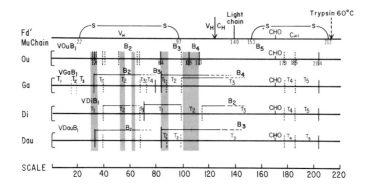

Fig. 3 Schematic alignment of the CNBr fragments of the Fd portion of the μ heavy chain of human IgM proteins Ou, Gu, Di, and Dau. Methionine residues are denoted by vertical, solid lines, arginine by dotted lines, tryptic peptides by T1, T2 etc., and CNBr fragments by B1, B2 etc. Vertical shaded lines identify regions of sequence that are hypervariable in the V region of all heavy chains. From Florent et al. (15).

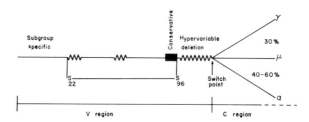

Fig. 4 Schematic diagram of the structural features common to μ, γ, and α heavy chains. See the text for explanation. From Florent et al. (15).

14

the class is initiated at the switch point located at the juncture of the V and C regions. It was at first predicted that the switch point would contain an amino acid sequence common to all heavy chains. This prediction was based on the assumption that the amino acid sequence at the switch point reflected a nucleotide base sequence that served as a recognition signal for the union of the postulated V and C genes by some kind of a translocation ligase. The sequence Val-Ser-Ser at first appeared to be common to the switch point of all human heavy chains, but two of these residues have been substituted in other μ chains that have since been sequenced. Thus, the amino acid sequence gives no evidence for a recognition signal in the nucleotide base sequence of the DNA.

Although the class character of heavy chains is expressed only in the C region because of the sharing of the same variable sequence groups by all classes of heavy chains, the variable regions of light chains are characteristic of the type of the light chain. That is to say, Vκ sequences are always associated with Cκ and Vλ with Cλ. Presumably the V and C genes for κ chains are on a different chromosome than the V and C genes for λ chains.

Only a single substitution in the C region of human κ chains has been reported, an allelic interchange of leucine and valine at position 191. However, a surprising number of isotypic interchanges in the C region of human λ chains have been identified. In addition to the five previously summarized (18), Anthony Infante in my laboratory has independently discovered three new amino acid substitutions in the C region of a single human λ chain (Burke) at positions 113, 115, and 164. These have been identified independently in the human λ chain McG by Fett and Deutsch (19), who use a slightly different numbering system. As shown in Fig. 5, two of the substitutions occur close to the beginning of the Cλ region. This is all the more interesting because these two substitutions occur in a pentapeptide sequence adjacent to the V/C switch point that is common to both human κ and λ light chains, i.e., the sequence Ala-Ala-Pro-Ser-Val. This emphasizes the difficulty of assigning a precise switch point. As more and more light and heavy chains of different classes have been sequenced, the switch point moves slightly towards the C-terminus.

DEFECTIVE CHAINS AND DELETION VARIANTS

The V/C region is apparently critical in that it is the

15

V$_\lambda$–C$_\lambda$ Switch Region in Human λ Light Chains

Protein	Subgroup			100				105			V$_\lambda$ → C$_\lambda$		110					115		
HA	I	PHE	GLY	GLY	THR	GLN	LEU	THR	VAL	LEU	ARG	GLN	PRO	LYS	ALA	ALA	PRO	SER	VAL	THR
NEW	I	PHE	GLY	GLY	THR	LYS	**VAL**	THR	VAL	LEU	GLY	GLN	PRO	LYS	ALA	ALA	PRO	SER	VAL	THR
BO	II	PHE	GLY	GLY	THR	LYS	LEU	THR	VAL	LEU	**ARG**	GLN	PRO	LYS	ALA	ALA	PRO	SER	VAL	THR
VIL	II	PHE	GLY	GLY	THR	LYS	LEU	THR	VAL	LEU	GLY	GLN	PRO	LYS	ALA	ALA	PRO	SER	VAL	THR
SH	III	PHE	GLY	GLY	THR	LYS	LEU	THR	VAL	LEU	GLY	GLN	PRO	LYS	ALA	ALA	PRO	SER	VAL	THR
BAU	IV	PHE	GLY	GLY	THR	LYS	LEU	THR	VAL	LEU	GLY	GLN	PRO	LYS	ALA	ALA	PRO	SER	VAL	THR
KERN	IV	PHE	GLY	GLY	THR	LYS	LEU	THR	VAL	LEU	**SER**	GLN	PRO	LYS	ALA	ALA	PRO	SER	VAL	THR
X	IV	PHE	GLY	GLY	THR	**ARG**	LEU	THR	VAL	LEU	SER	GLN	PRO	LYS	ALA	ALA	PRO	SER	VAL	THR
BURKE	II	PHE	GLY	**THR**	THR	LYS	VAL	**LEU**	VAL	**ILE**	GLY	GLN	PRO	LYS	ALA	**ASN**	PRO	**THR**	VAL	THR
MCG	II	PHE	GLY	**GLY**	THR	LYS	VAL	THR	VAL	LEU	GLY	GLN	PRO	LYS	ALA	**ASN**	PRO	**THR**	VAL	THR
GRAY	II	PHE	GLY	GLY	THR	LYS	VAL	THR	VAL	LEU	GLY	GLN	PRO	LYS	ALA	ALA	PRO	SER	VAL	THR

Fig. 5 Amino acid sequence of the V$_\lambda$–C$_\lambda$ switch region in human λ light chains. HA, BO, and SH are from our laboratory (12). NEW, VIL, BAU, KERN, and X are from other workers; see (18) for references. BURKE is from unpublished data of A. Infante and F. W. Putnam, MCG from Fett and Deutsch (19) and GRAY from unpublished data of F. C. Wong and F. W. Putnam.

16

most frequent locus of genetic aberrations at the DNA level that lead to defective light or heavy chains (20). These errors suggest misalignment of V and C genes during a translocation and joining event. A number of the defective heavy chains have deletions of a hundred or more amino acids including the V/C region, and the deletions often end precisely at position 216 in the hinge region of the constant sequence. Other deletions involve an entire domain, usually the last domain of the C region. We are studying one such deletion variant of the IgA type that lacks approximately the last 100 amino acids. The spontaneous mutations found by Milstein et al. (21) in tissue culture of clones of myeloma cells accumulate in the C region with deletions of entire domains. These, too, include deletions at or near position 216 in the hinge region. It will be very important to learn what gives the stop and restart signals in these deletion variants. The loss of the final domain in human and mouse α chains may be the result of a chain termination; it does not appear to be a proteolytic phenomenon.

The large deletions in the C region are quite different from the very short gaps of one to five residues that often occur in the V regions of light and heavy chains. The C region deletions occur between domains, involve entire domains, and appear to reflect recombinational events that involve cistronic segments the size of the postulated primitive gene that coded for about 110 amino acids. It is as if the C region deletions are invoking the forbidden memory of recombinational events early in evolution that led to the divergence of genes for the different classes of light and heavy chains.

EVOLUTION OF IMMUNOGLOBULIN CHAINS

Some of the facts suggesting that genetic recombinational events throughout evolution have given rise to the different classes of immunoglobulin chains are the following:
1. The strong homology in primary structure of all the V and C region domains of all of the light and heavy chains that have been sequenced, regardless of class of chain or species origin (3,4,18).
2. The great similarity in three-dimensional structure of the light chains and Fab fragments of human and mouse myeloma proteins that have been determined by high resolution X-ray crystallography (13).
3. The unusually high homology (50% or greater) of the C-terminal domains of the human μ and α chains, including the C-terminal tail which is absent in γ and ε chains (Fig. 6).

This structural homology is all the more striking because it occurs between the fifth domain of the μ chain and the fourth of the α chain. It is as if an internal C region domain was lost or added to one or the other of the two chains during the course of evolution.

4. The deletions in heavy chain disease proteins, all of which affect the hinge region or whole domains both in V and C regions and in Fd and Fc regions (20).

5. The deletion in the α2 hinge region and the duplication in the α1 hinge region of a short segment of sequence in human IgA proteins.

6. The variability in length of the hypervariable deletion region of heavy chains and the evidence for mismatching of V and C joining in the heavy chain disease proteins.

7. The identification of hybrid allotypic variants of the human γ chain suggestive of recombination between γ1 and γ3 C region genes.

8. The very fact that all Ig chains consist of tandem domains varying in number from 2 in light chains, 4 in γ and α heavy chains and 5 in γ and ε chains suggests recombination of tandem genes coding for single domains. The fact that C-terminal domains may be absent as in some half length chains or in the α chain suggests that there may still be separate genes for each domain.

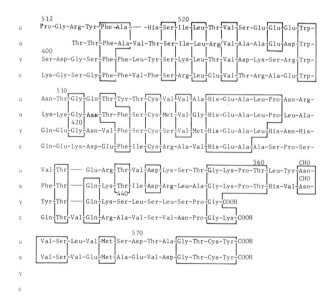

Fig. 6 Structural homology of α, μ, γ, and ε chains (6,7).

REFERENCES

(1) F. W. Putnam, in: Protides of the Biological Fluids, Vol. 20, ed. H. Peeters (Pergamon Press, Oxford, 1973) p. 29.

(2) F. W. Putnam, Physiol. Rev. 37 (1957) 512.

(3) F. W. Putnam, Science 163 (1969) 633.

(4) F. W. Putnam, in: The Plasma Proteins, Vol. 2, ed. F. W. Putnam (Academic Press, New York, 1975) in press.

(5) F. W. Putnam, G. Florent, C. Paul, T. Shinoda, and A. Shimizu, Science 182 (1973) 287.

(6) F. W. Putnam, T. Low, V. Liu, H. Huser, E. Raff, F. C. Wong, and J. R. Clamp, in: The Immunoglobulin A System, ed. J. Mestecky and A. R. Lawton III (Plenum Press, New York, 1974) p. 177.

(7) T. Low, V. Liu, Y. Tsuzukida, A. Toraño, and F. W. Putnam, Federation Proc. (1975) in press.

(8) G. M. Edelman, B. A. Cunningham, W. E. Gall, P. D. Gottlieb, U. Rutishauser, and J. M. Waxdal, Proc. Nat. Acad. Sci. USA 63 (1969) 78.

(9) E. M. Press and N. M. Hogg, Biochem. J. 117 (1970) 641.

(10) J. D. Capra, C. Chuang, R. D. Kaplan, and J. M. Kehoe, in: The Immunoglobulin A System, ed. J. Mestecky and A. R. Lawton III (Plenum Press, New York, 1974) p. 191.

(11) F. W. Putnam, K. Titani, and E. Whitley, Jr., Proc. Roy. Soc. (London) Ser. B 166 (1966) 124.

(12) F. W. Putnam, T. Shinoda, K. Titani, and M. Wikler, Science 157 (1967) 1050.

(13) D. R. Davies, E. A. Padlan, and D. M. Segal, Ann. Rev. Biochem. 44 (1975) in press.

(14) J. J. Cebra, P. H. Koo, and A. Ray, Science 186 (1974) 263.

(15) G. Florent, D. Lehman and F. W. Putnam, Biochemistry 13 (1974) 2482.

(16) J. Florent, D. Lehman, D. Lockhart and F. W. Putnam, Biochemistry 13 (1974) 3372.

(17) J. D. Capra and J. M. Kehoe, Proc. Nat. Acad. Sci. USA 71 (1974) 845.

(18) F. W. Putnam, J. Human Evolution 1 (1972) 591.

(19) J. W. Fett and H. F. Deutsch, Biochemistry 20 (1974) 4102.

(20) B. Frangione and E. C Franklin, Seminars in Hematology, 10 (1973) 53.

(21) C. Milstein, R. G. H. Cotton and D. S. Secher, Ann. Immunol. (Inst. Pasteur) 125C (1974) 287.

This is Contribution No. 989 from the Zoology Department of Indiana University. This work was supported by research grants from the National Cancer Institute (CA 08497), the Damon Runyon–Walter Winchell Cancer Fund (DRG–1235), and the American Cancer Society (IM–2B).

DISCUSSION

B. Becker, Purdue University: You passed briefly over the carbohydrates on the μ chains, are these all oligosaccharides?

F. Putnam, Indiana University: Yes.

B. Becker: And can you tell me whether arabinose is included as one of the residues?

F. Putnam: Would you put that last slide on again, please? No arabinose to my knowledge has ever been identified in the carbohydrates of any of the immunoglobulin heavy chains. There are a series of different carbohydrates; in essence they're hetero-oligosaccharides. In the instance of the μ chain, there are two kinds, which we call complex and simple. The complex ones have galactose, fucose, sialic-acid, glucosamine and mannose in them, but the simple ones have only mannose and glucosamine. Now, there is a difference in the number; there are, five in the case of the μ chain, six in the ε chain, three or four in the α chain and only one in the case of the γ chain. These are not generally in homologous positions. There is one homologous carbohydrate, perhaps the identical carbohydrate in the C-terminal domains of the μ and α chain, but in general they are not in homologous positions. They are just sited by the recognition by the transglycosidases of a particular sequence. The unique carbohydrate of the α chain is galactosamine; that's attached to the hinge region.

B. Becker: Thank you.

F. Putnam: Any more questions?

A. Nisonoff, University of Illinois: Dr. Putnam, is there any evidence as yet for a hinge region in IgM?

F. Putnam: I guess it depends upon how you define the hinge region. In the instance of IgM, cleavage by trypsin involves the excision of the third domain. There is no

21

region in IgM which is identical in terms of the frequency of both prolines and of inter and intra-chain disulfide bonds to the hinge region one finds in the α chain and in the γ chain. We have experiments that indicate that there is a conformational lability in the μ chain. That is, one can dissect out the third domain by cleavage with trypsin at 25° in the presence of urea. So, there is what might be called a flexible area that is more confirmatinally labile, but it is not hinged in the sense that it is compact, full of disulfide bonds and full of prolines, and carbohydrates.

A. Nisonoff: I believe that there are a few differences in amino acid sequence between your μ chain and that sequenced by Hilschmann's group. Has that been pinned down to a difference in allotype or sub-group or is it possibly just experimental error?

F. Putnam: I think that both Dr. Hilschmann and I agree that these differences are largely technical in nature. They involve the location or reversal of several residues. Some of them involve an amide position. I think that there are also still some unresolved differences in the human γ chain between sequences that have been found by the Rockefeller group and the Oxford group. As yet, we have no evidence that these involve genetic differences. We have not been able to detect such differences in the sequencing of other μ chains, or in the sequencing of the Fc region of normal IgM.

SYNTHETIC APPROACHES TO SOME APPLIED ASPECTS OF ANTIGENICITY

MICHAEL SELA
Department of Chemical Immunology
The Weizmann Institute of Science
Rehovot, Israel

INTRODUCTION

The knowledge of antigenic structure, and the use of the synthetic approach for proper antigen design, have been of great help for the understanding of the molecular basis of antigenicity as well as of such immunological phenomena as, e.g., tolerance, antigenic competition and genetic control of immune response. With the recent progress in cellular immunology, antigen design will be crucial for a molecular understanding of cellular phenomena. In this lecture I intend to present several examples of the use of synthetic antigens in some applied medical aspects of immunology, and to discuss also one example of covalent modification of antibodies.

The three topics discussed will deal with a synthetic basic copolymer capable of suppressing experimental allergic encephalomyelitis, with a synthetic peptide corresponding to the amino-terminal segment of the carcinoembryonic antigen of the colon, and with anti-cancer drugs attached covalently to antibodies.

SUPPRESSION OF ALLERGIC ENCEPHALOMYELITIS WITH A SYNTHETIC BASIC COPOLYMER

Experimental allergic encephalomyelitis (EAE) is an auto-immune disease induced in animals such as guinea pigs, rabbits and monkeys by injection of a basic protein of the myelin sheath in complete Freund's adjuvant. The induction of the disease is consistent and reproducible, and thus EAE provides a reasonable and sensitive biological model for studying the immunological phenomena which are relevant to demyelinating diseases, including multiple sclerosis (MS).

The experimental disease is associated with clinical manifestations of paraplegia and necrosis of the hind legs and with histological manifestations of inflammatory lesions of the brain and spinal cord, occurring usually 2-3 weeks after the injection of the nervous tissue or of the purified encephalitogen, a basic low molecular weight protein which is a major constituent of myelin. The disease may be transferred passively with sensitized lymphocytes, and it correlates with delayed hypersensitivity (possibly only to some unique determinants) rather than circulating antibodies (1-4).

The basic encephalitogen (BE) of various species has been purified (1,3,5-7) and characterized as a protein with a molecular weight of 18,500, exhibiting an open conformation without appreciable secondary or tertiary structure. Its complete amino acid sequence was determined (8,9), and the regions responsible for the encephalitogenic activity in several species have been identified (10-12). Injection of 1-10 μg of BE in complete Freund's adjuvant induces clinical EAE in guinea pigs.

BE, if given in high doses in incomplete Freund's adjuvant, is highly effective in preventing EAE in guinea pigs when administered before sensitization, or in suppressing EAE if given after the sensitization (13,14). In monkeys, suppression of EAE was achieved after unmistakable signs of the disease were observed (15). In view of these findings, we have synthesized in our laboratory several random basic copolymers, of amino acid composition approaching to a certain extent that of the natural encephalitogen, and tested their activity in either inducing or suppressing EAE. The polymers were prepared from the N-carboxyanhydride derivatives of the respective amino acids. None of these synthetic materials possessed any encephalitogenic activity, but some of them showed high efficacy in suppressing the onset of the disease (16).

Most of our work has been carried out with a copolymer, denoted Cop 1, composed of L-alanine, L-glutamic acid, L-lysine and L-tyrosine, in a residue molar ratio of 6.0:1.9: 4.7:1.0, with an average molecular weight of 23,000. This copolymer did not exert any encephalitogenic activity when injected into guinea pigs in doses of 10 μg up to 5 mg. On the other hand, it had marked suppressive effect on EAE, when injected either in incomplete Freund's adjuvant or in aqueous saline solution, after initial challenge with a disease-inducing dose of BE. The most effective suppression was achieved with 3 successive intravenous injections of Cop 1, given at 5-day intervals, commencing as late as 5 days following the challenge. Under these conditions the copolymer reduced the clinical incidence of encephalomyelitis in guinea pigs from 64% in the control group to 22%. The histological lesions were also decreased both in prevalence and in severity. The suppressive effect of EAE attained by Cop 1 is of the same order of magnitude as that of BE. The effect of Cop 1 is specific, since neither an acidic amino acid copolymer, nor unrelated basic proteins, had any suppressive action. On the other hand, independently prepared additional batches of Cop 1 showed activity identical to the first batch. Two additional copolymers related to Cop 1, one in which glutamic acid was replaced with aspartic acid, and another devoid of tyrosine, were also effective in suppressing EAE, but less so than Cop 1 (17).

Results of very recent experiments showed that the amount of 1 mg of Cop 1 arbitrarily used in the above experiments is an overdose. Three intravenous injections of as low a dose as 10 μg of Cop 1 in aqueous solution sufficed for efficient suppression of EAE. In guinea pigs thus treated only 21% showed clinical symptoms of the disease, and the severity of histological damage to the brain was much lower than in the control group (unpublished data).

All the above-mentioned experiments were performed in guinea pigs, using bovine BE for induction of EAE. Cop 1 was as effective when the disease was induced in guinea pigs with human BE - it reduced the clinical incidence from 63% in the control group to 22% in the experimental group, and was at least as efficient when the experiment was carried out in rabbits. In the latter case the clinical incidence in the Cop 1-treated group was only 19% compared to 70% in the untreated one, and their brains were almost free of any histological lesions (17). It is thus demonstrated that Cop 1 does not manifest species specificity, neither for the source of the encephalitogen nor for the test animal.

In contrast to the efficiency of Cop 1 in suppression of EAE, it was completely ineffective in preventing the disease. In other words, prior injection of the copolymer in aqueous solution did not affect the incidence of disease induced by a subsequent injection of the natural basic protein in complete Freund's adjuvant. On the other hand, guinea pigs in which the disease was successfully suppressed by Cop 1, remain protected against a repeated injection of BE. Thus, out of 20 guinea pigs surviving EAE following suppressive treatment with Cop 1, upon rechallenge with 10 μg BE in complete Freund's adjuvant 4 to 7 weeks following the last injection of Cop 1, none showed any clinical symptoms of EAE.

In this experiment, protection against EAE was very efficient, but the necessary initial exposure to a disease-inducing dose of BE still resulted in 28% of the animals succumbing to the disease. In subsequent experiments we demonstrated that this danger could be avoided if the initial exposure was to a sub-effective dose of BE. Thus, the administration, in complete Freund's adjuvant, of 0.1 μg of BE, a dose much too low to provoke any clinical symptoms or histological lesions of EAE, followed by an intravenous injection of an aqueous solution of Cop 1, efficiently protects the experimental animals against a subsequent challenge of the disease (18). The protection against EAE consists in this case of two stages, neither of which involves any encephalitogenic exposure or general immunosuppressive activity.

Bearing in mind that EAE is a disease of autoimmune nature, and apparently a manifestation of sensitization to BE, we have tested for immunological cross-reactivity between Cop 1 and BE as a possible explanation for the specific suppression of EAE by Cop 1. Indeed, a significant extent of cross-reactivity exists between BE and several basic copolymers which have a suppressive effect on EAE (19). This has been conclusively established at the cellular level, both in vivo by means of delayed hypersensitivity skin tests, and in vitro using transformation of sensitized lymphocytes, as measured by incorporation of radioactive thymidine. A limited extent of cross-reactivity was observed also at the humoral level: guinea pig anti-Cop 1 antibodies cross-reacted in the passive cutaneous anaphylaxis assay with the bovine basic encephalitogen. It seems thus that immunological cross-reactivity of BE with several basic amino acid copolymers may serve as a basis for explaining their suppressive effect on EAE.

The next stage was to find out whether Cop 1 is efficient in suppressing EAE in monkeys as well. Our experiments so far, although carried out in a limited number of animals, seem encouraging. Monkeys differ from other species in the detailed manifestation of the disease, both clinically (involving ataxia and disorientation rather than paralysis, and typical damage to the optic nerve) and histologically (involving more of the demyelination process, and thus resembling more the demyelinating diseases in man).

Our first set of experiments (20) included five rhesus monkeys, 2 serving as experimental group and 3 as controls (Table 1). All the monkeys were injected with BE and all of them developed symptoms of EAE between 16 and 24 days after sensitization. Two monkeys received suppressive treatment with Cop 1 in incomplete adjuvant. Daily injections were initiated with the onset of clinical symptoms and continued over 15 days with gradually decreasing doses. Both of these monkeys evinced noted improvement around 4 days after beginning the suppressive treatment, and they both appeared completely normal after the first 9 injections.

In the control group two monkeys were treated with incomplete adjuvant alone. These monkeys showed steady decline, ending in death 5 and 9 days after onset of clinical symptoms.

26

Table 1: Suppression of EAE in rhesus monkeys by Cop 1

| Monkey number[a] | Onset of symptoms | Treatment[b] | Clinical observation | | Histological damage |
			Course of disease	Result	
1 (control)	Day 16	none	Rapid decline	Death (day 20)	Positive
2 (experimental)	Day 19	Cop 1 in ICFA	Steady improvement starting after 5 injections	Recovery[c] (day 29)	Positive
3 (experimental)	Day 20	Cop 1 in ICFA	Steady improvement starting after 4 injections	Recovery (day 29)	Negative
4 (control)	Day 24	ICFA alone	Steady deterioration in condition	Death (day 29)	Positive
5 (control)	Day 24	ICFA alone	Steady deterioration in condition	Death (day 35)	Positive

[a]All the monkeys were injected with 5 mg BP in CFA at day 0.

[b]Treatment was initiated on the day of onset of clinical symptoms. Daily injections were administered intramuscularly over a period of 15 days or until death occurred.

[c]Monkey No. 2 suffered from relapses at day 67, and day 86 subsequently died at day 91 (see text).

ICFA - incomplete Freund's adjuvant; CFA - complete Freund's adjuvant.

One monkey did not receive any treatment whatsoever. Within 2 days after onset of symptoms it was prostrate in its cage and, following rapid deterioration, died two days later.

One of the monkeys that received Cop 1 treatment and fully recovered from the initial bout of EAE evinced a relapse 35 days after the termination of the suppressive treatment. Injections of Cop 1 were reinstated and continued over a period of 10 days when the appearance of the monkey was once again completely normal. However, 10 days later the monkey suffered a second relapse and died. This finding seems of interest, since in this respect monkeys differ from rodents, being capable of succumbing to relapse. This phenomenon might indicate a somewhat closer relationship between EAE in monkeys and the known remission - relapse state situation so typical of multiple sclerosis in man.

Histopathological examination of the central nervous tissue was performed on all the monkeys. All four monkeys that died of EAE, namely, the three controls and the monkey which died after recurrent relapses, had histological damage typical of this disease. In contrast, the monkey which fully recovered from EAE had no histological damage whatsoever. Many serial sections of various portions of the cerebrum, cerebellum and medula oblongata were examined in minute detail and no pathological findings were observed. The significance of this finding awaits confirmation in a larger number of monkeys.

In a recent second experiment in monkeys, essentially the same effects were observed. Control animals that received no treatment or incomplete adjuvant alone after appearance of symptoms deteriorated very rapidly and died within 3-4 days of onset of symptoms. In the experimental group, one monkey, treated with 5 mg Cop 1 in incomplete adjuvant for 15 days, reverted to completely normal behaviour and remained normal and apparently healthy. Another monkey received daily 5 mg injections of Cop 1 in saline for 30 days. This monkey appeared healthy and completely normal as well until termination of the experiment, over a month after treatment ceased.

We have recently demonstrated (21) that lymphocytes from a proportion of MS patients receiving steroids showed sensitivity towards BE, as measured by specific transformation in vitro. These were, without exception, those patients who failed to respond clinically to steroid therapy. While our findings may lead to new concepts about the efficacy and desirability of indiscriminate steroid therapy for MS patients, they also show that some MS patients indeed manifest immunological reactivity at the cellular level with the encephalitogenic protein of the central nervous system, and that -

whatever the etiology of multiple sclerosis - its expression
includes autoimmune aspects related to BE. Thus, our work on
suppression of EAE may be relevant to MS. Should BE and Cop
1 be effective in desensitization treatment of human patients,
it seems to us that there would be obvious advantages in the
use of synthetic materials over that of the natural encephalitogen. These include the fact that the synthetic substances are non-encephalitogenic, and that they can be readily
prepared on a relatively large scale in a reproducible manner.

SYNTHETIC AMINO-TERMINAL PEPTIDE OF CARCINOEMBRYONIC ANTIGEN
OF THE COLON

Another area in which we used a synthetic approach is of
possible interest for the diagnosis of some types of cancer.
Carcinoembryonic antigen of the colon (CEA) was shown to be
present in elevated amounts in the serum of patients of
cancer of the colon and some other related cancers, but not
in the sera of normal individuals (22,23). CEA is a heterogeneous molecule of a molecular weight around 200,000, and
containing 50-75% sugars (24). Efficient radioimmunoassays
for CEA have been developed, and the suggestion has been made
that they may develop into useful tools for cancer diagnosis
(25-27).

The amino acid sequence of the amino-terminal part of the
polypeptide chain of CEA has been established by Terry et al.
(28) to be: Lys-Leu-Thr-Ile-Glu-Ser-Thr-Pro-Phe-Asn-Val-Ala-
Glu-Gly-Lys-Glu-Val-Leu-Leu-Leu-Val-His-Asn-Leu. We decided
to synthesize an amino terminal segment of this sequence, and
use it for preparation of specific antibodies (R. Arnon, M.
Bustin, E. Calef, S. Chaichik, J. Haimovich, N. Novik and M.
Sela, unpublished data). We were encouraged to pursue this
approach by our previous experience in synthesizing a portion
(the "loop") of the hen egg white lysozyme molecule, which -
when attached to the right carrier - leads to the formation
of antibodies reacting efficiently with a unique, conforma-
tion-dependent region of the native lysozyme (29). We thus
hoped that the CEA segment might encompass an antigenic
region of the native molecule, or of its partial fragmenta-
tion products; alternately, we hoped that at least antibodies
to the synthetic peptide might recognize it in CEA.

We synthesized a peptide corresponding to the first 11
residues of CEA sequence, with Leu replacing Val in the 11th
position. The synthesis, depicted below, was performed by
the solid phase method according to Merrifield (30), using
the appropriately blocked t-butyloxycarbonyl (t-Boc)

derivatives of the required amino acids.

The synthetic CEA(1-11) peptide was attached by means of a water-soluble carbodiimide reagent to multichain poly-DL-alanine as well as to bovine serum albumin. Both macromolecular conjugates provoked in rabbits anti-CEA(1-11) peptide antibodies (Table 2). At this stage we could ask ourselves

Synthesis of the 11-residue
N-terminal peptide of CEA

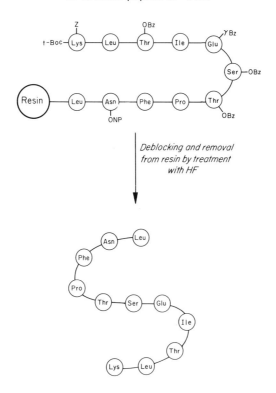

Bz - benzyl; NP - nitrophenyl

whether antisera against CEA react with the synthetic CEA (1-11) peptide, and whether antisera against the peptide are capable of reacting with CEA. As seen in Table 2, anti-CEA sera hemagglutinate CEA(1-11)-coated sheep red blood cells. Moreover, this reaction is efficiently inhibited with the free CEA(1-11) peptide. Thus, at least some of the anti-CEA

TABLE 2

Hemagglutination experiments with CEA(1-11)-A--L coated SRBC

Antiserum against	Hemagglutination titer	Inhibitor*
CEA(1-11)-A--L	1:128	CEA(1-11) (1 μg/ml) Crude CEA (200 μg/ml)
CEA(1-11)-BSA	1:32	CEA(1-11) (10 μg/ml) Crude CEA (500 μg/ml)
Pure CEA	1:64	CEA(1-11) (1 μg/ml)
Crude CEA	1:16	CEA(1-11) (100 μg/ml) Crude CEA (30 μg/ml)
BSA	1:4	n.d.
T4-bacteriophage	-	n.d.
Hexosaminidase	-	n.d.

* The inhibition experiments were done with serum concentration twice that of the hemagglutination titer; the numbers
  in parentheses indicate the lowest concentration of inhibi-
  tor which still prevents agglutination.

antibodies are directed against an antigenic determinant
including the amino-terminal segment, and we are able to
recognize this region of CEA molecule.

Concerning the question whether CEA reacts with antipep-
tide antibodies, we observed no such cross-reaction, using
either hemagglutination assay or the chemically modified bacteriophage technique. On the other hand, a semipure preparation of CEA, obtained through the courtesy of Dr. Sabine von
Kleist and Dr. Pierre Burtin, cross-reacted with antibodies
directed towards the CEA(1-11) peptide. Thus, an antiserum
against CEA(1-11) bovine serum albumin hemagglutinated weakly
semipure-CEA-coated sheep red blood cells, and the hemagglutination was inhibited with the free peptide.

The immunological CEA(1-11) peptide system was investigated also, making use of the chemically modified bacteriophage
technique (31,32). The peptide was attached to bacteriophage
T4 by means of glutaraldehyde. The CEA(1-11)-coated phage
was efficiently inactivated with antisera obtained with CEA
(1-11) macromolecular conjugates, and the inactivation reaction could be totally inhibited with the free peptide. The
semipure CEA could also inhibit the phage inactivation, but

31

less efficiently.

Based on the above results, we decided to test sera of some cancer patients for their capacity to inhibit the inactivation of CEA(1-11)-coated phage by means of anti-CEA(1-11) antiserum. The results are given in Table 3. As can be seen it appears that anti-CEA(1-11) antibodies recognize something present in the sera of most adenocarcinoma patients, but not other neoplasias nor in normal individuals. These results should be considered as strictly preliminary. The fact that many sera are positive in this test, even though intact CEA is negative, may imply that some patients may possess in their serum intact CEA, others may possess partial degradation products of CEA, while still others could contain both. It is possible that antisera against the CEA(1-11) peptide recognize only such degradation products. This hypothesis is now being investigated.

TABLE 3

Inhibition of CEA(1-11)-T4 inactivation by sera of patients*

Disease	Positives (>30% inhibition)	Total	% Positives
Colonic, rectal and stomach adenocarcinoma	23	29**	80
Pancreas adenocarcinoma	2	2	100
Breast adenocarcinoma	5	6	83
Lung tumors	0	3	0
Other neoplasias	1	8	12
Non-related diseases	0	2	0
Normals (25-40 years old)	2	26	8
Normals (over 65 years old)	5	13	38

 * Conditions: 0.05 ml patient's serum; 0.05 ml of antiserum (diluted 1:5000); 500 p.f.u. of modified phage.
** Three of the negative sera belonged to patients with complete remission of the tumor after chemotherapy.

DRUG-ANTIBODY CONJUGATES CYTOTOXIC TO TUMOR CELLS

Another area of immunological research with possible applied medical aspects, which we started actively investigating recently, is the covalent linkage of anti-cancer drugs to immunoglobulins containing antibodies with specificity directed preferentially to anti-tumor cells.

Agents which are effective in killing neoplastic cells usually also have detrimental effects on normal cells, particularly the rapidly proliferating ones of the gastrointestinal tract and bone marrow, and cancer chemotherapy is ultimately limited by its toxicity to these normal tissues. One possible approach for increasing the effectiveness of anti-tumor drugs would be to find methods of altering their distribution in the body to increase their local concentration at the tumor cell sites. In this way the selectivity of their toxicity for the tumor cells might be enhanced.

Several non-covalent complexes of alkylating drugs with immunoglobulins (e.g. 33, 34) and other macromolecules (35) have been studied. It was also shown that cytotoxic drugs of low molecular weight may retain their activity after covalent linkage to macromolecules (36-38). We have now investigated covalent conjugates of daunomycin and adriamycin, two potent cancer chemotherapeutic agents, with immunoglobulins containing anti-mouse tumor antibodies (E. Hurwitz, R. Levy, R. Maron, M. Wilchek, R. Arnon and M. Sela, unpublished data). The most suitable method for binding of the drugs to the antibodies was periodate oxidation of the drug, followed by the linking of the oxidized drug to the immunoglobulin, and subsequent reduction of the product with sodium borohydride.

The activity of the drug-antibody conjugates was tested in vitro on tumor and normal cell cultures, and was found to be similar to that of the free drug. A significant amount of antibody activity was retained, as found both with anti-bovine serum albumin antibodies, assayed by inactivation of bovine serum albumin-coated bacteriophage T4, and with rabbit anti-mouse B leukemia cells (39), assayed by C'-dependent cytotoxicity. In the last case, 64% of the activity was retained for the conjugate with 2 moles drug per mole antibody. In a second preparation, with 6 moles per mole, only 25% of the antibody activity remained.

The activity of daunomycin is based on their ability to bind to DNA, intercalating between the base pairs and inhibiting its template activity for DNA and RNA polymerase (40, 41). They must, therefore, enter the cell as well as the nucleus to exert their effects. It is possible that the drug-conjugates are effective because they may enter the cells by pinocytosis and be digested intacellularly to liberate either free drug or small drug-peptide conjugates.

The conjugates of daunomycin with immunoglobulins containing antibodies against either the previously mentioned carcinogen-induced B cell leukemia in SJL/J mice (39) or a mineral oil induced plasmocytoma (PC5) in BALB/c mice (42), were tested for their toxic effects on various tumor target cells as measured either by their inhibition of RNA synthesis or by their reduction of the growth of the tumor cells after transplantation (R. Levy, E. Hurwitz, R. Maron, R. Arnon and M. Sela, unpublished data). Tables 4 and 5 illustrate some of the results.

TABLE 4

Specific cytotoxicity of daunomycin linked to anti-B-leukemia

Incubated with	% Inhibition of $[^3H]$-uridine incorporation			
	Test cells			
	B-leukemia	YAC	PC5	Rat lymphoma
Daunomycin-anti-B-leukemia	38^a	42^a	17^b	9^b
Daunomycin-anti-BSA	1^b	0^b	4	9
Daunomycin-anti-BSA + Anti-B-leukemia	18^c	0^d	n.d.	n.d.
Free daunomycin	17	49	33	41

0.6 µg drug either as the protein conjugate or free drug was incubated with 10^6 cells in a total volume of 100 µl for 5 minutes at 37^oC. Medium was then removed, cells were washed and resuspended in fresh medium and pulsed with $[^3H]$-uridine at the end of two hours of further incubation.

Difference between [a] and [b] p <.001 by the Student's test.

Difference between [a] and [c] p <.05.

Difference between [a] and [d] p <.001.

TABLE 5

Specific cytoxicity of daunomycin linked to anti-PC5
immunoglobulin

	% Inhibition of $[^3H]$-uridine incorporation		
Incubated with	Test cells		
	PC5	Rat lymphoma	YAC
Daunomycin-anti-RPC5	60^a	63^a	20^b
Daunomycin-anti-BSA	7^b	14^b	n.d.
Daunomycin-anti-B-leukemia	16^b	14^b	62^a
Free daunomycin	32^c	53	67

1.5 µg of drug was used, other conditions were identical to
those in Table 1.

All [a] different from all [b] by p <.001, Student's T test.

[a] different from [c] by p <.001.

As is seen clearly in these Tables, the drug-conjugate
preferentially affected the target cells which the attached
antibody could recognize. These daunomycin-antibody conjugates are, therefore, sufficiently toxic and selective in their
effects to be potentially useful in in vivo therapeutic
studies.

CONCLUDING REMARKS

The common denominator of the three studies discussed
here is that all of them are based on synthetic approaches,
all of them use immunology, all of them have a medical application as a goal, and none of them have yet reached the stage
of such an application. It is also pertinent to remark that
these studies are a natural extension of our basic interest
in the molecular nature of antigens and antibodies, and the
use of proper antigen design for a better understanding of
immunological phenomena.

35

REFERENCES

(1) M.W. Kies, Ann. N.Y. Acad. Sci., 122 (1965) 161.

(2) P.Y. Paterson, Adv. Immunol., 5 (1966) 131.

(3) E.H. Eylar, J. Salk, G. Beveridge and L. Brown, Arch. Biochem. Biophys., 132 (1969) 34.

(4) E.C. Alvord, Jr., C.M. Shaw, R.P. Lisak, G.A. Falk and M.W. Kies, Int. Arch. Allergy Appl. Immunol., 38 (1970) 403.

(5) A. Nakao, W.J. Davis and E. Roboz-Einstein, Biochim. Biophys. Acta, 130 (1966) 163.

(6) P.R. Carnegie, B. Bencina and G.L. Lamoureux, Biochem. J., 105 (1967) 559.

(7) T. Hirshfeld, D. Teitelbaum, R. Arnon and M. Sela, FEBS Letters, 7 (1970) 317.

(8) E.H. Eylar, Proc. Natl. Acad. Sci. U.S., 67 (1970) 1425.

(9) P.R. Carnegie, Nature, 229 (1971) 25.

(10) E.H. Eylar, S. Brostoff, G. Hashim, J. Caccam and P. Burnett, J. Biol. Chem., 246 (1971) 5770).

(11) L.P. Chao and E. Roboz-Einstein, J. Biol. Chem., 245 (1970) 6397.

(12) R.F. Kibler, P.K. Re, S. McKneally, R. Shapira and M.E. Keeling, J. Biol. Chem., 247 (1972) 969.

(13) E.C. Alvord, Jr., C.M. Shaw, S. Hruby and M.W. Kies, Ann. N.Y. Acad. Sci., 122 (1965) 333.

(14) E. Roboz-Einstein, J. Csejtey, W.J. Davis and H. Rauch, Immunochemistry, 5 (1968) 567.

(15) E.H. Eylar, J. Jackson, B. Rothenberg and S. Brostoff, Nature, 236 (1972) 74.

(16) D. Teitelbaum, A. Meshorer, T. Hirshfeld, R. Arnon and M. Sela, Eur. J. Immunol., 1 (1971) 242.

(17) D. Teitelbaum, C. Webb, A. Meshorer, R. Arnon and M. Sela, Eur. J. Immunol., 3 (1973) 273.

(18) D. Teitelbaum, C. Webb. A. Meshorer, R. Arnon and M. Sela, Nature, 240 (1972) 564.

(19) C. Webb, D. Teitelbaum, R. Arnon and M. Sela, Eur. J. Immunol., 3 (1973) 279.

(20) D. Teitelbaum, C. Webb, M. Bree, A. Meshorer, R. Arnon and M. Sela, J. Clin. Immunol. Immunopathol., in press.

(21) C. Webb, D. Teitelbaum, O. Abramsky, R. Arnon and M. Sela, Lancet, II (1974) 66.

(22) P. Gold and S.O. Freedman, J. Exp. Med., 122 (1965) 467.

(23) C. Banjo, J.M. Gold, J. Shuster and P. Gold, Israel J. Med. Sci., 10 (1974) 856.

(24) J. Krupey, P. Gold and S.O. Freedman, J. Exp. Med., 128 (1968) 387.

(25) D.M. Thomson, J. Krupey, S.O. Freedman and P. Gold, Proc. Natl. Acad. Sci. U.S., 64 (1969) 161.

(26) M.L. Egan, J.T. Lautenschleger, J.E. Coligan and C.W. Todd, Immunochemistry, 9 (1972) 289.

(27) P. Lo Gerfo, J. Krupey, H.J. Hansen, New England J. Med., 285 (1971) 138.

(28) W.D. Terry, P.A. Henkart, J.E. Coligan, C.W. Todd, J. Exp. Med., 136 (1972) 200.

(29) R. Arnon, E. Maron, M. Sela and C.B. Anfinsen, Proc. Natl. Acad. Sci. U.S., 68 (1971) 1450.

(30) R.B. Merrifield, Science, 150 (1965) 178.

(31) J. Haimovich, E. Hurwitz, N. Novik and M. Sela, Biochim. Biophys. Acta, 207 (1970) 115.

(32) J. Haimovich, E. Hurwitz, N. Novik and M. Sela, Biochim. Biophys. Acta, 207 (1970) 125.

(33) T. Ghose and S.P. Nigam, Cancer, 29 (1972) 1398.

(34) J.H. Linford, G. Froese, I. Berczi and L.G. Israels, J. Natl. Cancer Inst., 52 (1974) 1665.

(35) M. Szekerke, R. Wade and M.E. Whisson, Neoplasma, 19 (1972) 211.

(36) G. Mathé, Ba Loc Tran and J. Bernard, Compt. rend. Acad. Sci. (Paris), 246 (1958) 1626.

(37) R. Magnenat, R. Schindler and H. Isliker, Eur. J. Cancer, 5 (1969) 33.

(38) M. Szekerke, R. Wade and M.E. Whisson, Nature, 215 (1967) 1303.

(39) N. Haran-Ghera and A. Peled, Nature, 241 (1973) 396.

(40) E. Calendi, A. Di Marco, M. Reggiani, B. Scarpinato and L. Valentini, Biochim. Biophys. Acta, 103 (1965) 25.

(41) W.J. Pigram, W. Fuller and L.D. Hamilton, Nature New Biol., 17 (1972) 235.

(42) M. Potter and C.L. Robertson, J. Natl. Cancer Inst., 25 (1960) 847.

Studies on experimental allergic encephalomyelitis and multiple sclerosis were supported by the Freudenberg Foundation and by the American Multiple Sclerosis Society Grant 841-A-1, while the synthetic approaches to the carcinoembryonic antigen were supported by Contract No. NIH-NCI-G-72-3890. M.S. is Established Investigator of the Chief Scientist's Bureau, Ministry of Health, Israel.

DETECTION OF CELL SURFACE ALLOANTIGENS*

F.H. BACH, M.L. BACH, B.J. ALTER, K.F. LINDAHL,
D.J. SCHENDEL and P.M. SONDEL
Departments of Medical Genetics and Surgery, Pediatrics and
The Immunobiology Research Center
The University of Wisconsin, Madison

Abstract: Antigens of the major histocompatibility complex
can be divided into two genetically and functionally
distinct categories. The immunological reaction which
antigens of these two types evoke may provide models
for our understanding of differentiation of cell
surface alloantigens.

The mixed leukoycte culture (MLC) test was described
ten years ago by Bain, Vas and Lowenstein (1) and by Bach
and Hirschhorn (2). Since that time it has been used for
immunogenetic analysis of histocompatibility antigens (primarily those of the major histocompatibility complex (MHC))
for clinical matching of donor and recipient for transplantation, for studies of lymphocyte cell populations and other
facets of cell-mediated immune reactions and for a variety
of biochemical studies. Four years ago a second test, the
cell-mediated lympholysis (CML) test (3-6), was added to
our armamentarium of in vitro models of cell-mediated immunity. Whereas the MLC test (usually assayed by studying
the incorporation of radioactive thymidine into dividing
cells in culture) can be thought of as an assay of recognition by T lymphocytes of alloantigenic differences leading
primarily to cell proliferation, the CML test is an assay
of cell destruction. We shall use the terms MLC and CML to
refer to the proliferative and cytotoxic reactions respectively unless otherwise noted.

Our purpose in this paper is to discuss recognition in
MLC and CML. This problem can be approached from several perspectives; we shall stress two: The complex genetic control
of alloantigenic differences which are recognized and the
cellular response that follows recognition. Studies which
bear on this topic have been performed primarily in mouse
and man; it appears in terms of the broad biological principles which may emerge from these studies that one can
freely extrapolate from one species to the other. A major
* The data published in this paper has been published elsewhere (Proc. of 9th Leukocyte Culture Conference, Novem-
  ber 1974, in press.)

focus of our discussion will be on the genetic control of
alloantigens which is more fully understood and more directly
analyzed in mouse.

The following terminology will be used. MHC will
refer to the major histocompatibility complex, HL-A in man
and H-2 in mouse. SD antigens are those antigens detected
serologically that are determined by MHC loci (LA, Four and
AJ in man; H-2K and H-2D in mouse) and which are present on
essentially all tissues of the body. LD determinants are
those differences of the MHC which lead to proliferation of
cells in MLC. Whether the LD differences are currently
being recognized serologically will be discussed later in
this paper. [The letters Hld (histocompatibility LD) are
used for the formal designation of H-2 loci governing the LD
antigens, since the letters LD have been used for another
locus in mouse.] Finally, we shall refer to the LD factors
as "antigens" on the basis that they elicit a clonal cellular
response(7-8), and that it has been possible to make animals
tolerant to LD (9).

GENETIC CONTROL OF ALLOANTIGENS

Genes Important in MLC Activation

Very early studies in man (10), mouse (11) and rat (12)
showed that the genes that led to proliferative events in MLC
were to a large extent restricted to the MHC, although it
must be noted that in mouse two other genetic systems can,
if different in two strains, lead to proliferation in MLC
(13,14). Since MHC antigens were first described by serological techniques in both man and mouse, it was assumed that
these serologically defined (SD) antigens were responsible
for activation in MLC. It is now well established that there
are genes of the MHC, other than the SD genes, which are of
prime importance in leading to proliferation of lymphocytes
in MLC, the evidence for this in humans evolving over several
years (15-19). These are the MHC LD genes.

Studies by Widmer (20-22), using mouse strains developed
by Snell, Stimpfling and others, led to the mapping of the LD
loci in the mouse. Figure 1 gives the genetic maps of the
MHC in several species including mouse. There is one locus
(loci) in the I region of H-2 which is the strong Hld locus.
A second relatively weaker Hld locus has been formally mapped
between Ss and H-2D (23). It is quite likely, however, that
there are still other loci yet to be discovered in the H-2

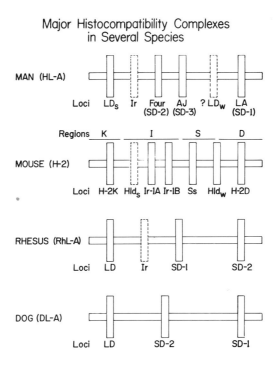

Major Histocompatibility Complexes in Several Species

Figure 1 legend. A schematic representation of the major histocompatibility complex in four species. In man, there are three loci identified, LA, Four and AJ, alleles of which determine the serologically defined antigens. The locus, differences at which lead to strong activation in MLC, is mapped as LD_S; the LD_W locus, if it does exist, maps between the AJ and LA loci. The Ir locus (loci are listed in a dotted line since the position of this locus is not known.

The mouse H-2 complex is divided into four regions, K, I, S, and D each designated by a marker locus, H-2K, Ir-1A, Ss and H-2D. The alleles of the H-2K and H-2D loci determine the classical serologically defined H-2 antigens. The loci, differences of which lead to MLC activation, are designated as Hld$_s$ and Hld$_w$ respectively; the Hld designation is used since the initials LD have been used for another locus in the mouse genome. The Ir-1A and Ir-1B loci determine immune response of the animal and the Ss locus controls the quantitative levels of a serum protein. Differences of the two LD loci result in activation of lymphocytes in mixed leukocyte culture and are associated with graft versus host reactions in vivo; the alleles of the Hld$_s$ locus are relatively stronger in this regard than alleles of the Hld$_w$ locus. The Hld$_s$ locus has not been formally separated from the Ir-1A locus.

The order of loci in rhesus and dog are shown. The existence of immune response loci in the RhL-A chromosome of rhesus has been documented; at least two of them map outside the SD region of RhL-A probably close to the strong MLC locus but separate from it by recombination. Only in mouse is the position of the centromere known.

---

complex that should be designated as Hld loci on the basis of their being associated with stimulation in MLC. An analysis of the data obtained in these studies shows the following: first, strong stimulation was observed in strain combinations differing for only the I and S regions, identical for the SD antigens; second, relatively weaker stimulation was seen when strains differed for only the SD antigens and were identical for the I and S regions (in some of these cases no stimulation was detected); third, when mice differed for the I region plus either K alone or plus other regions, there was on the average stronger stimulation than when there was no I region disparity. These results are shown in Table 1.

Table 1

Summary of MLC Responses

MHC Regions Which Are Different	Ratio of Stimulation	
	Range*	Average
K, Ir-1, Ss-Slp, D	1.2 - 33.6	7.2
K, Ir-1, Ss-Slp	1.4 - 15.7	6.1

K, Ir-1, D	3.3 - 20.5	7.0
K, Ss-Slp, D	1.5 - 8.6	3.3
Ir-1, Ss-Slp, D	2.7 - 15.1	8.3
K, Ir-1	3.2 - 18.3	6.6
K, Ss-Slp	No experiments	
Ir-1, Ss-Slp	2.7 - 12.8	5.8
K, D	3.0 - 3.8	3.4
Ir-1, D	No experiments	
Ss-Slp, D	0.7 - 4.7	2.0
K	0.8 - 2.2	1.4
Ir-1	No experiments	
D	0.8 - 5.4	1.8
Ss-Slp	0.6 - 4.9	2.0
None	0.6 - 1.9	1.2

*These numbers represent the lowest and highest ratios of stimulation noted.

These studies, which were confirmed by Meo, Shreffler et al. (24,25), in aggregate suggested that LD differences in the I region were of the greatest import in leading to MLC activation and that the SD antigens were either not stimulatory at all or only weakly so. More recent work using heat treatment of the stimulating cells (to be discussed later) demonstrates that it is possible to differentially inactivate the stimulating cell so that it no longer induces a proliferative reponse but the SD antigens are still expressed. We would not want to conclude from these data that the SD antigens are, in the absence of concurrent LD differences, unable to lead to a proliferative response in MLC; however, it would seem that if they can do so, they are certainly weaker in this regard than the LD differences.

Genes Important in CML

At first examination, in culture systems which were less sensitive than those used now, H-2 LD differences in the presence of SD identity led to excellent stimulation in MLC but no cytotoxicity in CML. More recently, using a more sensitive MLC technique (26), Peck, Schendel and Alter (27-30) have demonstrated low level CML in some of these combinations. We shall return to a discussion of this later.

Rather than using LD as the prime target in CML, lymphocytes activated in MLC to both LD and SD differences appeared to recognize primarily the SD antigens themselves or the products of genes very closely linked to those determining the SD antigens as the targets in CML. Because of this genetic inseparability, we shall refer to the CML targets as the SD antigens. Data from an experiment demonstrating this phenomenon are shown in Table 2, confirming similar findings in a human family (31). Cells activated to LD plus SD differences become cytotoxic to those target cells carrying the SD antigens but not to those carrying LD.

Recent experiments of K.F. Lindahl (32) using xenogeneic combinations are an example of differential cytotoxicity on LD and SD which dramatically demonstrates the difference between these two determinants leading to CML. In these experiments human lymphocytes sensitized to mouse cells are tested for their ability to lyse different mouse target cells. Combinations were selected to analyze whether both LD and SD antigens could function as targets or whether one was predominant in this regard. The results show that the SD antigens serve as excellent xenogeneic CML targets; in contrast there was no evidence that LD antigens were recognized by the xenogeneic effector lymphocytes. An example of such an experiment is given in Table 3. Human lymphocytes were sensitized to each of four different mouse strains, B10.A(4R), B10.A(1R), AQR and B10.T(6R). Since the prime targets in such xenogeneic CML tests are H-2 determined (32) we can focus on the H-2 phenotypes of these four strains. The two combinations of 4R-1R and AQR-6R are SD identical but differ for LD. AQR and 1R are I and S region identical and SD different. Human effector cells sensitized to AQR or 6R, for instance, are highly cytotoxic to AQR. These two strains are SD identical. On the other hand, the same human lymphocytes sensitized to 1R do not lyse AQR target cells, demonstrating the I and S region components of 1R which are shared by AQR are not recognized as targets. Results on the three other target cells are consistent with those on AQR.

LD-SD COLLABORATION IN CML

While LD differences by themselves or SD differences by themselves on the stimulating cells in MLC do not lead to strong CML on any target cell, the presence of both LD and SD

TABLE II

	MCL (mean cpm ± SD)	MCL Sensitization		CML Assay		
		Responding Cell (Effector)	Stimulating Cell (Sensitizing)	Target Cell	^{51}Cr released (mean cpm ± SD)	% CML
A[1]	14,819 · 1406	B10.A (kkdd)	AQR (qkdd)	B10.A (kkdd)	469 ± 11	- 4.6
				AQR (qkdd)	372 ± 36	- 3.6
	44,777 ± 5237	B10.A (kkdd)	B10.T(6R) (qqqd)	B10.A (kkdd)	484 ± 21	- 1.4
				B10.T(6R) (qqqd)	534 ± 19	37.5
				AQR (qkdd)	623 ± 19	42.6
				C57BL/10 (bbbb)	383 ± 33	13.8
	14,487 ± 846	B10.A (kkdd)	B10.A (kkdd)	B10.A (kkdd)	417 ± 54	-15.4
B[2]	13,725 ± 2236	B10.A(2R) (kkdb)	B10.A (kkdd)	B10.A(2R) (kkdb)	532 ± 142	- 4.9
				B10.A (kkdd)	552 ± 13	5.3
	79,236 ± 6902	B10.A(2R) (kkdb)	B10.D2 (dddd)	B10.A(2R) (kkdb)	889 ± 67	24.9
				B10.D2 (dddd)	1541 ± 140	72.3
				B10.A (kkdd)	1041 32	78.5
				C57BL/10 (bbbb)	1232 ± 43	40.6
	10,423 ± 623	B10.A(2R) (kkdb)	B10.A(2R) (kkdb)	B10.A(2R) (kkdb)	434 ± 7	-13.1

The % CML is based on the following spontaneous release (SR) and maximum release (MR) values (mean of triplicates ± SD) for each target cell:

[1] B10.A SR = 491 ± 20 MR = 974 ± 61; AQR SR = 391 ± 24
MR = 935 ± 45; B10.T(6R) SR = 328 ± 25 MR = 877 ± 66;
C57BL/10 SR = 721 ± 73 MR = 1978 ± 30.

The haplotype nomenclature is explained in note C to Table 7.

45

Table 2 - continued

[2] B10.A(2R)   SR = 591 ± 23   MR = 1786 ± 60;   B10.A   SR = 516 ± 14   MR = 1184 ± 59;   B10.D2   SR = 684 ± 47   MR = 1869 ± 34;   C57BL/10   SR = 721 ± 73   MR = 1978 ± 30.

Table 3

SD Specificity of Human Effector Cells

Human lymphocytes sensitized to	H-2 haplotype				% CML on targets from			
	K	I	S	D	4R	1R	AQR	6R
B10.A(4R)	k	k/b	b	b	43.4 ± 6.9	29.4 ± 10.0	8.8 ± 7.3	6.5 ± 12.4
B10.A(1R)	k	k	d	b	46.3 ± 6.2	23.5 ± 6.3	- 6.8 ± 11.5	- 1.4 ± 14.2
AQR	q	k	d	d	32.5 ± 6.1	16.2 ± 8.9	43.8 ± 11.3	31.3 ± 11.5
B10.T(6R)	q	q	q	d	24.9 ± 4.4	13.5 ± 7.2	36.6 ± 11.2	34.6 ± 12.4

CML assay was carried out for 3 hours with 70 effector cells:1 target cell. All assays were done in triplicate.

$$\text{\% CML} = \frac{\text{Exp. release} - \text{control release}}{\text{Max. release} - \text{control release}} \times 100$$

Control release is the amount of ^{51}Cr released with unstimulated (HH_{lu}) effector cells.

4R: M.R. - 944 ± 50 cpm; C.R. - 500 ± 18 cpm;
1R: M.R. - 1265 ± 28 cpm; C.R. - 556 ± 43 cpm;
AQR: M.R. - 1133 ± 48 cpm; C.R. - 571 ± 60 cpm;
6R: M.R. - 1309 ± 26 cpm; C.R. - 621 ± 89 cpm.

does allow the effective generation of cytotoxic cells. This has been referred to as LD-SD collaboration. This collaboration is most easily studied in three-cell experiments where the determinants are presented on separate stimulating cells. An example of such a three-cell experiment is presented in Table 4. B10.T(6R) is the responding population and LD sensitization is provided by AQR_m cells. $B10.G_m$ cells present SD determinants; in this case SD disparity is associated with H-2D locus differences. Sensitization of B10.T(6R) to only LD (AQR_m) produces strong proliferation but generates no CML. SD sensitization by $B10.G_m$ alone shows minimal proliferation and cytotoxicity. In three-cell cultures where both LD and SD determinants are used for simultaneous sensitization, one observes both MLC proliferation and CML. Following the consistently seen pattern, cytotoxic activity is only detected when effector cells are incubated with B10.G (SD-different) targets.

TABLE IV

A Three-Cell Experiment

Effector combination	Genetic stimulation	MLC (mean cpm ± SD)	AQR	% CML (mean ± SD) B10.T(6R)	B10.G
B10.T(6R) + AQR$_m$ (qqqd) (qkdd)	LD	16,817 ± 763	-3.1 ± 2.2	-3.9 ± 0.91	
B10.T(6R) + B10.G$_m$ (qqqq)	SD	5,852 ± 480	-1.4 ± 2.0		4.3 ± 1.5
B10.T(6R) + AQR$_m$ + B10.G$_m$	LD + SD	24,334 ± 508	-0.48 ± 2.6	-1.9 ± 1.9	-21.4 ± 2.2
B10.T(6R) + B10.T(6R)$_m$	--	2,473 ± 152		-2.2 1.4	

This experiment provides an example of a situation in which sensitization by either LD or SD antigens alone does not stimulate strong cytotoxic potential, but together they collaborate to generate specific CML which is directed towards SD targets. This experiment, together with others previously described (33) demonstrates LD-SD collaboration with SD antigens of either H-2K or H-2D stimulating cyto-toxic effector cells.

 Initial studies with many SD combinations differing only
at K or D failed to generate cytotoxic lymphocytes. Using
altered culture techniques it is now possible to obtain CML
effectors in most SD combinations. Even in situations where
stimulation by SD alone can lead to CML, a collaborative effect with stimulation by both LD and SD during the MLC sensitization phase produces an enhanced CML response compared
to that detected when only SD differences are used for stimulation. Figure 2 illustrates the cytotoxic potential of
cultures stimulated by SD region differences alone (AQR +
B10.A and LD plus SD differences (AQR + B10.T(6R)$_m$ +
B10.A$_m$). Data from AQR + B10.T(6R)$_m$ cultures (LD alone) are
not presented, as no significant CML response is detected.

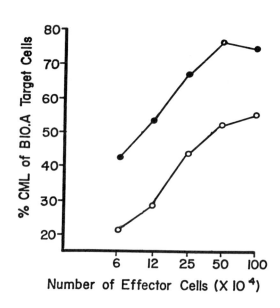

Figure 2 legend. The cytotoxic activity of effector cells stimulated by an SD region alone (o) and stimulated by LD + SD (●). Different numbers of effector cells are combined with a constant number of target cells (1×10^4).

At any effector-to-target-cell ratio, stimulation with (LD + SD) differences causes approximately 20% more CML of SD targets. The number of effectors required to cause 50% lysis of a given number of targets is 4.2-fold less in LD enhanced cultures compared to the cultures sensitized to SD alone. Not only is the specific activity of effector populations different in the two cultures, but there is also a two-fold difference in the number of effector cells recovered per culture. Using the preceeding two values, approximately eight-fold more effector cells are generated in this experiment by LD + SD stimulation compared to SD stimulation alone.

Is collaboration by LD an essential event or only a helper effect? Examples have been cited where neither LD nor SD alone stimulate CML but combined sensitization does; such results would indicate an obligate need for LD. However, stimulation by SD region differences alone can also produce CML responses under some conditions (figure 2). It must be emphasized again that when we speak of two strains having SD differences we are speaking of strains that differ for entire SD regions, and certainly only part of the genetic material contained in such a region is coding for SD antigens. Clearly, SD region differences alone are not totally incapable of activating MLC proliferation (34). The SD regions themselves may determine quantitatively weaker LD differences that can both stimulate proliferation and collaborate with SD antigens of the same region to produce CML. We have obtained evidence from one series of experiments which provide data consistent with the hypothesis that there are in fact LD-like determinants in the K region of B10.A which are recognized by AQR and collaborate with SD antigens to produce CML (28) as described below.

In human CML studies Eijsvoogel et al. (34) demonstrated that heat treatment of an allogeneic stimulating cell destroyed its ability to cause strong MLC proliferation but left its ability to sensitize for CML, provided an LD difference was supplied by another non-heat-treated cell. In addition, heat treatment has been shown to have no effect upon the ability of cells to absorb anti-SD antibody. These results indicate that heat treatment may inhibit or eliminate LD stimulatory potential but leave SD relatively unaffected. We have studied effects of heat treatment in the three-cell system. We wished to focus particularly upon the question of whether AQR and B10.A (SD region different) have weak LD differences determined by the SD region which collaborate to produce CML effectors.

The rationale of the experiment was to use heat treatment to damage any LD differences on the B10.A stimulating cell while leaving SD antigens intact. One could then determine whether SD antigens themselves produce CML effectors. Table 5 shows results of such a heat treatment experiment. The

TABLE V

The Effect of Heat-Treatment of Stimulating Cells

on the Generation of Cytotoxic Responses

Effector combination	MLC activation* (mean cpm ± SD)	% CML** (mean ± SD)
AQR + B10.A$_m$	4113 ± 190	-21.8 ± 2.2
AQR + B10.A$_m$ + B10.T(6R)$_m$	8292 ± 309	40.4 ± 2.8
AQR + B10.A$_\Delta$***	4332 ± 89	3.1 ± 1.9
AQR + B10.A$_\Delta$ + B10.T(6R)$_\Delta$	5771 ± 301	-3.2 ± 2.6
AQR + B10.A$_m$ + B10.T(6R)$_\Delta$	8771 ± 287	25.3 ± 3.5
AQR + B10.A$_\Delta$ + B10.T(6R)$_m$	17375 ± 426	42.7 ± 2.9

* The AQR + AQR$_m$ cultures gave 2926 ± 254 cpm and AQR + AQR$_\Delta$ gave 2316 ± 107 cpm.

** The % CML of the B10.A target cell is presented.

*** Δ = 45°C for 60 mins.

first set of data shows control values for the normal experimental system using mitomycin C to inactivate stimulating cells. The SD combination under these conditions gives positive proliferation and cytotoxicity, and CML is enhanced in the three-cell combination where both LD and SD are used as stimuli. When heat treatment is substituted for mitomycin C inactivation essentially all CML activity is lost. The last two lines show responses when both treatments are combined. When the LD stimulating cell is heat treated and the SD stimulating cell is inactivated with mitomycin C, CML is not significantly different from that seen with SD stimula-

tion alone in the normal system (25% vs 22%). More interestingly, though, when the SD stimulating cell is heat treated
and the LD stimulating cell is mitomycin C inactivated, CML
is as high as that seen in normal three-cell cultures (43% vs
40%). Cell populations stimulated by heat treated lymphocytes differing by SD alone or by both LD and SD are not cytotoxic, but CML can be restored by adding back a normal LD
stimulus on a mitomycin C treated cell. This indicates that
in AQR + B10.A the SD region difference is still expressed in
such a manner that it can sensitize for target recognition,
but it is critically affected in its ability to produce cytotoxic effector cells without an added normal LD stimulus.
Thus heat treatment may actually be damaging an LD difference
which is controlled by a locus closely linked to the H-2K
locus of B10.A and located within the SD (K) region. If
this interpretation is correct it would suggest that collaboration between LD and SD is essential in generation of CML.
Alternatively one could argue that heat treatment affects
only one molecule (i.e. that carrying the SD determinants).
Under this model heat treatment would cause relatively little
change of the SD antigens which are important targets
for cytotoxic cells but would inactivate LD-like determinants
on the same molecule. Lastly one must rule out that the SD
determinants per se are responsible for both reactions.
Nevertheless heat treatment allows operational separation of
LD and SD-type activity.

THE H-2 MUTANTS

The most perplexing findings in relation to the genetic
control of MLC and CML comes from studies with two mutants.
One mutant, discovered by Dr. Donald Bailey, carries a spontaneous mutation in the H-2^b chromosome of the C57BL/6By
mouse which leads to reciprocal skin graft rejection with its
parent strain; nevertheless, upon reciprocal immunization no
antisera defining SD-type antigens had been evoked. Recent
evidence suggests that the amount of the H-2K SD antigen in
the two strains is different (35) or there may even be a
qualitative difference (36). It is difficult to account for
the two-way MLC stimulation and CML on the basis of quantitative differences in the amount of the H-2K SD antigen, however. This mutant could be interpreted as showing that LD
differences lead to strong cytotoxicity. Similarly the mutant of Egorov, a spontaneous mutation apparently affecting
the H-2D locus product of the H-2^d chromosome, evokes both
MLC reactivity and skin graft rejection with the parental
strain (37). This might be taken as pure SD-type differences

51

causing strong proliferation. One must be cautious in inter-
preting these mutations as simple events affecting only LD or
SD. It is conceivable that these mutations, while spontaneous, are not point mutations but represent something more
complex which affects multiple closely-linked loci. Alternatively LD and SD phenotypic products may interact at the
molecular level. Such an interaction could lead to allosteric phenomena whereby a change in configuration of one
molecule could lead to a configurational change in the second
molecule. Based on the above arguments the mutants may well
fit into the LD-SD model we have presented in this paper; by
themselves they do not help us critically dissect the relative roles of LD and SD.

CELLULAR BASIS OF THE MLC AND CML RESPONSES

The LD-SD dichotomy discussed above posed a problem regarding the cell populations responding to the two types of
stimuli. It is known that both the response to LD stimuli as
measured by proliferation in MLC and the cytotoxic response
in CML are clonally distributed. LD-SD cooperation may involve two subpopulations of lymphocytes. Given two separate
responding subpopulations, we might postulate that one population, a proliferating helper cell, responds primarily to
LD-type stimuli; this response may then enable a second population, the eventual cytotoxic lymphocyte, to react to the
appropriate target (38-40). Whether it is proliferation of
the first population or a separate response (which might be
distinct from the proliferative events themselves) which is
essential to allow the second population to respond is a subject for further experimentation.

The cooperative response to LD and SD could be based on
a single responding cell population, since the two-cell model
has not been critically proven (40). One could either hypothesize that a single responding cell has two types of receptors, one recognizing LD differences and the other SD differences, or that a single receptor recognizes both LD and
SD. LD recognition and response might be essential before
the cell can recognize SD differences and develop into a cytotoxic lymphocyte. Given this model adsorption studies suggest (39) that within the responding population to any one
allogeneic stimulus there are many cells which respond to LD
differences, only a fraction of which differentiate to become
cytotoxic lymphocytes. Alternatively one might hypothesize,
as M. Cohn has done for antibody production, that an associative recognition takes place. The LD different stimulating

52

cell may <u>recognize</u> the eventual cytotoxic effector cell and give it a signal which permits it to recognize the SD difference.

Since MHC LD differences appeared to function as a less effective target for cytotoxic lymphocytes, the question arose whether this was true because LD did not effectively stimulate lymphocytes to become cytotoxic effector cells or whether the cytotoxic cells did develop, but the LD antigens did not serve as a good "target". Alternatively, the LD antigens may be present on so few cells that the destruction of these cells is not detected in CML; this will be discussed later. Alter (41) has used the system developed by Forman and Müller (42) in an attempt to answer this question. These authors demonstrated that lymphocytes sensitized to alloantigens in MLC are cytotoxic not only to target cells carrying those same antigens, but even to isogeneic (self) targets if phytohemagglutinin (PHA) is added to the mixture of sensitized cells and target cells during the cytotoxicity assay (PHA-dependent cytotoxicity). This autokilling is presumably due to agglutination of the killer cell with the target and not to recognition of self-antigens. To the extent that PHA-dependent cytotoxicity can be used as a model for assessing the presence of cytotoxic lymphocytes in CML, we have used this system to determine whether proliferative responses to LD antigens alone can "generate" cytotoxic cells.

Results of two of the six experiments performed are shown in Tables 6 and 7. In Table 6 are given results with PHA stimulated blast cells as target cells; in Table 7, fresh lymphocytes are used. In each table MLC results are given using cells from strains differing by H-2 LD and SD factors and MLC mixtures differing by LD factors alone. The cytotoxic assay is carried out either as in normal CML tests or in the presence of PHA (columns 1 and 2, respectively, under "percent cytotoxicity").

Cultures activated with cells which differ for both LD and SD components generate cytotoxic lymphocytes active against the specific target. In spite of significant and similar MLC activation, combinations which differ only by LD show little if any lysis of specific "targets (AQR or B10.T(6R)) or of unrelated targets bearing LD and SD differences from the sensitizing cells in CML.

The level of self killing when PHA is added to the cultures during the three-hour incubation depends upon the gene-

Table 6. PHA Dependent Cytotoxicity with PHA-Blast Lymphocytes as Targets

MLC[a]	Sensitization of Effectors[b]	Target	% Cytotoxicity ± SD[d]	
			No PHA Added During CML Assay	PHA Added During CML Assay
	LD + SD			
19819 ± 439	B10.T(6R) + C57BL/10$_m$[c]	AQR	2.3 ± 2.4	36.3 ± 3.6
		B10.T(6R)	-8.0 ± 1.7	31.8 ± 4.7
		C57BL/10	68.2 ± 4.1	77.9 ± 3.5
13303 ± 1075	AQR + C57BL/10$_m$	AQR	0.6 ± 0.8	40.1 ± 0.9
		B10.T(6R)	-7.1 ± 1.7	36.8 ± 2.6
		C57BL/10	71.8 ± 4.4	68.9 ± 4.0
	LD			
12205 ± 604	B10.T(6R) + AQR$_m$	AQR	-4.4 ± 1.6	1.7 ± 1.2
		B10.T(6R)	-14.7 ± 1.7	-3.1 ± 1.7
		C57BL/10	-11.4 ± 3.6	-1.6 ± 5.4
14771 ± 756	AQR + B10.T(6R)$_m$	AQR	-4.9 ± 1.8	5.4 ± 2.4
		B10.T(6R)	-9.5 ± 1.7	2.8 ± 2.5
		C57BL/10	-11.2 ± 3.8	1.4 ± 5.1

[a]Mean cpm of triplicate values ± SD; control values are B10.T(6R) + B10.T(6R)$_m$ = 761 ± 86; AQR + AQR$_m$ = 1577 ± 47.

[b]We refer to the four regions of the MHC as K,I,S,D. The loci, alleles of which determine the SD antigens are in the K and D regions; the strong LD locus appears to be in the I region. AQR = qkdd; B10.T(6R) = qqqd; C57BL/10 = bbbb.

[c]Reciprocal combinations (not shown) were also done with a comparable pattern of results.

[d]Percent cytotoxicity is calculated $\dfrac{ER - SSR}{MR - SSR} \times 100$

where experimental release (ER) represents mean counts per minute (cpm) released from ^{51}Cr labeled target cells incubated with effectors sensitized to either LD or LD + SD differences; specific spontaneous release (SSR) is the mean cpm released from the target when incubated with cultured cells syngeneic to the target, e.g., AQR + AQR$_m$/AQR target; maximum release (MR) represents the mean cpm released from target cells after rapid freeze-thaw treatment.

Target AQR, MR = 2063 ± 5.6, SSR = 570 ± 9.5, SSR (PHA added during CML assay) = 355 ± 13.4. Target B10.T(6R), MR = 2967 ± 162.3, SSR = 818 ± 21.0, SSR (PHA added during CML assay) = 571 ± 28.5. Target C57B1/10, MR = 2582 ± 66.0, SSR = 823 ± 52.5, SSR (PHA added during CML assay) = 549 ± 104.9.

Table 7. PHA Dependent Cytotoxicity with Fresh Lymphocytes as Targets

MLC[a]	Sensitization of Effectors	Target	% Cytotoxicity ± SD[e]	
			No PHA Added During CML Assay	PHA Added During CML Assay
	LD + SD			
16145 ± 826	B10.T(6R) + C57BL/10$_m$[d]	AQR	2.1 ± 4.6	37.0 ± 5.7
		B10.T(6R)	-1.0 ± 4.5	28.4 ± 4.4
		C57BL/10	55.4 ± 5.0	70.5 ± 2.8
9391 ± 433	AQR + C57BL/10$_m$	AQR	5.3 ± 3.3	40.0 ± 5.1
		B10.T(6R)	3.4 ± 4.4	37.1 ± 2.9
		C57BL/10	52.0 ± 7.1	59.2 ± 5.9
	LD			
10097 ± 274	B10.T(6R) + AQR$_m$	AQR	1.4 ± 4.7	10.8 ± 6.7
		B10.T(6R)	-4.4 ± 5.6	5.0 ± 3.9[b]
		C57BL/10	3.1 ± 6.2	7.6 ± 5.5
8253 ± 317	AQR + B10.T(6R)$_m$	AQR	0.4 ± 4.6	5.8 ± 4.7
		B10.T(6R)	8.7 ± 4.1	12.4 ± 3.0
		C57BL/10	3.7 ± 4.5	12.6 ± 5.6

[a]Mean cpm of triplicate values ± SD; control values are B10.T(6R) + B10.T(6R)$_m$ = 1128 ± 88; AQR + AQR$_m$ = 2223 ± 64.

[b]Percent cytotoxicity of duplicate values; all other data reflect triplicate values.

[c]We refer to the four regions of the MCH as K,I,S,D. The loci, alleles of which determine the SD antigens are in the K and D regions; the strong LD locus appears to be in the I region. We refer to the genotype of each strain with four lower case letters designating the H2 haplotypes from which the K,I,S and D regions are derived. AQR = qkdd; B10.T(6R)= qqqd; C57BL/10 - bbbb.

[d]Reciprocal combinations (not shown) were also done with a comparable pattern of results.

[e]Percent cytotoxicity is calculated $\dfrac{ER - SSR}{MR - SSR} \times 100$

where experimental release (ER) represents mean counts per minute (cpm) released from ^{51}Cr labeled target cells incubated with effectors sensitized to either LD or LD + SD differences; specific spontaneous release (SSR) is the mean cpm released from the target when incubated with cultured cells syngeneic to the target, e.g. AQR + AQR$_m$/AQR target; maximum release (MR) represents the mean cpm released from target cells after rapid freeze-thaw treatment.

Target AQR, MR = 664 ± 27.1, SSR = 212 ± 10.1, SSR (PHA added during CML assay) = 215 ± 19.0. Target B10.T(6R), MR = 689 ± 18.5, SSR = 239 ± 18.3, SSR (PHA added during CML assay) = 244 ± 11.0. Target C57BL/10, MR = 712 ± 314, SSR = 239 ± 14.0, SSR (PHA added during CML assay) = 233 ± 24.1.

---

tic differences existing during the MLC activation phase in the experiment: LD + SD activated cultures generate greater PHA-dependent cytotoxic activity than when the MLC is activated by LD differences alone, despite equivalent levels of proliferative response.

These data demonstrate that if both SD and LD differences are present during the MLC sensitization phase, the effector cells generated are cytotoxic not only to specific target cells in CML but also to isogeneic and other target cells in PHA-dependent cytotoxicity. However, with only LD differences present during the MLC sensitization procedure (identity for the SD antigens) despite an approximately equivalent proliferative response in MLC, the cells are only minimally cytotoxic to any target cells, even in the presence of PHA. This is true both with target cells stimulated three days previously with PHA and with fresh target cells. To the extent that PHA-dependent cytotoxicity can be used to argue about cytotoxic lymphocyte formation in general these results suggest strongly that LD differences present during MLC sensitization do not alone lead to the effective generation of effector cells.

SEROLOGICAL DEFINITION OF THE LD ANTIGENS

In both mouse (43-45) and man (46) there is evidence that products of the MHC genes other than the SD antigens can elicit antibody formation. In mouse, I region products defined with antisera have been called the Ia antigens. It is tempting to hypothesize a priori that these Ia antigens are the stimulatory products in MLC. Furthermore, Meo and his collaborators have recently shown that anti-Ia antisera block the stimulating cells in MLC (47) which is certainly consistent with the Ia antigens being LD. It must be stressed, however, that these studies do not prove that the two types of antigens are one and the same; until definitive proof is available it is probably advisable to maintain them as potentially separate entities. The work in humans is similarly inconclusive; however, if it can be shown that the LD antigens can be defined serologically, this would represent an important and major advance.

IN VIVO RELEVANCE

The relative roles of MHC LD and SD loci in vivo have been recently reviewed (48). In brief, it appears that H-2 LD differences are associated with proliferative graft-versus-host reactions and, in some cases, skin graft rejection; H-2 SD differences are relatively weaker in eliciting a proliferative graft-versus-host reaction and in some cases do not do so but lead to skin graft rejection. In both of these analyses it is important to remember that we are speaking of differences for whole regions of H-2 which include either a known SD locus or LD locus; there is always the possibility in the case of the SD region that there are, in addition, LD-type loci or differences included in that region. Results obtained in man are, insofar as testing permits, consistent with the above findings in mouse. There is no evidence yet available which answers the question whether there is LD-SD collaboration in vivo as there is in vitro.

The clinical usefulness of LD matching with MLC and SD typing has been the subject of intense investigation. The results have also recently been reviewed in detail (47).

THE CONCEPTUAL SEPARATION OF LD AND SD?

Do the experimental findings to date justify a conceptual distinction between LD and SD as two functionally distinct MHC antigenic systems, or might these all be H an-

tigens which function similarly in MLC and CML? The findings
discussed in previous sections of this paper suggest to us
that there are differences between LD and SD components of
the MHC which support a model which considers each as a separate system within the MHC. This has been challenged (35)
by the argument that in fact the differences are only quantitative, suggesting that the distinctions between them are
therefore not justified. We would have to take exception to
such a view on two grounds. First, to state that differences
are quantitative rather than qualitative is only worthwhile
when referring to very specific comparisons. Two gene products that differ only quantitatively in one assay could be
both structurally and functionally (qualitatively) distinct.
Second, it is well established that quantitative differences
are often the basis of differential biological function. The
validity of the conceptual separation of LD and SD depends on
their differential recognition in these two test sytems.

This question can be discussed under three headings,
basically those which have led to the suggestion of dichotomy.
First, is there a difference between LD and SD in leading to
lymphocyte proliferation in MLC? Second, do these two types
of antigens function differently in leading to the development and expression of positive CML reactions? Third, is
there a difference in their function in the LD-SD collaboration?

With respect to stimulation of proliferation in MLC, LD
is of course defined on the basis of this parameter. Speaking for the separation are those studies in mouse and man
which show that the LD differences are much stronger in
leading to proliferation than are the SD differences. This
is true in the studies of Widmer (20-22) quoted earlier as
well as the data obtained confirming those studies. Perhaps
even more impressive are those human families in which recombinational events occurred between the SD loci and the LD
locus and where those siblings that are presumably LD identical but differ for one HL-A SD haplotype stimulate very
little, if at all, in MLC (18,19,43). The results obtained
with _in vivo_ proliferative graft-versus-host reactions parallel the proliferative studies in MLC (50-52). Thus even _in
vivo_ at least some K region different mouse strains fail to
provide a proliferation stimulus under conditions where LD is
very potent.

Arguing against the separation on this basis are the
findings with the Egorov mutant (37) already discussed, as

well as the finding that mouse strains differing by only the D region do stimulate in MLC. It could be argued that this rather low stimulation (see Table 1) is due to the SD anti- gens themselves; likewise one could argue that at least some of these cases are due to concurrent differences for the weak Hld locus located between Ss and H–2D. As already mentioned, given the data we have to date, the Egorov mutant is not uni- quely interpretable. Nevertheless it should serve as a sig- nal that the biological function of the MHC may be far more complex than the rather simplistic LD-SD model currently envisioned.

The difference between LD and SD as a target in CML is also a complicated issue. Supporting the dichotomy are the findings in man and mouse which show that there is a differ- ence in the extent to which these differences function as targets in CML or, on the basis of the PHA-dependent cyto- toxicity studies mentioned in this paper, do lead to the generation of cytotoxic lymphocytes. The studies with xeno- geneic effector cells further support this concept. On the other hand, the finding of very strong cytotoxicity with the Bailey mutant (H(zl)) is once again not easily understood, as we have already discussed. Also, it has been found in some studies using human cells that an SD antigen apparently does not serve as a good target in CML (53). This would suggest that some SD antigens do not function well as a CML target.

It is somewhat disturbing that the two exceptions which seem to argue against the data obtained with recombinant families in man or recombinant mouse chromosomes are both spontaneous mutations of H-2. Various interpretations of these mutations, as discussed above, are however consistent with the LD-SD dichotomy. Clearly, more work must be done with these mutants.

Last, there is the LD-SD interaction which appears to suggest a dichotomy. LD differences in some culture systems, as already reviewed, do not lead to any cytotoxicity on any target cell. Yet, these same genetic differences potentiate the development of cytotoxicity against an SD target. In contrast, however, the opposite is not true.

It would seem to us that the differences summarized a- bove more than justify our working model of LD and SD anti- gens as separate systems of the MHC. It would be foolhardy to speak of this separation without recognizing the similar- ities also; the similarities to some extent are not unex-

pected when considering the similar function of all arms of
the immune system, i.e. recognizing and responding to antigenic differences. Rather, we have found it intriguing to
note the differences which seem to be present, suggesting to
us that for whatever reasons the products of the LD and SD
loci can be distinguished by their ability to stimulate distinct phases of cell-mediated responses in vitro. A number
of reasons can be suggested to explain the dichotomy, both
at the level of antigenic expression and cellular recognition,
including the molecular configuration, the rate of turnover,
the density or topographical location of the antigens on the
cell, the nature of specific responding subpopulations, or
other factors.

Why does LD not function as a strong target? Any of the
reasons just given could be the basis for the inability. In
addition there is the possibility that LD is expressed on
only a very small subpopulation of all the lymphocytes and
that even though these are killed we do not detect it in the
assay. This, of course, could be one basis for the LD-SD
difference in at least some tissues. If this is true, then
we would stress even more the strong nature of LD as a stimulus to MLC proliferation as compared with SD, which is present on all lymphocytes.

Why does SD not function as an efficient stimulant to
lymphocyte proliferation? One possibility would be that the
frequency of cells responding to SD is so small that we do
not detect a large increase in thymidine incorporation. If
this small population of SD-responsive cells contains the
cytotoxic cell precursors, then the LD stimulus is having a
marked effect in collaboration. Alternatively, this hypo-
thetical SD-responsive population may not consist of cytotoxic cell precursors but rather of helper cells similar to
those responding to LD; the small size of this SD-responsive
population may not be able to provide the level of collaboration needed for the development of cytotoxic lymphocytes.

PROBLEMS FOR THE FUTURE

It would be presumptuous to give a list of problems
which most need to be investigated in this very large area.
Our purpose here is rather to pin-point some of the areas
which seem to us to be of great import.

First, we would have to list an understanding of the
mouse mutant strains, one of which was in fact the basis on

which many of the studies referred to here were started (22). Second, there is the need to determine whether the LD antigens are the same as the Ia antigens, and whether the target for the cytotoxic lymphocytes in CML are the same SD antigens recognized serologically.

More work on the cell populations involved in both the stimulatory events and in the response is clearly needed. We would, for instance, like to study in CML a population of target cells which are all known to carry LD determinants. Likewise it is important to resolve whether there are two completely separable T cell populations which are involved in MLC and CML.

The in vivo relevance of the various reactions tested in vitro must be studied further, most of all the question whether the LD-SD cooperation in vitro also exists in vivo. However, questions such as the in vivo relevance of the CML test in various allograft systems must also be further evaluated.

Last, we might try to incorporate the findings with these in vitro models of the allograft reaction which have been related to the MHC with the many other systems now related to H-2, including the immune response genes and the I region products which are important in T-B cell cooperation (perhaps a model of cell interactions in some respects not different from MLC). Even the further development of the cellular techniques and new protocols using them will, it seems to us, not provide satisfying answers until some of the MHC products involved in this wide spectrum of reactions are isolated in a functional state.

REFERENCES

(1) Bain, B., Vas, M.R., and Lowenstein, L., Blood, 23:108, 1964.

(2) Bach, F.H., and Hirschhorn, K., Science, 143:813, 1964.

(3) Hayry, P., and Defendi, V., Science, 168:133, 1970.

(4) Hodes, R.J., and Svedmyr, E.A.J., Transplantation, 9: 470, 1970.

(5) Solliday, S., and Bach, F.H., Science, 170:1406, 1970.

(6) Lightbody, J.J., Bernaco, O., Miggiano, V.C., Ceppellini, R.G., J. Bact. Virol. Immunol. 64:273, 1971.

(7) Zoschke, D.C., and Bach, F.H., Science, 170:1404, 1970.

(8) Thorsby, E., Hirschberg, H., Helgesen, A., Transpl. Proc, V:1523, 1973.

(9) Wilson, D.B., Blyth, J.L., and Nowell, P.C., J. Exp. Med. 128:1157, 1968.

(10) Bach, F.H., and Amos, D.B., Science 156:1506, 1967.

(11) Dutton, R.W., J. Exp. Med., 123:665, 1966.

(12) Silvers, W.K., Wilson, D.B., and Palm, J., Science, 155: 703, 1967.

(13) Festenstein, H., Abbasi, K., Sachs, J.A., Oliver, R.T.D., Transpl. Proc., II:219, 1972.

(14) Peck, A.B., Bach, F.H., and Boyse, E.A., Transpl. Proc., V:1611, 1973.

(15) Amos, D.B., and Bach, F.H., J. Exp. Med., 128:623, 1968.

(16) Bach, F.H., Albertini, R.J., Amos, D.B., Ceppellini, R., Mattiuz, P.L., and Miggiano, V.C., Transpl. Proc., I: 339, 1969.

(17) Plate, J.M., Ward, F.E., Amos, D.B., Histocompatibility Testing 1970, (ed. P.I. Terasaki), p. 531, 1970.

(18) Yunis, E.J., and Amos, D.B., P.N.A.S. (U.S.), 68:3031, 1971.

(19) Eijsvoogel, V.P., du Bois, M.J.G.J., Melief, C.J.M., de Groot-Kooy, M.L., Koning, C., van Rood, J.J., van Leeuwen, A., de Toit, E., Schellekens, P.Th.A., Histo-compatibility Testing 1972 (ed. J. Dausset and J. Colombani), p. 501, 1972.

(20) Bach, F.H., Widmer, M.B., Segall, M., Bach, M.L., and Klein, J. Science, 176:1024, 1972.

(21) Bach, F.H., Widmer, M.B., Bach, M.L. and Klein, J. J. Exp. Med., 136:1430, 1972.

(22) Widmer, M.B., Alter, B.J., Bach, F.H., Bach, M.L. and Bailey, D.W., Nature New Biology 242:239, 1973.

(23) Widmer, M.B., Peck, A.B., and Bach, F.H., Transpl. Proc., V:1501, 1973.

(24) Meo, T., Vives, J., Miggiano, V., Schreffler, D., Trans. Proc., V:377, 1973.

(25) Meo, T., David C.S., Nabholz, M., Miggiano, V., Shreffler, D.C., Transpl. Proc., V:1507, 1973.

(26) Peck, A.B., and Bach, F.H., J. Immunolog. Methods, 3: 147, 1973.

(27) Alter, B.J., Schendel, D.J., Bach, F.H., Bach, M.L., Klein, J., and Stimpfling, J., J. Exp. Med., 137:1303, 1973.

(28) Schendel, D.J., and Bach, F.H., J. Exp. Med., 140:1346, 1974.

(29) Peck, A.B., and Bach, F.H., Eur. J. of Immunol., in press.

(30) Schendel, D.J., and Bach, F.H., Eur. J. of Immunol., submitted for publication.

(31) Eijsvoogel, V.P., du Bois, M.J.G.J., Melief, C.J.M., et al. Transpl. Proc. V:1301, 1973.

(32) Lindahl, K.F., and Bach, F.H., Nature, submitted for publication.

(33) Schendel, D.J., Alter, B.J., Bach, F.H., Transpl. Proc. V:1651, 1973.

(34) Eijsvoogel, V.P., du Bois, M.J.G.J., Meinesz, A., Bier-horst-Eijlander, A., Zeylemaker, W.P., and Schellekens, P.Th.A., Transpl. Proc., V:1675, 1973.

(35) Klein, J., J. Exp. Med., 140:1127, 1974.

(36) Apt, A.S., Blandova, Z., Dishkant, I., Shumova, T., Vedernikov, A.A., and Egorov, I.K., Immunogenetics, in press, 1974.

(37) Egorov, I.K., Immunogenetics 1:97, 1974.

(38) Bach, F.H., Transpl. Proc. V:23, 1973.

(39) Bach, F.H., Segall, M., Zier, K.S., Sondel, P.M., Alter, B.J., and Bach, M.L., Science, 180:403, 1973.

(40) Bach, F.H., Zier, K.S., Sondel, P.M., Transpl. Proc., V: 1717, 1973.

(41) Alter, B.J., and Bach, F.H., J. Exp. Med., 140:1410, 1974.

(42) Forman, J., and Möller, G., J. Exp. Med., 138:672, 1973.

(43) David, C.S., Shreffler, D.C., and Frelinger, J.A., P.N. A.S., 70:2509, 1973.

(44) Götze, D., Reisfeld, R.A., and Klein, J., J. Exp. Med., 138:1003, 1973.

(45) Sachs, D.H., and Cone, J.L., J. Exp. Med., in press, 1974.

(46) van Leeuwen, A., Schuit, H.R.C., and van Rood, J.J., Transpl. Proc. V:1539, 1973.

(47) Meo, T., presented at International Transplantation Conference, Jerusalem, 1974.

(48) Bach, F.H., and van Rood, J.J., N. Engl. J. Med., in preparation.

(49) Bonnard, G.D., Chappuis, M., Glauser, A., Mempel, W., Baumann, P., Grosse-Wilde, H., and Albert, E.D., Tranpsl. Proc. V:1679, 1973.

(50) Livnat, S., Klein, J., and Bach, F.H., Nature New Biology, 243:42, 1973.

(51) Klein, J., and Park, J.M., J. Exp. Med., 137:1213, 1973.

(52) Elkins, W.L., Kavathas, P., and Bach, F.H., Transpl. Proc., V:1759, 1973.

This study was supported by NIH grants GM;15422, CA-14520, AI-08439, AI-11576, NF-MOD grant CRBS 246; MLB is a recipient of the American Cancer Society Faculty Research Award; DJS was an NIH Trainee supported by NIH grant GM-00398. This is Paper No. 1821 from the Laboratory of Genetics and Paper No. 19 from the Immunobiology Research Center, The University of Wisconsin, Madison, Wisconsin 53706.

DISCUSSION

W.D. Terry, National Cancer Institute, NIH: Fritz, in
your presentation you considered LD as separate from Ia, but
then toward the end allowed that they may actually be identical. I would like to turn the question around and ask what
the compelling evidence is there for thinking that they are
different, that is, do you have any genetic or other evidence
that indicates that what you have been referring to through
your whole presentation is that LD is not identical to Ia.
This of course complicates things since Ia is clearly serologically definable and well as definable in terms of lymphoid reactions.

F.M. Bach, University of Wisconsin: Let me deal with
the last part of your question first. To me LD and SD could
just as well be called MD and CD which would stand for MLC
definable and CML definable. Whether something is serologically definable or not or definable by a lymphocyte reaction is not the question which I believe to be important.
I would like to ask, "Are there functional differences at
some level between what we call LD and DS"? If the answer to
that question is "yes", which I believe it is, I think the
two should be thought of separately at some level. Ia, if it
is the same as LD, has a very different tissue distribution
from the SD antigens. That in itself would lead me to refer
to it as something which is different from SD. With respect
to your question of compelling evidence for thinking that LD
and Ia are different, I think there is no such evidence.
The question whether to use a dual terminology is really a
matter of philosophy. The Ia and LD systems were described
by very different methodologies. Genetically they map together. The fact that two things map together however certainly does not prove that they are the same. At the very
end of my presentation I suggested that it seems very likely
that the Ia and LD antigens are the same. The evidence which
leads me to this conclusion is based on the work of several
individuals who have demonstrated that anti-Ia antibodies
block the stimulating cells in MLC. Even this to me does
not prove that Ia and LD are the same since many antibodies
block MLC reactions and it could well be that these two
molecules are generally close to one another on the membrane.

There is evidence, which is disturbing to me if Ia and LD are the same, which van Rood has obtained in humans. Van Rood has demonstrated that antisera which block MLC also stain what appear to be B cells by immunofluorescence. When he uses these antisera to define what may be the LD antigens (and are almost certainly the counterpart of the mouse Ia antigens) he finds that he gets a pattern which has a high degree of correlation with the LD antigens as they are defined with homozygous typing cells. However, and this is the important point, there is a dissociation which occurs about once in five to once in ten times. One possible interpretation of these data is that the Ia and LD antigens are not the same molecule, however the genes determining these two antigens are very close together and in very high disequilibrium. From the philosophical point of view thus I would continue to separate the Ia and LD antigens until we have a molecular isolation and the question is properly resolved.

P. Maurer, Jefferson Medical College: Fritz, as you described the H-2 complex controlling the major cell surface proteins, do you think there is any possibility that the findings of the immune response genes might be just fortuitour in terms of the kinds of cross-reaction which might be occurring between other kinds of cell surface proteins and that this whole thing is sort of a red herring at the present time in immune response genes?

F.M. Bach: I am too deeply immersed in the field of immunogenetics that I could think of any of the phenomena as being a red herring. Let me more directly answer your question. McDevitt and his colleagues, have shown, at least to my satisfaction, that the immune response gene is not functioning on the basis of cross-reactivity between the antigens being tested and the histocompatibility antigens. This lack of cross-reactivity between the histocompatibility antigens and the antigens related to the immune response genes has been demonstrated for the MHC SD antigens. It is still possible that the antigens being tested cross-react with the LD or Ia antigens of the major histocompatibility complex, although I tend to doubt this. I would rather think that the immune response genes in some way control cell surface structures, once again, which in a way which we do not at present understand modifies the overall recognition by that cell of a different antigen. I would not tend to think that the immune response gene codes for the primary T cell receptor. Similar speculations have recently been advanced by Katz and Benacerraf.

G. Warchalowski, Rutgers University: I was interested in the third model system that you had up on the board with the associative recognition. Are you saying that the target cell is producing an associative molecule which is then triggering the cytotoxic lymphocyte into destroying it?

F.M. Bach: No. Let me first deal with the model first. It seems possible that the responding lymphocyte, which is the eventual cytotoxic effector cell, recognizes only the SD antigen and that the LD stimulus actually acts in reverse. That is the responding lymphocyte would not recognize the LD differences on the stimulating cell; rather the LD antigens on the responding lymphocyte would be recognized by the stimulating cell. This would be similar to the associative recognition which has been proposed by Cohn for antibody production. Whether the molecule can be released and one can do it with a soluble factor is not a question which has yet been answered. Of course the model of T-T cell collaboration which fits the LD-SD dichotomy about which I have spoken is quite similar to the T-B cell collaboration and thus the associative recognition must be considered as a possibility. I would think that the factors which can be used to substitute for the T cells would probably also substitute for the LD requirement in the LD-SD interaction. The general problem of cell interaction is, of course, csomething which has been with us for a long time in biology and simply has not been solved. It will be interesting to see whether the same kind of genetic restrictions which seem to exist in macrophage-T cell interactions and in T-B cell interactions will exist in this particular case also.

R. Hiramoto, University of Alabama: You have shown that you can separate or dissociate transformation from cytotoxicity based on differences of LD and SD. Do you have any information whether these dissociations could also be shown for the in vitro and in vivo correlates of immunity--cell mediated immunity like MIF and DTH and graft rejection.

F.M. Bach: No. I have no information of that. Dr. William Elkins in Philadelphia has been studying that kind of problem however I do not have any information about the results he has been obtaining. The question to be asked in vivo, of course, is whether the reaction against SD can be potentiated by the LD difference.

L. Muschel, American Cancer Socity: I have a very simple question. Isn't it conceivable that the position of the LD antigen plays a role in its ineffectiveness as target for killing?

F.M. Bach: Oh, absolutely. I think the question of why LD by itself is relatively ineffective in terms of generating cytotoxic cells and/or acting as a target is totally unsolved. There is every possibility that the position of the LD mole- cule in the membrane, the turnover or shedding rates of LD from the membrane, the requirement for a molecular movement of LD in the membrane might influence the function of LD as a cytotoxic-inciting target. It could be, further, that the density of LD on the surface is the most important consider- ation. The most direct experiment which is informative is the one done by Barbara Alter in PHA dependent cytotoxicity which I discussed. This experiment suggests very strongly that, insofar as we can extrapolate from PHA dependent cyto- toxicity to a normal CML test, that LD is ineffective in generating cytotoxic cells.

B. Becker, Purdue University, Fort Wayne: This is a general question concerning the mechanism of cytotoxicity. Are the cell surface antigens also on the surface of the membranes for organelles like lysosomes, golgi, mitochondria, nuclear membrane etc.

F.M. Bach: I think the evidence is that the SD anti- gens are present on the plasms membranes only.

B. Becker: Only?

F.M. Bach: Yes. I think the evidence is very strong for that but I hope that somebody will correct me if there is additional information available. I should say that it is our assumption that the SD antigen is the cytotoxic tar- get. There are in fact some experiments which suggest that the target may be a molecule determined by genes very closely linked to those determining the SD antigens. This in itself is a question which as of yet has not been resolved.

NEW ANTIGEN MARKERS FOR PREMALIGNANT CELL POPULATIONS IN LIVER CANCER

E. FARBER, K. OKITA and L.H. KLIGMAN
Fels Research Institute and
Departments of Pathology and Biochemistry
Temple University School of Medicine
Philadelphia, Pa.   19140

Abstract: An apparently new protein antigen has been found
in premalignant hepatocyte populations during the induction of liver cancer in three strains of rats by one
of five different chemical carcinogens. This antigen is
cytoplasmic and has been found by double diffusion and
by immunofluorescence microscopy to appear in the ear-
liest identifiable new hepatocyte population and to be
present apparently exclusively in all new nodular hepatocyte populations and in all primary hepatocellular carcinomas. Its occurrence in transplanted hepatomas is
variable. The antigen has been partially purified. The
antigen appears to be intimately related to the state of
differentiation of premalignant hepatocytes and disappears when such hepatocytes differentiate into mature
liver early in carcinogenesis. The new antigen may be
related either to some fundamental disturbance in differentiation or to the possible presence of viruses. It
appears to be a reproducible marker for premalignant hepatocytes.

INTRODUCTION

The appearance of cancer, especially of epithelial origin, in many organs or tissues in both man and animals is
almost constantly preceded by a long period of development or
cellular evolution in which new focal cell populations appear regularly and progressively (1,2,3). This prolonged
period of premalignancy is often characterized by one or more
early populations that can undergo apparent regression or
differentiation and later populations that persist as such
and that act as immediate precursors for cancer. In principle, this type of neoplastic development has been found in
skin, liver, urinary bladder, breast, kidney, cervix, res-
piratory tract and other organs (see (1) and (2) for ref-

erences).

The common occurrence of such a premalignant history forces us to consider seriously whether the many properties associated with any population of cancer cells are acquired in a single transformation event or accummulate progressively during the cellular evolution from the original non-neo-plastic precursor cells to a malignant cell population (2). The major emphasis in cancer research during the past two years has been on the attempt to characterize the essential attributes of populations of cancer cells derived in vivo or in vitro with heavy concentration on collections of cells already transformed. The heavy commitment early to biochemi-cal and metabolic analysis and the increasing commitment more recently to immunologic characterization rests on the unstated hypothesis that the cancer cell has a minimum num-ber of variables associated with its malignant biological be-havior and that these can somehow be characterized and under-stood by concentrating on an end state, namely cancer. Ac-cording to this hypothesis, the new populations that are seen regularly in the premalignant time phase during carcinogene-sis would appear to be due to phenomena parallel but basical-ly unrelated to the malignant transformation of target cells (Fig. 1).

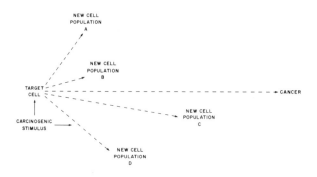

Fig. 1. Diagrammatic representation of car-cinogenesis in which the production of different cell populations is due to parallel but basically unrelated phenomena.

The rapid transformation of virtually a whole population of cells by some strains of Rous sarcoma virus and the turning on or off coincidentially by temperature modulation of many properties characteristic of cells transformed by some temperature-sensitive mutants are consistent with this hypothesis and even perhaps favor this formulation.

However, an alternate hypothesis, the progressive acquisition by succeeding cell populations of properties that in composite enable a population of malignant cells to behave biologically as a cancer should behave (Fig. 2) is perhaps more consistent with what we know today about the development of cancer in vivo. According to this view, an individual malignant neoplasm behaves at any moment in its life history in a manner which reflects the many and varied properties it has acquired progressively and seriatim since it began to evolve from initiated target cells. However, the more rigorous testing of this hypothesis is closely dependent upon the finding of specific markers that may enable the study of functional and ultimately genetic relationships between the major putative premalignant cell populations and cancer cells. Such markers might also facilitate the identification of these different cells when isolated from tissues during carcinogenesis and hopefully grown in vitro.

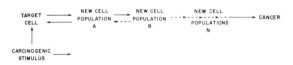

Fig. 2. Diagrammatic representation of carcinogenesis in which different cell populations are sequentially related to each other in the form of a progression to cancer.

Attempts to characterize premalignant populations biochemically or histochemically have concentrated heavily upon

the liver and have yielded several interesting findings.
These have been summarized (4,5). However, the key biochemical observations are all negative, e.g. decrease or loss of
one or more of the properties characteristic of normal liver
cells, such as glucose-6-phosphatase, ATPase, glycogen phos-
phorylase or uptake of iron. These various studies pointed
clearly to the need for positive markers that appear during
carcinogenesis.

PRENEOPLASTIC (PN) ANTIGEN

The simplest approach to exploring such a possibility
seemed to be immunologic. Basic to this study was the availability of a system to obtain putative premalignant cell
populations in sufficient quantity. This we had developed
several years ago (6). By increasing the concentration of
the carcinogen (2-acetylaminofluorene or ethionine) in the
diet and by allowing for periodic intervals free of the carcinogen, we could regularly obtain gram quantitites of hyperplastic nodules.

Crude microsomal antigen preparations from normal rat
liver or from hyperplastic nodules were injected into rabbits.
The antiserum so produced reacted reproducibly with the antigenic preparations from nodules after exhaustive absorption
with antigenic preparations from normal adult liver, fetal
liver and a variety of normal tissues including kidney,
spleen, lung, heart, gastrointestinal tract or brain (7,8).
With Ouchterlony double diffusion, a sharp precipitation line
was regularly found with such absorbed serum with hyperplastic nodules and with primary hepatomas. Absorption with
nodule or hepatoma preparations abolished the reaction with
either interchangeably. Normal rat serum proteins and alpha-
fetoprotein ($\alpha_1 F$) (8) are negative. The precipitation lines
with the antigenic preparations from hyperplastic nodules and
primary liver cancer appear to be identical.

A method for purifying the antigen from hyperplastic nodules has been developed. This involves sephadex G-200, DEAE-
cellulose and preparative acrylamide gel electrophoresis.
Since the only assay so far available is double diffusion in
agarose gel, the method is still cumbersome. Hopefully, as
larger amounts of purified antigen become available, the possibility of development of a sensitive radioimmunoassay should
facilitate the purification procedure. Also, the availability
of purified antigen will allow studies on its essential chemical and biochemical nature. The antigen appears to have a

molecular weight of over 100,000 daltons and to contain carbohydrate.

LOCALIZATION OF PN ANTIGEN BY IMMUNOFLUORESCENCE

The new antigen has been localized in tissue sections and in cell monolayers in culture by immunofluorescence using the indirect method (7,8). Intensive staining, abolished by absorption with antigen preparations from hyperplastic nodules or from primary hepatomas, has been observed in all early and late hyperplastic nodules and in all primary hepatocellular carcinomas. The nodules were induced in Fischer or in Wistar rats by ethionine (E) or by 2-acetyl-aminofluorene (2-AAF). The carcinomas were induced in Fischer, Wistar or Buffalo rats by E, 2-AAF, dimethylnitros-amine (DMN), diethylnitrosamine (DEN) or 3'-methyl-4-di-methylaminoazobenzene (3'-Me-DAB). The specific fluorescence appeared as fine granules in the cytoplasm. Nuclei were uniformly negative. Normal rat livers, fetal livers or cholangiocarcinomas were negative.

OCCURRENCE UNDER VARIOUS EXPERIMENTAL CONDITIONS

Using the Ouchterlony double diffusion method and the more sensitive immunofluorescence, PN antigen was found in two of five animals at 2 weeks after initiating a carcinogenic regimen with 2-AAF and in every animal thereafter (over 50 animals) at all time intervals up to 13 weeks. Ordinarily, nodules first become evident sometime between 1-1/2 and 3 weeks and remain throughout the process. The liver surrounding nodules or cancer is uniformly negative. Transplantable hepatomas are variable - some, e.g. Morris 7288, Sidransky and Reuber hepatomas are positive while many others are negative or almost so. The sera of animals bearing nodules or liver cancer have been uniformly negative.

The antigen could not be found at the current level of detection in livers of animals treated acutely with CCl_4, DMN or α-naphthyl-isothiocyanate (ANIT), in regenerating liver or in three other types of cancer - carcinoma of the ear duct induced by 2-AAF, renal carcinomas induced by DMN or DEN or in leukemic spleens from animals given 2-AAF. Thus, the PN antigen has a distribution quite different from that of fetal α-2-glycoprotein of Grabar et al. (9).

POSSIBLE NATURE AND SIGNIFICANCE OF PN ANTIGEN

Several possibilities exist concerning the origin and nature of this ostensibly new component that is common to all premalignant and primary malignant hepatocyte populations in the liver. These include: (a) it is normal liver constituent made in excess in premalignant and malignant tissue; (b) it is a normal multi-unit protein that has been altered during carcinogenesis; (c) it is a normal liver protein modified by interaction with the chemical carcinogens; (d) it is a protein from fetal liver or from another fetal tissue new reappearing in significant amounts in the new liver cell populations; (e) it is an antigen, again possibly fetal, that is appearing in response to a disturbance in liver cell differentiation; and (f) it is a viral antigen, either from an RNA (C-type particle?) or DNA virus, that is playing some role in carcinogenesis.

(a) The possibility that the PN antigen is a normal liver constituent being overproduced is not highly probable, since exhaustive absorption of antisera with normal liver preparations does not seem to remove the antigen. However, the exploration of this possibility will be facilitated when a highly sensitive assay is developed for pure antigen.

(b) A normal multi-unit protein may have an alteration or deficiency in one or more of its subunits, thus generating new antigenic sites. An attempt was made to study this by incubating crude extracts of hyperplastic nodules with similar extracts from normal liver at 37⁰ for 2 hours. As controls, each type of extract was incubated separately under the same conditions. All preparations containing extracts from the hyperplastic nodules gave equally strong reactions with antiserum to nodules and the presence of normal liver extracts had no observable influence.

(c) The possibility of the PN antigen being a liver protein modified by interaction with a chemical carcinogen is ruled out by finding it in altered hepatocytes induced by one of five chemically different compounds and by its presence in some hepatomas which have been transplanted up to 150 times over a period of 15 years.

(d) The possibility of the PN antigen being a fetal protein is very strong. However, so far, no evidence in support of this possibility has been found. It is definitely not alpha-fetoprotein (α_1F) by several criteria (8) including comparison with pure rat $\alpha_1 F$ and anti-rat-$\alpha_1 F$ anti-serum. Also, whole 10 or 12 day old fetuses, fetal liver (14, 16, 18 or 20 day old) newborn liver and amniotic fluid obtained at different times between 10 and 20 days were all negative. A careful study of many time intervals before 10 days has yet to be done since it appears quite possible that the antigen may appear only transitorily during fetal development in the liver or elsewhere.

(e) The possibility that the PN antigen might appear in response to a disturbance in differentiation of premalignant hepatocytes is attractive. There is now good evidence to suggest that hepatocarcinogens interrupt the differentiation or maturation of putative premalignant cells to mature liver. The PN antigen is present by immunofluorescence in the early nodule during carcinogen feeding but disappears when the nodule hepatocytes become more normal after the carcinogen is removed. Later nodules are consistently positive both in the presence and absence of exogenous carcinogen.

(f) The possibility that the PN antigen is a viral or virus-related antigen is also attractive. There is appearing a growing literature on the possible role of chemical carcinogens in favoring the appearance of oncogenic viruses, especially RNA viruses in cells in culture. Included in this are several reports on the possible role of viruses in the induction of liver cancer and their appearance in hepatomas (12-14). Conceivably, the PN antigen could be a viral-related antigen that is intimately related to the state of differentiation or maturity of new hepatocyte populations. Such a cell constituent could play a role in the subsequent development of liver cancer. Obviously, the purification of sufficient antigen will enable a rigorous test of its chemical relationship to known RNA (13,14) or DNA (12) viruses associated to date with liver cancer.

GENERAL CONSIDERATIONS

In regard to liver neoplasms, there are several reports of a marked decrease or loss of liver antigens in hepatomas (see 7 for references). Also, Weiler (15) showed the loss of specific liver antigens in focal islands of altered liver cells, considered to be a presumptive premalignant population. This is the only reported study of antigens in premalignant liver cells.

New antigens have been found in a variety of hepatomas, many induced by chemicals (see 16 for review). Some of these appear to be unique for each hepatoma or for groups of hepatomas induced by a single carcinogen while others are probably fetal in type, including, of course, $\alpha_1 F$. However, no antigen other than $\alpha_1 F$ apparently common to early and late premalignant hepatocyte populations and primary liver cancers has been described.

In general, the analysis of premalignant liver cells with any approach, but especially immunologic, has been neglected. One obvious reason for this has been the general unavailability of sufficient tissue for study.

However, several other organs or tissues have been studied. These include premalignant or benign neoplasms in the mammary glands (17-20), the colon (21), the skin (22,23) and the urinary bladder (24), all induced by chemical carcinogens. In the case of some of these studies (19-21, 24), cross-reacting "tumor antigens" were found among malignant neoplasms and between benign and malignant tissues. In other cases (17, 22, 23), apparently unique antigens were found in common between individual premalignant hyperplastic or papillomatous lesions and in the malignant neoplasms derived from them. Thus, with both syngeneic and xenogeneic systems, common antigenic components have been found in premalignant and malignant neoplasms of a single organ or tissue. Hopefully, such studies can be extended to the development of highly selective markers for the different cell populations seen in the premalignant time phase of carcinogenesis. Conceivably, such studies in depth might well generate new further insights into some of the biochemical and metabolic components involved in the development of cancer and could lead to the development of much needed new diagnostic procedures for early premalignant lesions in man.

In addition, the discovery of a general property of premalignant and malignant cell populations induced by several chemically different carcinogens offers a needed new perspective in the study of carcinogenesis. Many biochemical and immunologic studies over the past 25 years point on the whole to the uniqueness of individual neoplasms rather than to their similarities (e.g. see (2), Baldwin (16) and Weinhouse (25)). Even though the origin of many neoplasms from single cells by cellular evolution is highly probable, one cannot help being impressed by the many superficial similarities in the biological properties of malignant neoplasms. The observations of common antigens for premalignant and malignant neoplasms in any one carcinogenic process raises again the prospect of discovering other common unifying markers in the development of cancer and of ultimately utilizing such markers in either the prevention or cure of cancer.

REFERENCES

(1) L. Foulds, Neoplastic Development, Vol. 1 (Academic Press, New York, 1969).

(2) E. Farber, Cancer Res., 33 (1973) 2537.

(3) L.M. Shabad, J. Nat. Cancer Inst., 50 (1973) 421.

(4) E. Farber, in: Homologies in Enzymes and Metabolic Pathways and Metabolic Alterations in Cancer. Miami Winter Symposium, Vol.2, eds. W.H. Whelan and J. Schultz (North-Holland, Amsterdam, 1970) p. 314.

(5) E. Farber, in: Methods in Cancer Research, ed. H. Busch (Academic Press, New York, 1973) p. 345.

(6) S.M. Epstein, N. Ito, L. Merkow and E. Farber, Cancer Res., 27 (1967) 1702.

(7) K. Okita and E. Farber, Gann Monograph on Cancer Research, 14 (1975) in press.

(8) K. Okita, L.H. Kligman and E. Farber, J. Nat. Cancer Inst., in press.

(9) P. Grabar, M. Stanislawski-Birencwajg, S. Isgold and J. Uriel, UICC Monograph, 2 (1966) 20.

(10) E. Farber, Arch. Path., 98 (1974) 145.

(11) E. Farber, in: Liver Cancer, eds. K. Okuda and R.L. Peters (John Wiley, New York) in press.

(12) J.P. Anderson, K.J. McCormick, W.A. Stenback and J.J. Trentin, Proc. Soc. Exp. Biol. Med., 137 (1971) 421.

(13) I.B. Weinstein, R. Gebert, U.C. Stadler, J.M. Orenstein and R. Axel, Science, 178 (1972) 1098.

(14) J.S. Rhim, K.D. Wuu, M.L. Vernon, H.W. Chen, H. Meier, C. Waymouth and R.J. Huebner, Cancer Res., 34 (1974) 489.

(15) E. Weiler, Z. Naturforsch., 116 (1956) 31.

(16) R.W. Baldwin, Adv. Cancer Res., 18 (1974) 338.

(17) G. Slemmer, Nat. Cancer Inst. Monograph, 35 (1972) 57.

(18) G. Slemmer, J. Invest. Dermatol., 63 (1974) 27.

(19) J.A. Kellen and K.M. Anderson, Oncology, 25 (1971) 49.

(20) J. Ankerst, G. Steele, Jr. and H.O. Sjögren, Cancer Res., 34 (1974) 1794.

(21) G. Steele, Jr. and H.O. Sjögren, Cancer Res., 34 (1974) 1801.

(22) M.A. Lappé, J. Nat. Cancer Inst., 40 (1968) 823.

(23) M.A. Lappé, Nature, 223 (1969) 82.

(24) L.A. Taranger, W.H. Chapman, I. Hellström and K.E. Hellström, Science, 176 (1972) 1337.

(25) S. Weinhouse, Cancer Res., 32 (1972) 2007.

This investigation was supported in part by Public Health Service Research Grants Nos. CA-12227, CA-12218 and AM-14882 from the National Cancer Institute and the National Institute of Arthritic, Metabolic and Digestive Diseases and the American Cancer Society (BC-7Q) and by a contract (NO1-CP-33262) from the National Cancer Institute.

DISCUSSION

R.C. Leif, Papanicolaou Cancer Research Institute: In the changed cells or early changed cells, are they both ductular and hepatocytes and also is the new antigen found on both ductular cells and hepatocytes?

E. Farber, Temple University: The PN antigen has been found only in pre-malignant and malignant hepatocytes and not in bile ductular cells or proliferating ductular cells which are seen commonly early in the carcinogenic processes. Malignant neoplasms of bile ducts are negative.

E. L. Lloyd, Argonne National Laboratory: You showed some very beautiful pictures of C-type particles in neoplastic liver cells. I wondered if you'd looked at normal liver cells for C-type particles? The reason I ask this question is because we've been looking at bone tumor cells specifically, for C-type viruses. We found many of these. However, when we looked at normal bone from normal control mice we also found C-type particles.

E. Farber: In our hands its very variable. Some "normal" liver cell cultures, the first one I showed ostensibly normal, did show C-type particles but others are completely negative as far as one can tell. The latter are uniformly negative for this new antigen.

M.M. Sigel, University of Miami School of Medicine: Have you had the opportunity to determine whether the host manifests any form of cellular immunity to this antigen?

E. Farber: We've so far failed to show any recognition on the part of the host of this antigen. As whether its possible to immunize and whether we would have any effect on carcinogenes is something that must be explored further.

W.D. Terry, National Institutes of Health: I'd like to make a comment and ask for your return comment on it. One of the problems that has always bedeviled this general approach to looking for tumor associated antigens is the necessity for having quantitative assay systems. In a number of tumor systems, an antigenic substance that appeared to be present on tumor cells and absent from normal cells when assessed with qualitative assays, such as Ouchterlony analysis, were utimately found to be normal tissue components when quantitative assays were used. The difficulty is that the tumor cell may contain several thousand times as much of the substance as the normal tissue, and the normal tissue component can only be found with quantitative absorptions. It seems likely that the antigenic material you are studying may fall into this category.

E. Farber: I couldn't agree with you more, as I stressed in my presentation. Our own view is that we should concentrate on the purification of the antigen. That we think should receive the first priority.

R.E. Parks, Brown University: I would like to ask whether you have examined the phenomenon of co-carcinogenesis where you stimulate cells initially with a true carcinogen and then treat the tissue with a non-carcinogen? I wonder whether you could turn off antigen production by stopping crotin oil treatment or whether the co-carcinogen can actually cause antigen production?

E. Farber: This would be interesting. We haven't looked at skin at all and of course liver isn't a particularly good organ to study co-carcinogenesis.

R.E. Parks: Is there an experimental system in liver for studying co-carcinogenesis?

E. Farber: Not well.

R.E. Parks: I guess the phenomenon is best studied with skin carcinogenesis.

E. Farber: That's right. There probably are so called co-carcinogens for the liver but its not yet a clean system.

D. Axler, Battelle Memorial Institute: As you suggest, the possibility exists that the expression of this antigen may be due to activation of an endogenous virus by these chemicals. It's also well established that a number of the halogenated pyrimidines can induce the expression of these endogenous viruses. Have you ever treated tissue not demonstrating this angigen with BudR or IudR? A concommitant expression of virus and antigen would help establish this relationship.

E. Farber: The problem, of course, is we don't have a reproducible system in vitro. The few attempts in vitro with normal liver cells have not proved to be successful, but that doesn't rule it out by any means.

E.L. Springer, University of California: Dr. Farber, have you had an opportunity yet to correlate reverse transcriptase activity with the appearance of your PM antigen?

E. Farber: We're right in the middle of this. Some results look encouraging, but as you know the assay for reverse transcriptase has to be done extremely carefully with concomitant assays for the human DNA polymerases.

Z. Brada, Papanicolaou Cancer Research Institute: Dr. Farber, I would like to ask you, is the antigen present also in circulation or is it only hyperplastic nodules?

E. Farber: No.

Z. Brada: And is it possible to find it in other species than in rats?

E. Farber: I don't know yet. We've just examined one human liver cancer by immunofluorescene, using the anti rat antiserum, and it was negative.

Z. Brada: Is the antigen distributed in hyperplastic nodules uniformly in all cells or are some cells more labelled?

E. Farber: As far as the method allows, it seems to be uniform. We don't find any significant number of cells that don't stain, and as I stressed its present in every premalignant nodule.

G. Schiffman, State University of New York: Dr. Farber, would you like to guess which class of compounds your antigen might fall into? Is it protein, carbohydrate?

E. Farber: Its a protein containing carbohydrate.

GENETIC CONTROL OF HOMOGENEOUS ANTI-PHENYLARSONATE ANTI-BODIES PRODUCED IN STRAIN A MICE

A. NISONOFF and A.S. TUNG
Department of Biochemistry
University of Illinois at the Medical Center
and
J.D. CAPRA
Department of Microbiology
University of Texas, Southwestern Medical School

Abstract: All A/J mice immunized with KLH-p-azophenylarson-
ate (KLH-Ar) produce anti-Ar antibodies, 20 to 70% of
which share a cross-reactive idiotypic specificity (CRI).
Large amounts of anti-Ar antibodies were produced in individual mice by the induction of ascites fluids through
repeated intraperitoneal inoculations of KLH-Ar in complete Freund's adjuvant; over 100 mg of antibody was obtained from an occasional mouse. Molecules bearing CRI
were localized during preparative isoelectric focusing
in peaks with pI values of 6.7 and 6.9 ($\pm$ 0.05). Their
heavy chains were found to have an unblocked N-terminal
group, permitting analysis with a Beckman automatic se-
quencer. A single sequence was obtained through the
first hypervariable region; the degree of homogeneity
was comparable to that of a typical myeloma protein.
The same sequence was obtained with the heavy chains
from an individual A/J mouse or from a pool of 18 mice.
The recovery of amino acids in the first hypervariable
region was also consistent with the presence of a single
major sequence. Heavy chains of A/J anti-Ar antibodies
lacking CRI were then investigated. A single sequence
was obtained which was identical up to the first hypervariable region with that observed for antibodies with
CRI. Within the hypervariable region heterogeneity was

evident and the sequence differed from that of antibody
with CRI. A clear relationship between idiotype and
hypervariable sequence is thus established for an induced antibody.

INTRODUCTION

In its original usage the term idiotype referred to u-
nique antigenic determinants present on antibody of a given
specificity from one individual (1). This definition was
based on the observation that antibodies of the same specificity but from different outbred individuals generally do
not share idiotypic specificities (2-4). Idiotypic cross-
reaction are more frequent, although by no means universal,
among antibodies of the same specificity from partially inbred rabbits (5) or from mice of an inbred strain (6-9).
Whether such cross-reactions occur is dependent on the antigen and on the strain of mouse (10,11). Idiotypic determinants are present, as would be expected, in the variable domain of the Fab fragment (12). Inhibition of antiidiotypic
antibody by hapten (13) or by antigen specifically reactive
with the idiotypic antibody (14) has demonstrated that the
region of the combining site is generally a major idiotypic
determinant. This in turn would implicate sequences in hypervariable regions as factors determining idiotype (13-15).
One facet of the work to be described here provides direct
evidence supporting this conjecture.

Among the strongest intrastrain idiotypic cross-reactions which we have encountered are those involving the anti-
p-azophenylarsonate (anti-Ar) antibodies of strain A/J mice.
All A/J mice, when immunized with a conjugate of keyhole
limpet hemocyanin and p-azophenylarsonate groups (KLH-Ar)
produce antihapten (anti-Ar) antibodies some of which share
a cross-reactive idiotype (CRI). In a specifically purified
anti-Ar antibody population from an individual mouse, 20 to
70% of the molecules will, in general, share CRI although
the fraction is lower in an occasional mouse. For the studies to be described below, sera were chosen on the basis of
a high content of CRI. A second relevant factor was the
ability to induce in A/J mice ascites fluids containing high
concentrations of anti-Ar antibodies (16,17); this has made
feasible structural studies on antibodies from individual
mice, as well as from pools. The results of these investigations are presented here.

EXPERIMENTAL

Eight to 12-week old A/J mice were immunized with key-hole limpet hemocyanin to which p-azophenylarsonate groups were conjugated (KLH-AR); 500 μg quantities were emulsified with Freund's complete adjuvant and injected intraperitone-ally on a weekly basis for 5 weeks (16,17). An ascites fluid developed in most recipients after 3 to 4 weeks and was tapped over a period of 3 to 5 weeks. Concentrations of anti-Ar antibodies averaged about 8 to 10 mg/ml and the a-mount of ascites fluid obtained from individual mice varied from 2 to 40 ml with an average of about 6-8 ml. Mice whose ascites fluids were used for further studies were selected on the basis of 2 criteria: a high yield of anti-Ar anti-bodies and a high percentage of molecules bearing the cross-reactive idiotype in the isolated population of anti-Ar anti-bodies. The latter were specifically purified (8,16) from ascites fluids by precipitating with a bovine IgG-Ar conju-gate, dissolving the precipitate with p-arsanilate at pH 8, and passing the solution through DEAE-cellulose; the antibody and much of the hapten pass through the column while the antigen is retained. The hapten is removed from the antibody by exhaustive dialysis.

Antiidiotypic antibodies were prepared in rabbits by im-munization with immune precipitates comprising anti-Ar anti-bodies from an individual mouse and rabbit IgG-Ar. Precip-itates were dissociated at pH 3.5 and emulsified in Freund's complete adjuvant prior to injection. The rabbit antibodies were rendered specific for idiotypic determinants by absorp-tion with IgG from nonimmune A/J mice and with normal A/J serum. Tests carried out to prove the idiotypic specificity of the absorbed antibodies were based on the radioimmuno-assay discussed next and are described elsewhere (8,10).

The assay for antiidiotypic antibodies (8,10,16) utilized 10 ng of ^{125}I-labeled specifically purified anti-Ar antibody, 0.05 to 0.1 μl of the absorbed antiidiotypic antibody, 2 to 3 μl of rabbit antiovalbumin serum (added as carrier), and sufficient goat antirabbit Fc to precipitate all of the rab-bit IgG present. Antibodies with CRI in unknown samples were quantitated through their capacity to prevent precipi-tation of the radiolabeled ligand (8,10).

Isoelectric focusing (IEF) of specifically purified anti-Ar antibodies was carried out on a semi-preparative scale (250 μg protein) on cylindrical polyacrylamide gels (16). Antibody was eluted from the gels after IEF, in yields of 50 to 75%, by using a Savant "Autogel Divider". The antibody was lightly labeled with ^{125}I to permit subsequent

quantitation of the highly dilute protein that was eluted
(16). When such samples were assayed for their content of
CRI, the radioactive ligand used in the assay was labeled
with ^{131}I rather than ^{125}I. On a preparative scale, isoelectric focusing was carried out by a modification of the
method of Radola (16,18), which utilizes a flat bed of
"Superfine" Sephadex G-75 as the supporting medium. The size
of the slab was 30 X 15 X 0.5 cm and the amount of protein
applied was 50 to 75 mg. The protein was quantified by measurements of optical density after elution from the gel with
neutral buffer. In either method of isoelectric focusing,
freshly deionized urea was present at a final concentration
of 3.5 M.

For amino acid sequencing heavy and light chains were
prepared from antibodies isolated by isoelectric focusing
from preparations with a high content of CRI. A modification of the method of Bridges and Little (19) was used for
separating the chains. The modification consists of gel
filtration in 1 M propionic acid (lacking urea). Material
focusing in the major peaks (pI, 6.7 and 6.9 ($\pm$ 0.05)) was
used for these studies. The heavy chains were first totally
reduced in 5 M guanidine-tris HCl, pH 8.4, and alkylated
with ^{14}C-iodoacetamide. Sequences were obtained with the
Beckman Model 890C instrument by methods previously described (20-22). PTH derivatives were identified by gas
chromatography (23) thin-layer chromatography (24), counts
per minute of ^{14}C (25) and by back-hydrolysis with subsequent amino acid analysis. In the case of nonspecific H
chains the latter procedure was used only on selected residues and quantitation was based mainly on gas chromatography
and thin-layer chromatography. The results therefore are
estimates rather than precise quantitative values. In the
H chains of the anti-Ar antibodies isolated by isoelectric
focusing, no secondary amino acid residues were detected.
For the H chains of anti-Ar antibodies lacking CRI the product at each step was determined by gas and thin-layer
chromatography and quantitated by back hydrolysis and amino
acid analysis.

RESULTS

Isoelectric Focusing in Polyacrylamide Gels. This set
of experiments was concerned with localizing the antibody
possessing CRI after isoelectric focusing. Specifically
purified anti-Ar antibodies from individual mice were lightly labeled with ^{125}I for quantitation and focused over a pH
range of 5 to 8. Individual eluted fractions were tested

for their content of CRI by measuring their inhibitory capacity in the radioimmunoassay as described above. The
weight required to cause 50% inhibition is an inverse measure
of content of CRI. In Fig. 1 the antibody subjected to isoelectric focusing is the same as that which served as the
[131]I-labeled ligand in the radioimmunoassay, namely, anti-
Ar antibody raised in mouse 79.

The inhibitory capacity of individual fractions is indicated by the numbers above the graph, which specify the
weights of antibody, in the peaks directly below each number,
required to cause 50% inhibition of binding. Antibodies with
strong inhibitory capacity have pI values between 6.65 and
6.95, with major peaks at pH 6.67 and 6.87. Outside this
range of pH the inhibitory capacity per unit weight falls off
rapidly to values less than one-tenth of the maximum.

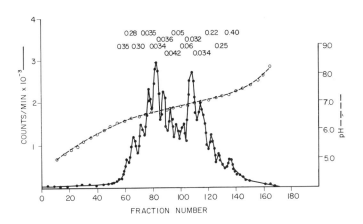

Fig. 1. Results of isoelectric focusing on polyacrylamide gel (pH range, 5 to 8) of 250 μg ^{125}I-labeled specifically purified anti-Ar antibody of mouse 79. The protein in
each peak was tested for its content of CRI by the standard
inhibition assay using the same antibody, labeled with ^{131}I,
as ligand. The antiidiotypic antibodies employed in the
assay were prepared against anti-Ar antibodies of mouse 79.
The weight of antibody in each peak, required to cause 50%
inhibition of binding, is indicated directly above the corresponding peak in the figure.

Results obtained with specifically purified anti-Ar
antibodies from 10 individual mice are shown in Figs. 2 and
3. The ligand used in the radioimmunoassay was ^{131}I-labeled
anti-Ar antibody of mouse 79. In each case maximum inhibitory capacity appears in the range of pI 6.65 to 6.95. However, the antibodies from individual mice show marked quantitative variation. This is particularly evident in Fig. 3,
where antibodies from 3 of the 5 mice show definitely less
inhibitory capacity, at the optimum pH, than the other 2
preparations. In Fig. 2, 4 of the 5 preparations are virtually identical and are essentially equivalent to that of the
donor mouse, #79. Actually, the data in Fig. 3 are more
representative, since the majority of mice produce anti-Ar
antibodies containing less CRI than mouse 79. Only anti-

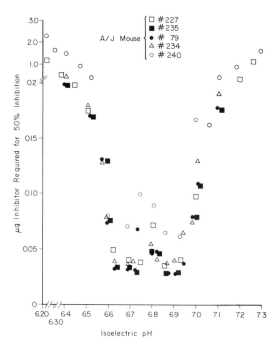

Fig. 2. Composite of data from several mice on the content of CRI in fractions obtained after isoelectric focusing
of specifically purified anti-Ar antibodies on polyacrylamide gels (pH 5 to 8). The ^{131}I-labeled ligand and the
antiidiotypic antibody are the same as in Fig. 1. Note that
the antibodies from 4 of the 5 mice appear to be idiotypically almost identical.

bodies with a high content of CRI were utilized in subsequent studies.

There is a direct correlation between content of CRI and the percentage of the total antibody which focuses in the range of pH, 6.65 to 6.95. For the strongest inhibitors at least 70% of the antibodies have pI values in this range.

When proteins in the major peaks were refocused, the pI values were found to be nearly identical to those observed in the first run (16). It was also shown that the micro-heterogeneity observed is not due to the presence of residual hapten in the specifically purified anti-Ar antibody. This was demonstrated by using an alternative method of purification that does not require hapten. No differences in the focusing patterns, or in inhibitory capacity of individual peaks, were noted in the 2 preparations (16).

In another set of experiments it was shown that the proteins in the 2 major peaks are idiotypically equivalent.

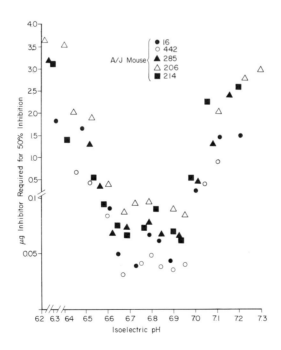

Fig. 3. See legend of Fig. 2. The results obtained with anti-Ar antibodies of 5 additional mice are shown here.

This was demonstrated by cross-inhibition experiments in which materials in the peaks with pI 6.67 and 6.87 were used as ligands or as inhibitors in separate experiments. Regardless of the preparation used as ligand, the antibody in each peak was quantitatively identical, within experimental error, with respect to inhibitory capacity (16).

Isoelectric Focusing on a Preparative Scale. The patterns obtained with a single preparation by the 2 methods of

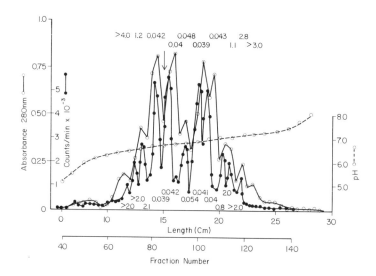

Fig. 4. Comparison of IEF profiles obtained with polyacrylamide gel (250 μg of protein, open circles) or with Sephadex G-75 "Superfine" (55 mg of protein, filled circles) as supporting medium. The protein is specifically purified anti-Ar antibody from mouse 672. The numbers shown in the graph indicate the weight of protein in the corresponding peak required to cause 50% inhibition of binding in the standard assay system (same system as in Fig. 1). The upper set of numbers refers to the upper curve (open circles); the lower set to the lower curve (filled circles). The length plotted on the abscissa refers to the distance measured along the length of the Sephadex slab; the fraction numbers refer to the polyacrylamide gel. The pH range in each case is 5 to 8. The arrow indicates the position of application of the sample in the Sephadex gel.

isoelectric focusing are shown in Fig. 4. Fifty-five mg of antibody was used in the preparative method (with Sephadex G-75 as supporting medium), and 250 μg was introduced into the polyacrylamide gel. It is apparent that the methods yield very similar patterns with respect to relative amounts of protein in each peak and their inhibitory capacities. IEF in polyacrylamide gel gives slightly higher resolution.

Class of Antibody Bearing CRI. The anti-Ar antibodies from the hyperimmunized mice which carry CRI were found to form precipitates in agar gel with monospecific antiserum to IgG1 but not with anti-IgG2, anti-IgM or anti-IgA.

Amino Acid Sequence of Pooled H Chains from Nonimmune Mice. These data are presented in Fig. 5. In the N-terminal framework (nonhypervariable) region (to position 30) only a single amino acid was detected at 20 positions. At 10 positions a small amount of one, or in one position, two other amino acids were observed. The percentages listed for these secondary amino acids (Fig. 5) are maximal values, since in some cases very small amounts were seen but were recorded as 10%. At most positions the quantitation of the second amino acid is quite exact (26). At position 9, a total of 3 amino acids was detected.

By contrast, several amino acids were detected at positions 31, 32, 33, and 35, in the hypervariable region; the symbol V is used to indicate this variability. Over 80% of the chains possess methionine at position 34. At position 36 to 38, beyond the hypervariable region, essentially all of the chains exhibit the same sequence (-Trp-Val-Arg-).

Sequence of H Chains from Anti-Ar antibodies with CRI. These studies were carried out with H chains of anti-Ar antibodies from a pool of ascites fluid from 18 mice or from an individual mouse (no. A12). The antibodies used were those with pI values between 6.7 and 6.9 (± 0.05). The results are shown in Fig. 5. Only a single amino acid could be identified at each position; this includes the first hypervariable region. The homogeneity is comparable to that observed with typical myeloma proteins. The same sequence was obtained with the H chains of antibodies from the individual mouse or the pool.

Sequence of H Chains of Anti-Ar Antibodies Lacking CRI. These antibodies were obtained from a pool of 7 mice whose anti-Ar antibodies contained a low percentage of molecules with CRI. In addition the antibodies used were those having pI values outside the 6.7-6.9 range. As a consequence the concentration of molecules with CRI was very low (less than 5%). In obtaining this sequence every thiazolinone derivative was subjected to back hydrolysis and quantitation with

$V_H I$ (Human) PCA VAL GLN LEU VAL GLU SER GLY ALA GLU VAL LYS LYS PRO GLY SER SER VAL LYS VAL

(position 10 above GLU ALA GLU; position 20 above VAL LYS VAL)

A/J Nonspecific Pool GLU ———— GLY GLY LEU VAL GLN ———— GLY ——— LEU LEU
(Asp 10%) (Gln(Gln 15%)20%) (Ala(Glu 20%)40%)(Pro 20%) (Ser 10%)(Val 20%)

A/J Anti-Ar (Idiotype) GLU ———— GLN GLN ———— LEU VAL ———— MET

A/J Anti-Ar (Lacking Idiotype) GLU ———— GLN GLN ———— LEU VAL ———— MET
(Val 20%) (Pro(Gly 20%)10%) (Gly 20%) (Leu 10%)

21
$V_H I$ (Human) SER CYS LYS ALA SER GLY GLY THR PHE SER V V V V V TRP VAL ARG

(position 30 above PHE SER; position 38 above VAL ARG)

A/J Nonspecific Pool SER LEU ———— PHE SER TYR ———— V ———— V V MET V
(Ala(Phe 20%)10%)(Ala 10%)

A/J Anti-Ar (Idiotype) SER ——— THR ——— TYR ———— SER TYR GLY LEU TYR

A/J Anti-Ar (Lacking Idiotype) SER ——— THR ——— TYR ———— V V V V V
(Lys 10%)(Ser 10%)(Phe 10%)

Fig. 5. Amino-terminal sequences of V_H regions. A solid line indicates identity at that position with the prototype (human $V_H I$) sequence. Secondary residues, when present, are shown in parentheses below the major sequence. The symbol V indicates marked heterogeneity.

94

the amino acid analyzer. In 22 of the first 30 positions a single amino acid was detected at each step. In the 8 positions where a secondary amino acid was seen, its yield did not exceed 20%. There was no indication of the presence of tyrosine at position 32 or leucine at position 34; these 2 amino acids are exclusively present at these 2 positions in the H chains of antibody possessing CRI, obtained either from a pool or from an individual mouse.

DISCUSSION

The data presented indicate the feasibility of producing antibodies of restricted heterogeneity within an inbred strain of mouse. The antibodies are isolated from ascites fluids of mice which produce substantial titers of anti-Ar antibodies containing a high percentage of molecules bearing a cross-reactive idiotype (CRI). The molecules with CRI are isolated by isoelectric focusing on a preparative scale, using a flat bed of Sephadex gel as the supporting medium (16). Large quantities of antibodies are obtained from the ascites fluids, which are induced by repeated injections of antigen in Freund's complete adjuvant. Data on H chain sequences are obtainable from antibodies of individual mice as well as from pools. About 1 mouse out of 10 produces enough antibody of restricted heterogeneity for N-terminal sequence analyses. Molecules isolated on the basis of shared idiotypic specificity contained H chains which appear homogeneous on the basis of amino acid sequence through the first hypervariable region.

Molecules with CRI were found to have pI values of 6.7 to 6.9 ($\pm$ 0.05), and a trough was generally seen between these 2 pI values. Upon refocusing, protein in each peak retained the same pI value, indicating homogeneity with respect to pI. However, on the basis of quantitative cross-inhibition tests, using a radioimmunoassay, the antibodies in the 2 peaks appeared idiotypically identical. The basis of this microheterogeneity is unknown, but may well be attributable to amino acid sequence differences in L chains (unpublished data); differences in amide and carbohydrate content may conceivably also be involved. The possibility was ruled out that residual hapten in the purified antibody is responsible for the microheterogeneity.

Although anti-Ar antibody preparations from different A/J mice may differ markedly in their content of CRI (per unit weight of anti-Ar antibody), molecules possessing the idiotype always focused within the same range of pI.

From amino acid sequence analysis it was found, first,

that all or nearly all the H chains of anti-Ar antibodies with CRI are unblocked at the N-terminus; this was true also of a substantial fraction (about 40%) of the H chains of nonspecific A/J IgG. This permitted sequence analysis on the automatic Beckman instrument. The H chains of anti-Ar antibodies possessing the CRI were found to be homogeneous by the criterion of sequence analysis. Only one amino acid could be detected at each position up to position 38, which includes the first hypervariable region.

The sequence of the H chain of anti-Ar antibody with CRI was quite different from that of the major sequence of the H chains of nonspecific A/J IgG (Fig. 5). At positions where the H chains of antibody and nonspecific IgG differ, the amino acid residue identified in the antibody H chains was present as a minor component in the nonspecific IgG; thus the data indicate that the H chains of the antibody with CRI belong to a minor V_H subgroup represented in the pooled nonspecific IgG. When sequences were compared with the prototypes of the human V_H subgroups, homology for the nonspecific mouse H chains was maximal with human V_{HIII}; for the H chains of the antibody with CRI, homology was maximal with the human V_{HI} subgroup; the homology with the H chain of human protein Eu (V_{HI}), excluding the first hypervariable region, was over 75%. The hypervariable region cannot be considered here because the nonspecific H chains gave a sequence reflecting great heterogeneity in this region; except at position 34, no single residue was present at a level exceeding 20% of the total yield.

Of considerable interest was the observation that H chains of anti-Ar antibodies lacking CRI belong to the same V_H subgroup as do the antibodies with CRI; the sequences are identical from positions 1 through 30. Thus, the anti-Ar specificity is associated with the same V_H subgroup, regardless of idiotypic specificity.

Within the hypervariable region, however, the similarity no longer obtains. In contrast to the H chains of anti-Ar antibody with CRI, those from antibody lacking CRI gave a sequence reflecting marked heterogeneity; no residue, between positions 31 and 35, was present in an amount exceeding 30% of the total yield at that position. (However, the yields of the major component at each position were somewhat greater than those obtained with H chains of nonspecific IgG.) It is noteworthy that the sequence of the H chains from antibodies with CRI was not detectable in the hypervariable region of anti-Ar antibody devoid of CRI. The observation of identity in the nonhypervariable region and nonidentity in the first hypervariable region provides strong support for the hypothesis that idiotype is largely dependent on sequences in hypervariable regions. A similar conclusion based on sequences in L chains of myeloma proteins rather than induced antibodies has been reached by Barstad et al. (27). However, similar H chain sequences were found in the first hypervariable region of myeloma proteins with similar antigen-binding specificity but of different idiotype (27).

Our findings are consistent with results indicating that the binding site itself is generally a major idiotypic determinant (13,14). (That a determinant can also be present outside the site is indicated by experiments in which immunization was carried out with complexes of a protein-hapten conjugate and antihapten antibody, prepared in antigen excess (28). In contrast to conventionally prepared antiidiotypic antibodies, those elicited by this method were not at all inhibitable by free hapten; however, the antiidiotypic antibodies elicited combined with a relatively small fraction of the donor (antihapten) antibodies, indicating that blocking of the active site reduced immunogenicity.)

Since the same sequence was present in the individual mouse and in the pool, the data can most readily be interpreted on the basis that the V_H region of anti-Ar antibodies with CRI is controlled either by a germ line gene or by a gene related to a germ line gene through a small number of somatic mutations, which occur in each A/J mouse.

The data indicate that the idiotype under investigation represents a well defined structure, rather than a group of related structures, at least with respect to the H chain. Sequences of L chains from antibodies with CRI are heterogeneous; the data will be presented in another report.

REFERENCES

(1) J. Oudin, Proc. Roy. Soc. Ser. B Biol Sci., 116 (1966) 207.

(2) H.G. Kunkel, M. Mannik and R.C. Williams, Science, 140 (1963) 1218.

(3) J. Oudin and M. Michel, C.R. Acad. Sci., 257 (1963) 805.

(4) P.G.H. Gell and A.S. Kelus, Nature, 201 (1964) 687.

(5) K. Eichmann and T.J. Kindt, J. Exp. Med., 134 (1971) 532.

(6) M. Cohn, G. Notani and S. Rice, Immunochemistry, 6 (1969) 111.

(7) M. Potter and R. Lieberman, J. Exp. Med., 132 (1970) 737.

(8) M.G. Kuettner, A.L. Wang and A. Nisonoff, J. Exp. Med., 135 (1972) 579.

(9) K. Eichmann, Eur. J. Immunol., 2 (1972) 319.

(10) L.L. Pawlak and A. Nisonoff, J. Exp. Med., 137 (1973) 855.

(11) A. Nisonoff, Annal. Immunol. (Inst. Pasteur), 125c (1974) 363.

(12) J.V. Wells, H.H. Fudenberg and D. Givol, Proc. Nat. Acad. Sci. U.S., 70 (1973) 1585.

(13) B. Brient and A. Nisonoff, J. Exp. Med., 132 (1970) 951.

(14) R.C. Williams, H.G. Kunkel and J.D. Capra, Science, 161 (1968) 379.

(15) J.D. Capra and J.M. Kehoe, Proc. Nat. Acad. Sci. U.S., 71 (1974) 4032.

(16) A.S. Tung and A. Nisonoff, J. Exp. Med., 141 (1975) in press.

(17) A. Nisonoff, A.S. Tung and J.D. Capra, Prog. Immunol. II, North-Holland, Amsterdam, 2 (1974) 17.

(18) B.J. Radola, Biochim. Biophys. Acta., 295 (1973) 412.

(19) S.H. Bridges and J.R. Little, Biochemistry, 10 (1971) 2525.

(20) J.D. Capra and H.G. Kunkel, Proc. Nat. Acad. Sci. U.S., 67 (1970) 87.

(21) J.M. Kehoe and J.D. Capra, Proc. Nat. Acad. Sci. U.S., 68 (1971) 2019.

(22) J.M. Kehoe and J.D. Capra, Proc. Nat. Acad. Sci. U.S., 69 (1972) 2052.

(23) J.J. Pisano and T.J. Bronzert, J. Biol. Chem., 244 (1969) 5597.

(24) M.R. Summers, G.W. Smythers and S. Oroszlan, Anal. Biochem., 53 (1973) 624.

(25) J.D. Capra, J.M. Kehoe, D. Kotelchuck, R. Walter and E. Breslow, Proc. Nat. Acad. Sci. U.S., 69 (1972) 431.

(26) J.D. Capra, A.S. Tung and A. Nisonoff, J. Immunol., in press.

(27) P. Barstad, S. Rudikoff, M. Potter, M. Cohn, W. Konigsberg and L. Hood, Science, 183 (1974) 962.

(28) S.B. Spring-Stewart and A. Nisonoff, J. Immunol., 110 (1973) 679.

ACKNOWLEDGMENT

This work was supported in part by grants from the National Science Foundation (GB-41530X) and the National Institutes of Health (AI-12127, AI-06281, and AI-10220).

DISCUSSION

E. Harber, Harvard Medical School: The data concerning
the hypervariable region of the heavy chains is certainly
very interesting and provocative, but I would like to make
a plea that you do not stop at sequencing the first hypervariable region. In data that we have accumulated on several
homogeneous rabbit antibody light chains there seems to be
very little variability among different antibodies in the
first hypervariable region of the heavy chain, whereas the
forth hypervariable region differ greatly among antibodies
in both length and sequence. It should be noted that Cebra
and his collaborators have not yet reported sequence data
on the third hypervariable region of the guinea pig antibody
heavy chain. The uniformity of amino acid sequence observed
in the first two hypervariable regions among antibodies of a
given specificity may not be borne out in the third.

A. Nisonoff, University of Illinois: Well, I don't
think that we are going to find very much heterogeneity in
the heavy chains because of the isoelectric focusing patterns
which are very restrictive once the idiotype is selected for.
Another point is that, there is great variability in the
hypervariable region, if one looks at the anti-arsonate
antibodies that lack the idiotype; they are very heterogeneous, so that the mouse is capable of generating many
different sequences in that first type of variable region,
even with respect to the anti-arsonate antibodies. In any
case, we are (Dr. Friedensen at the University of Illinois)
is hoping to sequence the entire V_H region. I wouldn't be
surprised if some heterogeneity were found. But really the
question is what kinds of information can you get with this
system, and the kind of information that we are most interested in has to do with the nature of variability in individual mice. Whether mutations can occur in the framework
regions? That's one type of information. And secondly,
the relationship between sequence in the hypervariable region and the specificity; particularly since the guinea pig
and the mouse utilize similar amino acids squences in the
first hypervariable region.

E.A. Kabat, Columbia University, New York: What are the proportions of the heterogeneous light chains, you say that there are at least three sequences? Is one of these three sequences predominate, or are they fairly equal because you can't be absolutely sure from the sequencing that you found a sequence for all of your heavy chains? It might represent only 70 or 80% of the heavy chains and if you have 70 or 80% of a single sequence of the light chains, still there might be differences.

A. Nisonoff: I think that Dr. Kabat's question has to do with the number of sequences in the light chain, since the heavy chain itself could conceivably contain another sequence. But first, Dr. Capra doesn't see another sequence; he only sees one amino acid in each position. And he is capable of detecting, he thinks, 5%; certainly 10% of another aminoacid by his methods. So, I think your value of 70% is probably an understatement of the degree of homogeneity. In terms of the heterogeneity of the light chains, this is an indeterminate value for the following reason; you can't really tell too much difference between the antibody light chains and non-specific light chains although even specific light chains are restricted in the sense that one aminoacid may tend to predominate in position, 5, 6 or what have you and all I can say is that at many positions shown there on the blackboard, there are at least two or three aminoacids present and this is the sort of thing you find in the non-specific light chains. So that this kind of sequence data can be consistent with three sequences, or maybe with fifty, because there may be small proportions of other light chains having a substitution accounting for 2% of the total that wouldn't be seen. I think that we can get at that a little bit more conclusively by isoelectric focusing, particularly if we sub-fractionate the anti-arsonate antibodies to start with. Then, after the light chains begin to appear more homogeneous by isoelectric focusing, the sequencing data might begin to be more meaningful on the light chains.

B. Becker, Purdue University: In this preparative separation method on a thin layer plate, the proteins don't go off the plate?

A. Nisonoff: No, they stay on the plate and in the appropriate pH range, then the granular gel is sliced immediately after the focusing run and the protein is eluted from the Sephadex.

101

THE IDENTIFICATION BY PLAQUE CYTOGRAM ASSAYS
AND BSA DENSITY DISTRIBUTION OF IMMUNOCOMPETENT CELLS

R.C. LEIF[a], J.L. HUDSON[b], G.L. IRVIN, III[b]
M.L. CAYER[a] AND J.T. THORNTHWAITE[a,c]

[a]Papanicolaou Cancer Research Institute
Miami, Florida 33123

[b]Veteran's Administration Hospital
Miami, Florida 33136

This chapter will describe our first efforts to establish a taxonomy of lymphocytes. Taxonomic studies of cells are to a large extent the product of Cytophysics which is the application of physical techniques in cellular studies. For lymphocytes, these applications primarily involve cellular characterization and separation. It would not be appropriate to review all of these cell separation and analysis techniques here since several comprehensive reviews have already been written (Leif 1970, Pretlow et. al. 1975, Shortman, 1972 Cutts 1970 , Hannig 1969 , Mullaney et al. 1975). Pretlow et. al. (1975) have described a very promising approach to separating cells by sedimentation utilizing a low speed centrifuge and isokinetic gradients. This procedure greatly decreases the time for the separations compared with unit gravity sedimentation and thus will facilitate both the maintenance of viability and multidimensional separation. Since this is a centrifugal procedure, these authors emphasize that the speed and temperature of centrifugation must be precisely controlled. These authors further state "it is our opinion that the use of discontinuous gradients is rarely justified and, in fact, most often results in the production of artifacts". The major problem of cell electrophoresis, ohmic heating, has apparently been solved by Zeiller et al. (1970) by the use of special low conductivity glycine based buffers. Most probably, electrophoretic mobility techniques are at present the best way to preparatively separate cells by type, e.g., T-cells from B-cells (Zeiller et al. 1972a, Zeiller et al. 1971, Zeiller et al. 1972b and Andersson et al. 1973).

Choi et al. (1974) have described an elegant solution to the problem of separating cells by immunologic affinity. Antibody specific for a hapten was adsorbed onto polystyrene

[c] In partial fulfillment for the Ph.D. degree in Chemistry at Florida State University.

tubes. This hapten was then in turn conjugated to either an antibody which was specific for a given type of cells, (e.g. B-cells) or a protein which was bound by a specific subpopulation of cells. In either case, the hapten acted as an intermediate link and bound the cells, via the antihapten antibody, to the polystyrene tubes. The cells could be desorbed by the addition of free hapten, which being non-specific for the cells was not deliterious and did not impair biological function. The technique is obviously general and could be extended to isolate specific allotype bearing cells. This technique, if perfected, should be an inexpensive alternative to the use of a sorter for many types of separations of specific immune cells where cell surface markers are to be utilized.

The current solution to the immunologic separation of cells is to employ a cell sorter. The original sorter design was by Fulwyler (1970) who perfected this technique for separating cells by volume. This design was then adopted to fluorescence by Herzenberg's group. The latest version of this sorter (Hulett et al. 1973) utilizes both a He-Ne laser for low angle light scattering measurements and an argon ion laser for fluorescence measurements. These measurements are performed on the cells while they are present in the center of a stream which is jetting down from an ultrasonic droplet former, but prior to the actual break-up of the stream into drops. This system is by far the most simple design for a sorter.

Lastly, in the case of counter current distribution, Walter et al. (1972) have found that all beef erythrocytes exhibited similar electrophoretic mobility despite differences in partition coefficients and sialic acid content. This result contradicts Walter's previous hyopthesis (Walter 1969) that counter current distribution basically separates by cell surface charge. These encouraging results mean that these two techniques can both be fruitfully applied to separating cells, since they do not separate by the same phenomenon.

After the cells have been separated a major problem presents itself, namely; how to monitor the composition of cells present in the fraction. Centrifugal Cytology (Leif et al. 1971) was specifically devised for this purpose. The major topic of this chapter will be the extention of Centrifugal Cytology to functional assays for immunocompetent cells.

Plaque Cytogram assay is a general term for a method utilized for the detection of several types of immune responses on a cellular level. Essentially, the technique involves utilizing Centrifugal Cytology (Leif et al., 1971) to form homogeneous monolayers of cells on a slide substrate with greater than 90% cell recovery (Leif et al. 1971, Gratzner et al. 1974, Thornthwaite et al. 1975a). The cells are concentrated enough on the restricted area of the slide to induce an immune cell-target cell interaction. The first cellular assay developed for immunocompetent cells was the enumeration and classification of plaque-forming cells (PFC) and rosette-forming cells (RFC) from the mouse spleen during the primary immune response against sheep red blood cells (SRBC). Since then, modifications of the Plaque Cytogram assay have been perfected for the analysis of spontaneous RFCs, complement-independent PFCs, and effector cells which can destroy tumor cells by a cell-mediated response. At the end of this chapter a summary will be given which shows the types of cellular immune assays that are being applied and will be developed utilizing the Plaque Cytogram method.

PREPARATION OF CELLS FOR LIGHT, SCANNING ELECTRON AND TRANSMISSION ELECTRON MICROSCOPY.

A special multipipetting machine as shown in Figure 1 was utilized for layering the various solutions (e.g. 10% guinea pig complement in the IgM PFC assay) and the glutaraldehyde fixative. During the addition of the glutaraldehyde, approximately 100 μl of 4% glutaraldehyde in 0.05M cacodylate-HCl (pH 7.4) buffer was layered 1 mm above the cell monolayer at a rate of 10 μl/min. Careful layering of solutions, especially when SRBC were used, prevented disruption of the homogeneous monolayer of cells on the slides.

Several stains were utilized in these studies. Benzidine (Leif et al. 1971) and the Papanicolaou (Papanicolaou 1954) stains were used to reveal the unlysed SRBC and spleen cells in the IgM-PFC Plaque Cytogram assay. Alcian blue (Yip and Auersperg 1972, Thornthwaite and Leif 1975b) was used for the cell viability studies. After glutaraldehyde fixation cells which were dead prior to fixation stain intensely, while cells which were viable prior to fixation stain very faintly but sufficiently well to be enumerated. Alcian blue became very useful in our efforts to develop a cellular assay (to be described later in this report) for the enumeration of effector cells binding to destroyed tumor cells. A lipase staining technique (Ansley and Ornstein 1970, Thornth-

waite and Leif 1974) was utilized for the detection of monocytes and macrophages.

Special gridded slides (W. Teledyne and L.E. Gurley Co.
Troy, New York) were utilized for the combined light and SEM
observation of the PFC and effector-tumor cell interactions.
Selected cells were photographed and their locations marked.
After leaving the slides in xylene overnight to facilitate
the removal of the Coverbond (Harleco Co.) coverslip medium,
the slides were either air dried from xylene (Leif et al.
1971) or placed in 100% acetone and critical point dried
utilizing CO_2 (Thornthwaite et al. 1975a). The slides were
then prepared for SEM observations by depositing a 100-200 Å
thickness of Au-Pd on the cell monolayers. After relocation
of the cells by SEM utilizing the grid coordinates, the same
cells photographed earlier for light microscope observation
were rephotographed for SEM visualization.

Cells to be utilized for transmission electron microscope (TEM) observation were centrifuged on to Thermanox
plastic slides (Lux Scientific Co.) and glutaraldehyde fixed.
Subsequently, the cells on Thermanox slides were stained
with 1% osmium tetroxide and dehydrated at five minute intervals through acetone (25%, 50%, 70%, 95%, 100%). From
100% acetone the slides were placed in Spurr (Polysciences,
Inc.) embedding resin for 15 minutes and then positioned in
silicone rubber molds. After removal of the Thermanox slide
from the hardened resin, the embedded cells were sectioned
en face. TEM observation of the effector-tumor interactions
was made possible by post fixing in 1% OsO_4 and staining for
five minutes in alcian blue. After dehydration through
acetone, the cells were embedded in a two mm thickness of
Spurr plastic. Selected areas of effector cell-tumor cell
interaction could easily be seen in the Spurr under a 10X
microscope objective. The area around these cells was circled with a sharp pin, cut out of the block and sectioned *en
face* for TEM.

LIGHT MICROSCOPY OF PLAQUE-FORMING (PFC) AND ROSETTE-FORMING
(RFC) CELLS.

Jerne and Nordin (1963) and Ingraham and Bussard (1964)
have described a method for enumerating antibody-producing
cells by the formation of hemolytic plaques in a physiologic
gel containing both lymphoid cells and target sheep red blood
cells (SRBC). Cunningham in 1965, perfected a "free suspension" technique for PFC (Plaque-forming cells) enumeration

by incubating lymphoid cells and SRBC in a monolayer inside a glass chamber.

In our laboratory a new assay for PFC and RFC (rosette-forming cell) has been developed (Thornthwaite and Leif 1974). The Plaque Cytogram assay is basically an adaptation for PFC and RFC of the free suspension technique of Cunningham (1965) to Centrifugal Cytology (Leif et al. 1971). Centrifugal Cytology differs from all other previous centrifugal techniques in that multiple dispersions can be produced on the same slide and the cells are not air dried. The Plaque Cytogram assay has been utilized to prepare glutaraldehyde fixed, stained dispersions of PFC and RFC on slides for morphologic analysis with the light microscope, on coverslips for surface morphology studies with the scanning electron microscope (SEM), and on Thermanox coverslips for subsequent embedding for transmission electron microscopy (TEM). The sensitized immune cells and target SRBC are centrifuged on to a restricted area of a microscope glass slide. This area, together with the spacer block of the Centrifugal Cytology bucket, forms a chamber volume to which subsequently can be added a more dense solution such as 10% guinea pig complement or glutaraldehyde. The cells can then be stained and mounted for light microscopy without air drying or prepared for SEM or TEM.

In the Plaque Cytogram assay (Thornthwaite and Leif 1974) (Fig. 1), 0.1 ml of 2×10^5/ml spleen cells from BALB/c mice injected i.v. four days previously with 4×10^8 SRBC was syringed into each of the 12 Centrifugal Cytology bucket chambers and the buckets were centrifuged at 1500 rpm (400xg) at 4^0C in an International PR2 centrifuge for 10 min. A 0.1 ml quantity of 4×10^7/ml SRBC was slowly added with a syringe onto the spleen cell monolayer and centrifuged under the same conditions. After the final centrifugation, 2×10^4 nucleated spleen cells and 4×10^6 SRBC formed a homogeneous monolayer of closely packed cells on each of the twelve 0.5-cm square areas of the slide surface. The special multi-pipetting machine was used to remove the supernatant down to 1 mm above the cell surface. The same pipetting machine was then utilized for slowly (5 min) layering 0.1 ml of 10% complement on each of the slide areas. The complement was added after formation of the monolayer because preliminary experiments had revealed that when complement was mixed with SRBC or spleen cells prior to centrifugation, there was inhomogeneity in the cell monolayers due to clumping of the SRBC. The buckets were incubated for 15 min in a level, 37^0C

PLAQUE CYTOGRAM ASSAY

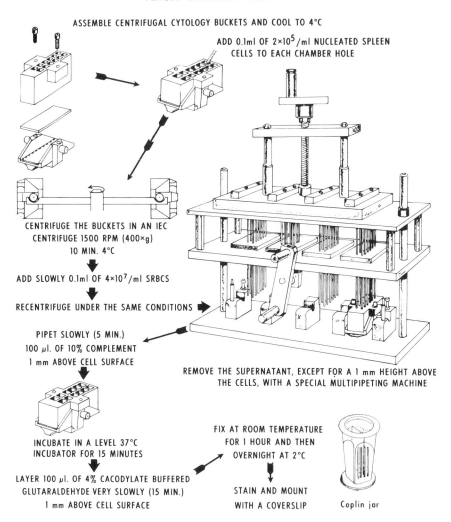

ASSEMBLE CENTRIFUGAL CYTOLOGY BUCKETS AND COOL TO 4°C

ADD 0.1ml OF $2×10^5$/ml NUCLEATED SPLEEN
CELLS TO EACH CHAMBER HOLE

CENTRIFUGE THE BUCKETS IN AN IEC
CENTRIFUGE 1500 RPM (400×g)
10 MIN. 4°C

ADD SLOWLY 0.1ml OF $4×10^7$/ml SRBCS

RECENTRIFUGE UNDER THE SAME CONDITIONS

PIPET SLOWLY (5 MIN.)
100 μl. OF 10% COMPLEMENT
1 mm ABOVE CELL SURFACE

REMOVE THE SUPERNATANT, EXCEPT FOR A 1 mm HEIGHT ABOVE
THE CELLS, WITH A SPECIAL MULTIPIPETING MACHINE

INCUBATE IN A LEVEL 37°C
INCUBATOR FOR 15 MINUTES

FIX AT ROOM TEMPERATURE
FOR 1 HOUR AND THEN
OVERNIGHT AT 2°C

LAYER 100 μl. OF 4% CACODYLATE BUFFERED
GLUTARALDEHYDE VERY SLOWLY (15 MIN.)
1 mm ABOVE CELL SURFACE

STAIN AND MOUNT
WITH A COVERSLIP

Coplin jar

Figure 1. The Plaque Cytogram assay for Immunocompetent cells.

incubator. After incubation, care was taken in handling the
buckets and performing the pipetting steps so the plaques
would not be disturbed. The supernatant, except for a 1 mm
height above the cell monolayer, was removed from each bucket compartment with the pipetting machine. Then 0.1 ml of

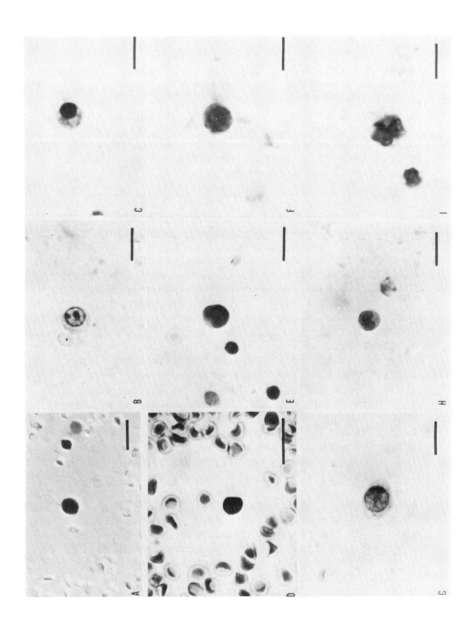

4% glutaraldehyde was slowly (15 min) layered on the cell monolayer at a distance of 1 mm.

(Caption of the composite from the previous page)

> Figure 2. (A), Plaque Cytogram showing the lysed SRBC around a central PFC using Nomarski optics. B-I, the eight types of PFC found in the spleen of a mouse 4 days after a single i.v. injection of SRBC as shown by light microscopy: B, plasmablast; C, plasma cell; D, small, E, medium, F, large lymphocyte; G, lymphoblast. H, cell with an eccentric, indented nucleus; I, binucleated cell (all scales 10 µ).

Figure 2 is a light microscope composite showing the eight morphologic PFC classes (Fig. 2B-I) identified by the Plaque Cytogram assay. PFC producing anti-SRBC IgM in the presence of guinea pig complement have lysed the surrounding SRBC so that a clear zone of lysis can be seen around each PFC due to the loss of hemoglobin from the lysed SRBC and subsequent lack of staining for hemoglobin with benzidine. The erythrocyte ghosts are made visible by utilizing Nomarski optics as shown in Figure 2A. The cell in Figure 2C appears to be a mature form of the cell in Figure 2B. These cells have dark, eccentric nuclei and are classified as plasma cells. Small, medium, and large lymphocytes are shown in Figure 2D-F. The smallest PFC are the small lymphocytes (Fig. 2D) while the largest PFC are the large lymphoblasts (Fig. 2G). In Figure 2H is an example of a general class of cells that have either indented or segmented nuclei. Large binucleated PFC with dark-bordered nuclei and a central nucleolus in each nucleus (Fig. 2I) are observed in a small percentage (Table Ii) of the PFC population.

Table I gives the results of the classification of eight distinct morphologic types of PFC from 250 PFC analyzed from one mouse during the primary immune response. The latter designation of each type in the table corresponds to the designation in Figure 2. Since the whole plaque can be observed, the relative amount of the antibody being produced by each PFC can be related to the hemolytic plaque diameter. The smallest plaques (30 µ) are formed by the small lymphocytes (Table Id), while the largest plaques (80 µ) are created by the binucleated cells (Table Ii). The rest of the PFC had similar average plaque diameters and no correlation between the maturity of a cell type (based on an in-

TABLE 1

Plaque-Forming cell types from one BALB/c mouse spleen injected i.v. four days earlier with 4×10^8 SRBCs. 250 PFCs analyzed.

	CELL DESCRIPTION	CELL DIAMETER (MICRONS)	PLAQUE DIAMETER (AVERAGE) (MICRONS)	PERCENTAGE
b.	Plasmablast - Eccentric, Dark Bordered Nucleus with Nucleoli Nucleus: Cytoplasm ratio 1:2	6-11	40-80 (70)	3
c.	Plasma Cell - Small, Dark, Eccentric Nucleus with Rough Cytoplasm Nucleus: Cytoplasm ratio 1:2	5-9	40-80 (60)	10
d.	Small lymphocyte - Concentric, Dark Nucleus, Little Cytoplasm	5-6	20-55 (30)	38
e.	Medium lymphocyte - Concentric Dark Nucleus, Little Cytoplasm	7-8	30-60 (55)	16
f.	Large Lymphocyte - Concentric, Dark Nucleus, Little Cytoplasm	9-12	50-80 (60)	9
g.	Lymphoblast - Concentric, Dark Bordered Nucleus With Condensed Chromatin, Little Cytoplasm	5-15	25-130 (60)	10
h.	Indented, Eccentric, Dark Nucleus or Segmented Nuclei	6-7	65-120 (70)	9
i.	Binucleated with Dark Bordered Nuclei with Condensed Chromatin	6-11	30-130 (80)	5

creasing ability to release more hemolytic antibody, thus forming a larger plaque) and morphology could be made. The small plaque-producing cells are not easily observed in either the agar gel or free suspension methods, but can be observed in the Plaque Cytograms using a 40X objective. Whether these PFC are producing plaques by cell-bound antibody only or actually producing soluble antibody is not known.

The RFC observed in the Plaque Cytogram assay do not include any cells producing hemolytic antibody. In the cell monolayers, every spleen cell is touching the surrounding SRBC, so that rosettes can be easily identified by the aggregated binding of seven or more SRBC. A third of the RFC could not be classified because of the large number of SRBC binding to their surfaces. In the observable RFC population, Table 2, about 82% are morphologically similar to lymphocyte types d, e, f, in Table I. In the Plaque Cytogram assay, there are 1.0 to 1.5 times as many RFC as PFC.

TABLE 2

Rosette-forming cell types from the same mouse spleen as in TABLE 1

CELL DESCRIPTION (Primed letters denote the same morphological lettered cell type as in Table 1)	DIAMETER (MICRONS)	PERCENTAGE
b' Plasmablast - Eccentric, Dark Bordered Nucleus with Condensed Chromatin Nucleus: Cytoplasm ratio 1:2	11	2
c' Plasma Cell - Eccentric, Dark Nucleus, Nucleus: Cytoplasm ratio 1:2	7-11	8
d' Small Lymphocyte - Concentric, Dark Nucleus, Little Cytoplasm	5-6	27
e' Medium Lymphocyte - Dark Nucleus, Little Cytoplasm	7-8	38
f' Large Lymphocyte - Concentric, Dark Nucleus, Little Cytoplasm	9-12	17
g' Lymphoblast - Concentric, Dark Bordered Nucleus with Condensed Chromatin, Little Cytoplasm	11	3
h' Indented, Eccentric Dark Nucleus	8-10	5

Table 3 is a summary of the results of staining cells for lipase activity (Ansley and Ornstein 1970; Thornthwaite and Leif 1974). Only cells staining a deep red-brown color were identified as lipase positive. RFC that stained with lipase were medium to large mononuclear cells (7 to 13 μ in diameter). No PFC in over 100 observed stained with lipase.

While an average of 85% of a spleen cell population was viable by alcian blue dye exclusion, the analysis of over 120 PFC showed 100% viability utilizing the alcian dye.

Light microscopy has been useful in classifying eight distinct morphologic types of PFC and seven types of RFC. These immune cells appear to be mature and immature forms of several distinct classes of cells. Limited TEM observation (Harris et al. 1966; Hummeler et al. 1972) of a few PFC found in the lymph nodes of rabbits demonstrated that these cells show signs of physiologic activity by having well marked condensed chromatin, much of which borders on the nuclear membrane. Figure 2 shows several types of PFC that have dark bordered nuclei. Several of the PFC observed by the Plaque Cytogram assay have dark-staining chromatin bridges running from the nucleoli to the periphery of the dark bordered nucleus, suggesting a communication between the RNA rich nucleolus and perinuclear envelope DNA.

TABLE 3

Summary of Lipase Stain Measurements of Various Cell Classes

Type Cell in the Mouse	Percent Stained For Lipase	Number of Cells Observed
Thymus[a]	0.1	500
Spleen[a]	6.0	500
Bone Marrow[a]	11.0	800
RFCs (Spleen)	27.0	100
PFCs (Spleen)	0.0	120

[a] similiar results were obtained from non-immunized mice

The observation that some PFC have indented or segmented nuclei (Fig. 2H, Table 1h) and some are binucleated (Fig. 2I, Table 1i) suggests that at least a small population of these cells are undergoing nuclear division or cell fusion as reported by Claflin and Smithies (1967). They reported observing by phase microscopy in a modified agar gel assay the fusion of two PFC in a plaque to form a single binucleated cell.

At least three types of RFC can be distinguished by the Plaque Cytogram assay. The first type of RFC are presumably phagocytes. Both macrophages and their precursors have been shown to be able to bind SRBC in both non-immunized and immunized animals (Abramson et al. 1970; Bach and Dardenne 1972). The Plaque Cytogram assay shows the number of macrophage-monocyte RFC can be found by enumerating the lipase positive RFC. The second class of RFC (Fig. 3) are the aggregated RFC, which release a type of soluble antibody which can bind surrounding SRBC but cannot lyse them in the presence of complement, and RFC in which aggregates of SRBC form around the central RFC but do not bind to it.

These are included in the enumeration of RFC even though they are probably immunoglobulin-producing cells which are releasing an antibody (IgG?) that is weakly hemolytic in the presence of guinea pig complement. The third cell type, which is

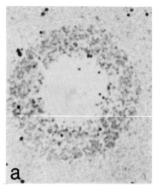 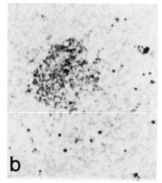

Figure 3. Two types of RFC which are releasing immunoglobulin. x 250. a, "Doughnut" shaped rosette in which the central RFC type causes aggregation of SRBC to which it is not directly bound ; b, aggregated RFC.

termed an antigen reactive cell, is the RFC that will not stain positive for lipase and does not form a plaque of lysed or unlysed SRBC but only a single layer of surface-bound SRBC. These cells are thought to be of thymic origin (Minowade et al. 1972; Gudat and Villiger 1973).

There are about 1300 PFC/10^6 nucleated cells in a BALB/c mouse spleen 4 days after a primary i.v. injection of SRBC, and the number of RFC is about 1 to 1.5 times more than the number of PFC, while about 27% of the RFC stain positive for lipase. Future experiments utilizing autoradiography will establish whether the morphological heterogeneity for the PFC and RFC are due to different stages of the cell cycle or whether the cells are different cell types.

DENSITY GRADIENT ANALYSIS OF PLAQUE-FORMING CELLS.

In recent years, primarily because of buoyant density separation data on PFCs, a controversy has arisen concerning the pleomorphic nature of PFC. In agreement with the results of electron microscopy (EM) observations of PFC (Harris et al. 1966; Bussard and Binet 1965; Fitch et al. 1965; Gudat et al. 1970) and the light microscopic observations by the Plaque Cytogram assay (Thornthwaite and Leif 1974) which indicate that these cells are pleomorphic, Haskill et al. (1969) have described a heterogeneous density population. However, Gorczynski et al. (1970) have critized the relia- bility of morphologic assessment because of the "unknown" effects of fixatives on cell morphology and heterogeneous density data (Haskill et al. 1969) because they (Gorczynski et al. 1970) believe varying osmolarity would probably account for the multiple density peaks. Their results obtained by volume (Miller and Phillips 1969) and density analysis with Ficoll (Gorczynski et al. 1970) have shown PFC to be homogeneous with respect to these two parameters. Therefore, they have concluded that PFC are a homogeneous cell type. In order to resolve this controversy, a study was performed in which both the morphology and density of PFC could be compared.

Immune spleen cells from a BALB/c mouse, that had been injected i.v. four days previously with 4×10^8 SRBC, were separated by bovine serum albumin (BSA), pH 6.8, linear buo- yant density gradient centrifugation as previously described (Thornthwaite and Leif 1975c). The Plaque Cytogram assay was utilized on the gradient fractions to identify the various morphological classes of plaque-forming cells (Thorn- thwaite and Leif 1974; 1975c).

Density distribution analysis of the gradients was analyzed by a Fortran V-Cell Type Program (S.B. Leif et al. 1973; Leif et al. 1975). The $F(\rho)$ and $G(\rho)$ are normalized distribution functions. $F(\rho)$ has been defined (Leif and Vinograd 1964, Leif 1970) to be

$$F(\rho) = \frac{\text{number of cells in the fraction}}{\text{number of cells recovered from the gradient} \cdot \Delta\rho}$$

$\Delta\rho$ is the density range of the individual fractions. $G(\rho)$ is a new function which is utilized for analysis of subclasses of cells.

$$G(\rho) = \frac{\text{number of cells of a specific subclass in the fraction}}{\text{number of cells of that general class recovered from the gradient} \cdot \Delta\rho}$$

Figure 4 shows a typical density distribution of white blood cells (WBC), RBC, and PFC from the spleens of immuniz- ed mice. The RBC peak is about 1.0804 $\text{gcm}^{-3} \pm 0.0006$ average deviation from the mean and the majority of the WBC are centered at 1.0637 $\text{gcm}^{-3} \pm 0.0011$ average deviation from the

mean. Also, in figure 4 is shown a typical PFC density profile. Three distinct peaks or shoulders have been seen in
at least three different PFC density gradient experiments.
In these three gradients each of the three peaks have an
average density deviation of ± 0.003 gcm^{-3} around the mean
densities at points a, b, and c of 1.060, 1.050, and 1.043
gcm^{-3}, respectively. The increase in number of PFC per fraction at the peaks in all three gradient experiments is a >
b > c.

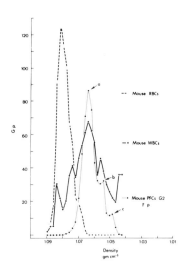

Figure 4. Density distri-
bution of WBCs, RBCs, and
PFCs from the spleen of a
BALB/c mouse 4 days after
a single i.v. injection of
sheep erythrocytes.

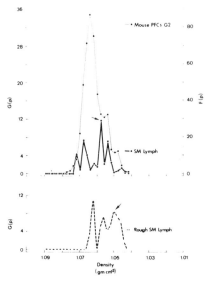

Figure 5. Density distri-
bution of small lymphocyte
and small rough lymphocyte
PFC.

Table IV shows the densities of the PFC density peaks
of three gradient experiments. The number of PFC in the
total WBC population at the PFC density peak was 0.1 to 0.8
PFC/100 WBC which resulted in a PFC enrichment between 1.0
and 2.9. The PFC enrichment was calculated by dividing the
concentration in terms of PFC per total WBC in a particular
fraction by the concentration recovered from the entire
gradient. The second (G2) gradient experiment was the one
analyzed in detail for PFC types. Over 1200 PFC were analyzed by the Plaque Cytogram assay in the second gradient
experiment. In gradient fractions between 1.075 and 1.045
gcm^{-3}, 50 to 200 PFC were analyzed for the differential count

Table IV. Peak Densities for Plaque-forming cells.

Gradient	$\rho - (gcm^{-3})$	Percent PFCs in a density fraction out of the total number of WBCs in that fraction	Enrichment of PFCs
G1 PFCs	a-1.0612	0.14	1.4
	b-1.0491	0.23	2.5
	c-1.0430	0.13	1.1
G2 PFCs	a-1.0637	0.17	2.2
	b-1.0538	0.11	1.5
	c-1.0479	0.70	1.0
G3 PFCs	a-1.0558	0.40	1.7
	b-1.0461	0.80	2.9
	c-1.0387	0.40	1.5

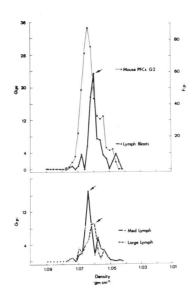

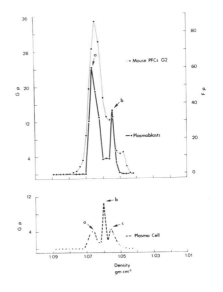

Figure 6. Density distribution of lymphoblast and medium and large lymphocyte PFC.

Figure 7. Density distribution of plasmablast and plasma cell PFC.

117

of each density fraction. Even though the other gradient experiments were not analyzed in as great detail for PFC type as the second gradient, they did show similar overall PFC density profiles as shown in gradient two. However, the density profiles of the specific types of PFC varied considerably, but still indicated that the different morphologic classes of cells were distinct entities.

The density distributions of some of the PFC types described in the first part of this chapter are shown in Figures 5 through 7. The corresponding densities of the arrow marked experimental points in the PFC density diagrams are shown in Table V.

Table V. Analysis of types of plaque-forming cells at their peak densities.

Plaque-forming cell types	$\rho(gcm^{-3})$	Percent [a] Cell Type	Percent [b] Total Cells	Enrichment [c] Factor
Small Lymphocyte	1.0597	26.9	24.7	2.9
Samll Rough Lymphocyte	1.0498	66.2	14.1	5.3
Medium Lymphocyte	1.0637	10.3	16.7	1.0
Large Lymphocyte	1.0597	5.8	6.4	0.7
Lymphoblasts	1.0597	17.3	40.4	1.0
Plasma Cells	a-1.0656	5.0	18.9	0.7
	b-1.0597	5.3	31.3	0.8
	c-1.0558	5.3	19.1	0.8
Plasmablasts	a-1.0656	34.2	25.2	1.8
	b-1.0538	44.9	15.1	2.3
Indented, Eccentric Nucleus	1.0676	16.7	26.9	2.8
Multinucleated	1.0617	7.7	38.7	2.3
Segmented Nucleus	1.0676	16.7	32.8	3.4
Aggregated Rosette-forming cell	1.0597	3.0	50.6	3.0
Rosette Plaque-forming cell	1.0577	7.3	28.7	4.3

[a] Percentage of a particular PFC type out of the total PFC types found at that density. [b] Percentage of a particular PFC type found at that density out of the total PFC of that type found in the whole gradient. [c] Percentage of a given type of PFC in terms of total PFC in a given fraction divided by the percentage of a given type of PFC in terms of total PFC recovered from the gradient.

As shown in Figure 5, among the PFC, the small lymphocytes in general are more dense than the small rough lympho-

cytes (as shown by SEM). In Figure 6, the large PFC lymphocytes are less dense than the medium PFC lymphocytes at their
respective peak densities of 1.0597 and 1.0637 gcm^{-3} (Table
V). Also, in Figure 6, lymphoblast PFC have a large peak
at a density of 1.0597 gcm^{-3} where 40% of the total lymphoblast PFCs (Table V) are found. Plasmablasts and plasma
cells (Figure 7) are the only PFC types in which significant
multiple peaks are found.

These results with the linear, pH 6.8 BSA density gradient technique of Leif and Vinograd (1964) and Leif (1970)
are in partial agreement with the BSA density separation of
CBA mouse spleen cells at pH 5.1 by the method of Shortman
(1969, 1972), which shows a broad lymphoid cell density distribution with a density maximum peak at 1.075 gcm^{-3} (Williams et al. 1972), compared with 1.0637 gcm^{-3} found in this
study. Also, the density of mouse erythrocytes is reported
to be 1.081 gcm^{-3} (Williams and Shortman 1972) compared to
1.080 gcm^{-3} (Figure 4). They show the PFC density profile is
broad with a maximum peak at 1.062 gcm^{-3}. However, when a
different gradient material is used, a quite different density distribution is obtained. Gorczynski et al. (1970) have
used Ficoll at pH 7.2 to describe the density distribution
of C3H mouse spleen cells as being a rather broad peak centered around 1.080 gcm^{-3}. With Ficoll, the density of the
mouse erythrocytes is 1.090 gcm^{-3} and the single narrow peak
for PFC is 1.070 gcm^{-3}. The 0.01 gcm^{-3} increase in the cell
density measurements with Ficoll is probably due in part to
the rapid decrease in water activity in Ficoll concentrations
between 10% and 30% (w/w) (Williams et al. 1972). The decrease in water activity, due to an increase of the amount
of water binding to the hydroxyl groups in Ficoll (polysuc-
rose), would create a hypertonic solution which would cause
the erythrocytes and lymphoid cells to shrink and band at a
heavier density than expected from the BSA gradient results.
Williams et al. (1972), obtained a 0.01 gcm^{-3} increase in
PFC density by varying osmolarity of the gradient from 269
to 314 milliosmolar. A general increase in lymphoid cell
density was also obtained.

The measurement of PFC enrichment at the PFC density
peaks has yielded up to 2.9-fold enrichment of PFC in terms
of WBC. This is in agreement with the enrichments found by
Haskill et al. (1969). Unfortunately, since the plaque
response is dynamically changing at 4 days, it will probably
be impossible to obtain completely reproducible profiles of
the differing morphologic species of PFC. Further studies

must await the development of an autoradiographic technique compatable with Centrifugal Cytology (Thornthwaite, Yopp, Dalmau and Leif, in preparation) which does not require air drying. It would then be possible by pulse labeling to determine the progenitor-progeny relationships of the PFC.

In correlation with the density heterogeneity of PFC, the Plaque Cytogram assay reveals considerable pleomorphism of PFC and the types of plaques they produce. The gradients are especially useful in identifying morphologically distinct PFC types since a particular PFC type can be enriched up to 66% (Table V) (small rough lymphocyte) of the total PFC found at a certain density. The combined morphology and density methods are able to separate the small rough lymphocyte PFC from the more dense small lymphocyte PFC.

Besides the small lymphocyte PFC, only the plasma and plasmablast PFC showed an apparent heterogeneity in density. No further attempt was made to differentiate these cells morphologically at their density peaks. It should be possible to utilize a pattern recognition microdensitometer system such as TICAS (Weid, et al. 1970) to objectively categorize the plaques for comparison with the subjectively identified morphologic buoyant density distribution of PFC.

The combination of the density gradient technique and the Plaque Cytogram assay have validated the findings from Shortman's laboratory (Williams et al. 1972; Shortman et al. 1970) that the density distribution of PFC is multimodal and have further established that this heterogeneity by density is at least substantially due to the presence of differing morphologic species.

SCANNING ELECTRON MICROSCOPY (SEM) OF PFC AND RFC

Figure 8a-g shows SEM pictures of the PFC. Three distinct types of plaques (Fig. 8a-c) are observed in the Plaque Cytogram assay. In Figure 8a are two typical plaques where the central PFC are lysing the surrounding SRBC. About a third of the small lymphocyte PFC form plaques (Fig. 8b, e) without detectable red cell ghosts. These are the only plaques observed (Fig. 8b) without the presence of complement. These complement-independent cells have very rough surfaces (Fig. 8e), while the other lymphocyte PFC (Fig. 8f) possess a much smoother surface. The complement independent (or rough small lymphocyte) PFC is discussed later in this chapter. The third type of plaque observed is

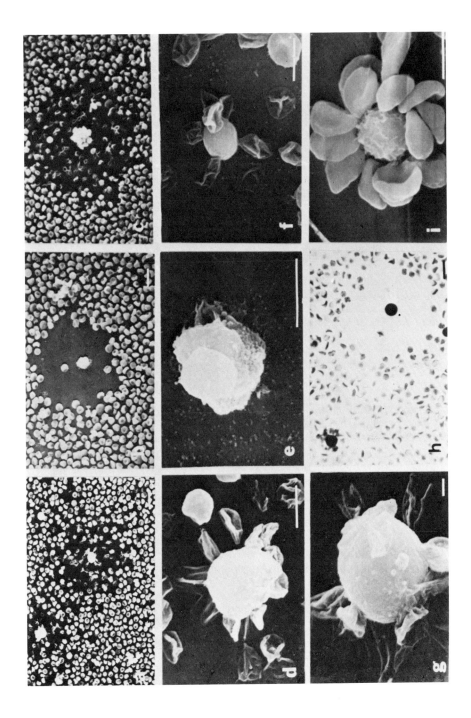

(Caption of the composite from the previous page)

Figure 8. Three types of plaques found in the Plaque Cytogram assay as shown by SEM (scale 10 μ): a, two typical
plaques with lysed SRBC surrounding the central PFC; b, PFC
with no lysed SRBC in the plaque; c, RFC forming a lysed
SRBC plaque around itself; d, higher magnification of the
PFC in the plaque on the left in Figure 8a; e, higher magnification of the rough surfaced PFC in Figure 8b; f,
smooth surface small lymphocyte PFC (d, e, f scale 5 μ);
g, high magnification of a typical PFC illustrating knob-
like structures and point-adhering lysed SRBC on a fairly
smooth surface (scale 1 μ); h, light microscopy picture
showing simultaneous PFC and RFC in the Plaque Cytogram
assay (scale 10 μ); i, rough surfaced RFC (scale 5 μ).

---

shown in Figure 8c. The central PFC has about 20 morphologically intact, benzidine positive SRBC binding to its surface while around the PFC is a large plaque of lysed SRBC.
These cells cannot be observed clearly through the red cell
cluster but appear to be medium or large lymphocytes by
light microscopy. The cell surface is smooth, at least on
the area that can be observed between the bound SRBC by SEM.
About 1% of the PFC observed formed these rosette-type
plaques. It has been shown (Donnelly and Sussdorf 1973)
that glutaraldehyde-fixed SRBC can be incubated with immunized spleen cells and cause rosette formation. These
rosettes can then be incubated in a Cunningham assay with
unfixed SRBC which result in plaque formation by some of
the antibody-producing cells that have fixed SRBC binding
to their surfaces. However, the SRBC binding in Figure 8c,
in what can be called a rosette PFC in the Plaque Cytogram
assay, are not fixed until plaque formation. A possible
explanation of why the released antibody would not lyse the
bound SRBC, while it is lysing a considerable number of SRBC
in the plaque area, could be that rosette-PFC are secreting
or have bound to their surfaces one or both of the two
inhibitors found in mouse sera which can inhibit guinea pig
complement components C1 and C3 and thus prevent lysis of
the cell-bound SRBC (Adolphs 1973).

Figure 8 (d-g) illustrates the pleomorphism of the PFC
by SEM. Point adherence of lysed SRBC onto the PFC membrane
is observed in all the PFC population with the typical
plaques (Fig. 8a). Diameters of PFC varied from 5μ small

lymphocytes (Figs. 2D, 8(e, f) and Table I) to 15μ large lymphoblasts (Fig. 2G and Table I). Under higher magnification, some surface detail such as small knob-like structures (Fig. 8g) can be seen on the PFC. However, essentially all of the complement dependent PFCs possessed surfaces which were smoother than any other type of cell previously observed except for erythrocytes.

Rosette formation can also be observed with the Plaque Cytogram assay; in fact, both PFC and RFC can be identified on the same slide as shown by the light microscopy photograph in figure 8h.

In Figure 8i is an SEM photograph of a RFC. This cell appears to be a small lymphocyte by its size (5 μ diameter) and has about 15 SRBC binding to its surface. An almost point-like adherence can be seen between the SRBC antigen and cell-bound antibody on the lymphocyte surface. In general RFC have rough surfaces.

There are two characteristics that distinguish the typical PFC by SEM. One feature of these cells is that they always have lysed erythrocytes bound to their surfaces (Fig. 8d, f, g). Secondly, the PFC have smooth surfaces when compared to RFC. The binding of the SRBC suggests that the first stage of plaque formation involves antigenic contact with the antibody-producing cell.

COMBINED LIGHT AND SEM OF PLAQUE-FORMING CELLS.

A useful method for establishing a correlation between the surface structure of cells and their identification by light microscope morphology has been developed (Leif, Zucker and Thornthwaite, unpublished results). In this part of the chapter, the PFC will be the only type of cell compared by light and SEM. Later on, the usefulness of this technique for establishing effector cell-tumor cell interaction by SEM will be presented.

Figure 9 shows a typical homogeneous monolayer of SRBC and immunized mouse spleen cells on a gridded slide. A similar sample by SEM can be seen in Figure 10. In both cases the gridded letter-numbered areas can be seen clearly by light and SEM. This enables one to observe the same cell by two morphological criteria. In Figures 11 and 12 are combined light and SEM photographs of PFCs. Figure 11a and b show a large lymphoblast PFC in which the adherance of

Combined light and SEM of plaque-forming cells is one example of the usefulness of this technique. Future work on comparing the surface architecture of mammalian cells to the internal structure will include human white blood cells, thymus and bone marrow cells.

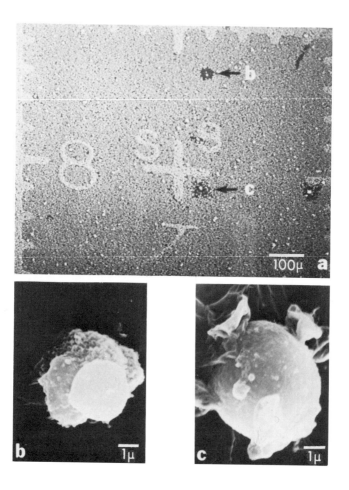

Figure 10. (a) SEM of lawn of SRBC and mouse spleen cells. (b) and (c) are the complement-independent and typical PFC, respectively.

lysed SRBC does not occur uniformily over the entire cell membrane. The SRBC are adherent to areas of the plasma membrane
which bound cytoplasmic constituents of the cell (e.g. golgi
apparatus, rough ER), but are not adherent to areas of the
membrane which closely bound the nucleus. Figures 11c and d
show the spatial arrangement of two PFC plaques. SRBC ghosts
can barely be seen in the light microcope photograph, while
the SEM photograph shows a network of lysed SRBCs in the
plaques. Combined light and SEM of a Rosette-PFC can be seen
in Figures 11e and f. Light microscopy can be used to show
that this cell has unlysed SRBC (benzidine positive) binding
to itself, while the number of unlysed SRBCs bound to this
antibody-producing cell can be enumerated utilizing SEM.
Higher magnification of PFCs by combined light and SEM can
be seen in Figure 12. Figure 12a and b shows a higher magnification of the lymphoblast found in Figures 11a and b.
A PFC in mitosis can be seen in Figures 12c and d and a
medium plasmablast in Figures 12e and f. The plasmablasts
were more flat and oblong than the lymphoblasts by SEM.

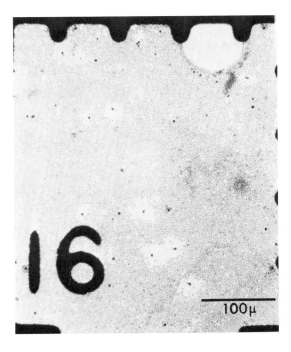

Figure 9. Light microscopy photograph of a lawn of
SRBC with complement independent PFC.

125

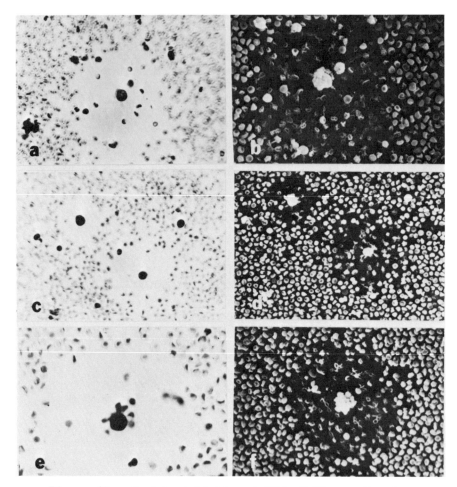

Figure 11.   Combined light and SEM of Plaque-forming
cells (a), (b) - lymphoblast (c), (d) - two plaques
(e), (f) - rosette-PFC.   1000X.

Since thousands of cells can easily be compared by light
and SEM, a statistical correlation between cell surface morphology and transmission light microscopy can be made.   The
utilization of SEM for the study of cell surface structure
permits a classification of cells independent of the previous light and transmission electron microscope morpho-
logies which are based on internal structure.   The correlation of the cell surface morphology with the internal morphology permits the determination of the surface structure of
presently known classes of cells and the utilization of

surface morphology descriptors to redefine and improve the present classification of cells.

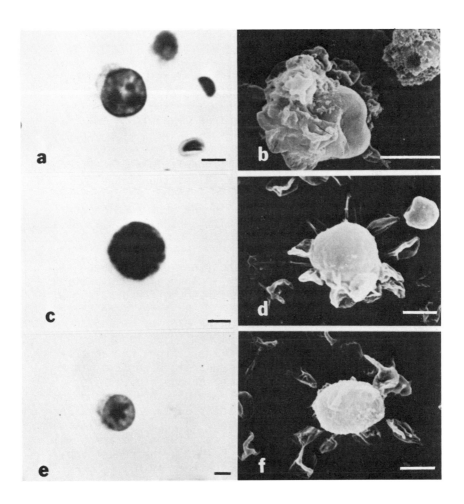

Figure 12.   Combined Light and SEM of Plaque-forming cells (a), (b) lymphoblast as in Fig. 11a, b (c), (d) - mitotic PFC (e), (f) - Plasmablast. Bar-5μ.

SPONTANEOUS ROSETTE-FORMING CELLS (SRFC)

As previously described in this chapter, the bone marrow derived PFC are relatively smooth surfaced when compared to the rough surfaced RFC which are believed to be thymus (T) derived. These results on the identification of B- and T-cells in the mouse spleen by SEM is contrary to the work of Polliack et al.(1973) and Lin et al. (1973). In studying B- and T-cells from human peripheral blood, these two groups of authors reported that the B-cells were "villous" or rough surfaced when compared to the "relatively smooth" T-cells. Since the previous cell surface studies reported here were limited to the mouse spleen, the Plaque Cytogram assay was extended to include the preparation of human peripheral blood lymphocytes (HPBL), for SEM observation to determine if the two T- and B-cell populations of HPBL could be distinguished from each other. Also, the Plaque Cytogram assay was utilized for preparing spontaneous rosette-forming cells (SRFC). These are T-cells in the HPBL population which form spontaneous rosettes with SRBC at 0°C (Lay et al. 1971; Wybran and Fudenberg 1973).

Human peripheral blood lymphocytes were obtained by either Ficoll-Hypaque or Plasmagel-nylon column separation and resuspended in Dulbecco's phosphate buffered saline with 0.2% bovine serum albumin (PBS-BSA). Rosettes were formed with sheep red blood cells (SRBC) and HPBL by mixing one ml each of 1×10^8/ml SRBC with 5×10^6/ml HPBL in either PBS-BSA or RPMI 1640 with 0.2% BSA. The mixture was centrifuged at 50xg in a PR-2 clinical centrifuge for two minutes at 4°C and then placed in ice for one hour. After incubation at 0°C the cells were carefully resuspended and portions of the rosetted cell suspension were added to the precooled (4°C) Centrifugal Cytology bucket. The cells were then centrifuged onto the restricted glass slide areas which were formed by the radial square holes in the bucket top. After centrifugation in a PR-2 centrifuge at 100 xg for 5 minutes at 4°C, the cells had to be brought to room temperature (about 21°C) for layering with glutaraldehyde. After fixation overnight at 2°C, the slides were critical point dried (Thornthwaite et al. 1975a).

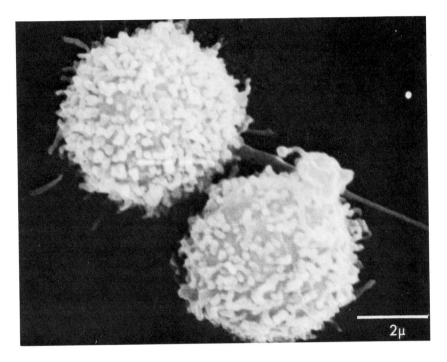

Figure 13. Two human lymphocytes separated by Ficoll-Hypaque and prepared for SEM.

Figure 13 shows two typical villous HPBL prepared by the Plaque Cytogram technique. Also, the SRFC were rough surfaced as shown in Figures 14 and 15. Figure 14 shows a SRFC completely surrounded by the SRBC. Except for SRBC binding to the T-cell in Figure 15, the rosetted and non-rosetted lymphocytes are indistinguishable by surface morphology alone. Essentially the same results were obtained after air drying the cells from xylene (Thornthwaite et al. 1975a).

Transmission electron microscopy (TEM) observations following *en face* sectioning of SRFC agree with the SEM data in that microvilli can be seen in the TEM sections attached to the target SRBC (Figure 16).

Smooth surfaced lymphocytes and SRFC can form on the microscope slides by allowing the centrifuged cells to come in contact with the slide substrate for 30 min. at 37°C (Figures 17 and 18). The SRFC go through a stage of having very long, sparse microvilli which are also lost by longer incubation at 37°C.

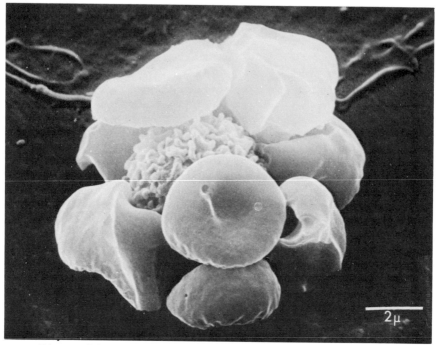

Figure 14.　Human T cell lymphocyte spontaneous rosette with SRBC.

In agreement with our observation that all of the lymphocytes from HPBL are villous, Kay et al. (1974) have reporting viewing "several hundred thousand normal human lymphocytes with SEM over the past 2 years and have found microvilli to be a constant characteristic of lymphocyte surfaces". Also, these authors showed that SRFC are villous lymphocytes. In agreement with our SEM and TEM results, Galey et al. (1974) support our results which show that HPBL and T-cell SRFC have numerous microvilli.

Wetzel et al. (1974) has shown that lymphocyte surface integrity was affected profoundly by the substrate utilized for supporting the cells. By aspirating HPBL onto Flotronic silver membranes or Nucleopore filters, they showed a loss of surface microvilli, unless the cells were initially fixed in suspension. This supports our observation (figures 17 and 18) that cells which are in prolonged contact with the slide substrate prior to glutaraldehyde fixation can lose their microvilli. These observations (Wetzel et al. 1974) could account for the discrepancies between Kay et al.

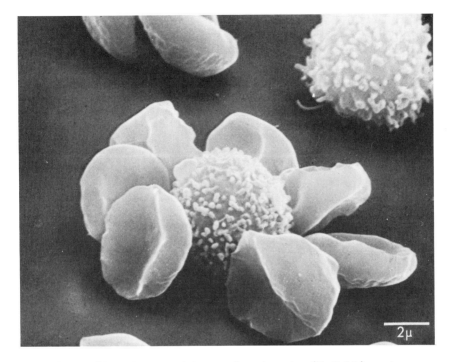

Figure 15.   Rosetted human lymphocyte (T-Cell) and non-rosetted cell (B-cell).

(1974) and our results and the results from Polliack et al. (1973) and Lin et al. (1973) who aspirate HPBL onto Flotronic membranes prior to fixation.

In any event, a gross morphologic classification of B- and T-cells by SEM would not necessarily be valid for "minor" cell populations which are 0.2 to 0.1% of the total lymphoid cell population as in the case of the B-cell PFC and T-cell RFC in the immune mouse spleen cell population (Thornthwaite and Leif 1974). Since the state of the cell surface evidently depends on prior treatment of the cells (Wetzel et al. 1974), it is perhaps best to describe the surface of cells operationally. For example, the cell surface phenomena described for SRBC immunized mouse spleen cells pertain only to the PFC and RFC performing their biologic functions. These studies of cells with specific biological activities may be more useful in the long run than studies on broad categories of lymphocytes such as B- and T-cells which will

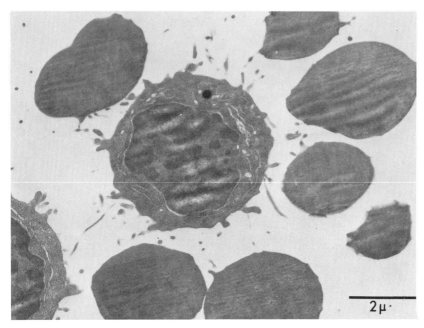

Figure 16. *En face* transmission electron microscope section of a villous T cell rosette from human lymphocytes.

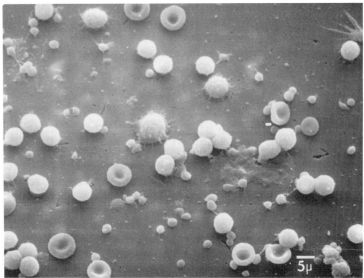

Figure 17. Human lymphocytes after being left for 30 min. at 37°C on a glass microscope slide.

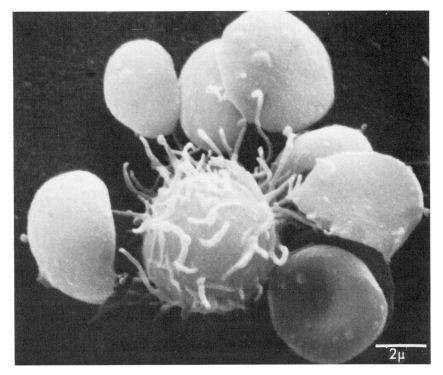

Figure 18. Human SRFC after being left for 30 min. at 37°C on a glass microscope slide.

in the future in any event have to be subdivided.

THE COMPLEMENT INDEPENDENT PLAQUE-FORMING CELLS (CIPFC)

This type of cell was first observed in the Plaque Cytogram assay (Thornthwaite and Leif 1974) as shown in Figures 8b, e and Figure 10b. These cells were originally referred to as small rough lymphocytes (Thornthwaite and Leif 1974; 1975c) due to their rough surface when compared to the typical smooth surfaced PFC as shown in Figure 10. These cells could easily be distinguished from the typical antibody producing PFC by light microscopy due to the fact that they formed clear plaques without detectable lysed SRBC in the plaque area (Figure 19). In the presence of 10% guinea pig complement only about one nucleated spleen cell from BALB/c mice in 9000 formed such a plaque (Figure 20a). However, approximately one cell in 50 formed a discernible clear plaque in the absence of complement as shown in

Figure 20b.   The CIPFC concentration of about 2% is about
the same for either SRBC immunized or non-immunized mice.
Thus far, the CIPFC has also been detected in BALB/c and
DBA/2 spleen and lymph node cell populations.   Further studies
are currently being performed to establish the mode of the
RBC destruction by the CIPFC.

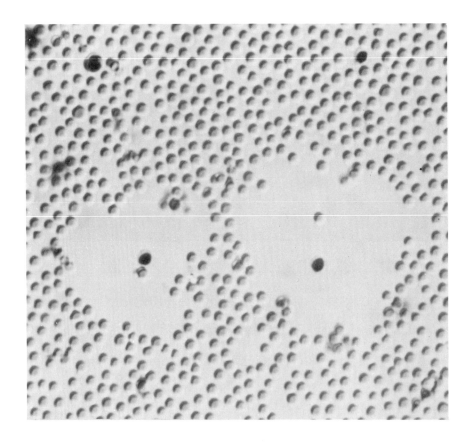

Figure 19.   Complement-independent PFC from an
unimmunized DBA/2J mouse which are completely destroying surrounding SRBC in order to form a clear
plaque.   900X.

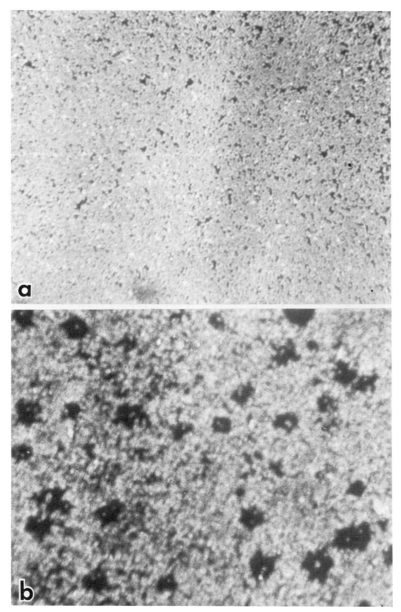

Figure 20. Dark field optics showing the SRBC-unimmunized DBA/2J cell monolayer 15 min. after incubation at 37°C (a) with and (b) in the absence of 10% guinea pig complement. 40X.

PLAQUE ASSAY FOR CELL MEDIATED IMMUNITY

By utilizing a modification of the Plaque Cytogram assay, we have been able to observe cell mediated immunity by light, scanning electron (SEM) and transmission electron microscopy (TEM). The basic technique is to form effector-target cell rosettes and centrifuge aliquots of these rosettes onto a restricted microscope slide area. During incubation, the target cells are destroyed by the cytotoxic lymphocytes. The cells are then fixed by slowly layering glutaraldehyde onto the cell monolayer. The alcian blue vital staining procedure is then utilized to detect killed tumor cells (stained) with cytotoxic lymphocytes (unstained) attached. Data on the cellular interaction between EL 4 ascites or P-815-X2 mastocytoma tumor and immune lymph node cells (ILNC) will be presented. It should be emphasized that the cytotoxic effect described below may not be entirely directly related to conventional measurements of stimulated cytotoxic activity such as the ^{51}Cr-release assay   since allogenic, non-stimulated (normal) lymph node cells (NLNC) produce reactions which are almost as large as the ILNC population. However, as will be described below, the Plaque Cytogram is measuring a true cytotoxic interaction.

Both MEBM (a modification of mouse embryo basal medium with 10 mM HEPES, 0.1g/L $NaHCO_3$, antibiotics, and 10% heat inactivated fetal calf serum (FCS), pH 7.2 and 290 MOSM) and RPMI-1640 (25 mM HEPES, Grand Island Biological Co.) with 0.2% bovine serum albumin were utilized in the effector cell assay. Dulbecco's phosphate buffered saline with calcium and 10% FCS (PBS-FCS) was utilized for harvesting and washing the cells.

EL 4 and P-815-X2 mastocytoma cells were harvested from the peritoneal cavities of C57BL/6J and DBA/2J mice, respectively, 7 days after a primary intraperitoneal injection of 10^7 tumor cells (0.1 ml) in PBS.

The effector immune lymph node cells were obtained from the efferent lymph nodes of mastocytoma injected C57BL/6J EL 4 injected DBA/2J mice 7-11 days after a subcutaneous injection of 10^7 tumor cells (0.04 ml) in PBS.

After filtration of the cell suspensions through a 70μ Nytex filter (Small Parts, Inc. Miami, Fla.) to remove cell debris, the cells were diluted up to 50 ml and washed in a PR-2 centrifuge (700xg, 10 min., 4oC).

In some of the experiments, the ILNC and NLNC were passed through a Leukopak column (LP-1 Leukopak, Fenwal Labs, Morton Grove, Ill.) to remove most of the B-cell population (Trizo and Cudkowicz, 1974). Basically, eight ml of either the ILNC or NLNC (3×10^7) were added to a 10 ml syringe which had been packed to the eight ml mark with 0.8 g of Leukopak material. The column was sealed with Parafilm and allowed to incubate at 37°C for 45 minutes. After incubation, 50 ml of PBS was poured through the column and the effluent collected. After washing, the cells were resuspended in tissue culture medium.

In order to form the initial contact between tumor and effector cells, various ratios of LNC to tumor cells were mixed with one ml of 3×10^6/ml LNC. Various aliquots of tumor cells (3×10^6/ml) were added to the LNC to form LNC/tumor cell ratios of 10/1, 20/1, 50/1, and 100/1. The best results were obtained when the ratio was between 20 and 50 ILNC per tumor cell. The cell mixtures, LNC and tumor cells, were

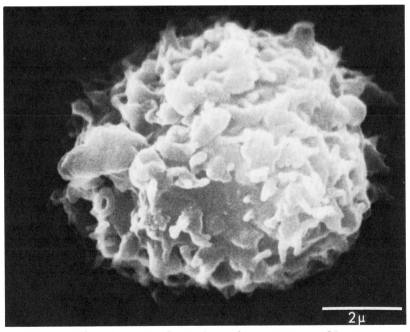

Figure 21. A typical EL 4 ascites tumor cell as revealed by SEM. These cells have prominent ruffles on their surface which are in contrast to the villous human and mouse lymphocytes described earlier in this chapter.

added to 35 mm diameter (Falcon 3001) dishes and rocked at room temperature for 15 minutes on a Bellco rocker at six RPM. Then, aliquots of the cells were gently removed from the dishes and added to each chamber of the 12 hole Centrifugal Cytology buckets. The buckets were incubated at 37°C for up to three hours. The cells, after centrifugation (5 min., 4°C, 100xg, PR-2 centrifuge), were fixed by layering 0.1 ml of 4% glutaraldehyde-0.05M cacodylate solution (pH 7.4) on to the cell monolayer utilizing the special multi-pipetting machine (Fig. 1). After fixation overnight at 4°C, the cells were stained with benzidine followed by alcian blue to reveal the destroyed target cells. After staining, these cells could be prepared for light microscope, SEM, combination of both light and SEM, or TEM observation by methods described at the beginning of the chapter.

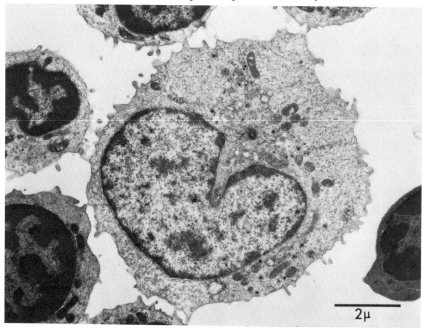

2μ

Figure 22. A typical rosette by TEM which results when ILNC and EL 4 tumor cells are initially rocked at room temperature. As shown in the figure, binding occurs between the microvilli of the lymphocytes and the tumor cell. When these rosettes are incubated at 37°C and later stained with alcian blue after glutaraldehyde fixation, select populations of ILNC can be seen binding to dead (stained) EL 4 tumor cells (Inserts to Figures 23 and 24).

By utilizing the special gridded slide technique described earlier in this chapter, we were able to observe the
effector cell-tumor cell interaction by combined light and
SEM. Selected rosettes between the effector cells of the LNC
and the target cells were located by light microscopy as
shown by the inserts in Figures 23 and 24. After SEM preparation of these samples, the same rosettes could be
relocated by the grid coordinates and subsequently photographed for SEM observation (Figures 23 and 24).

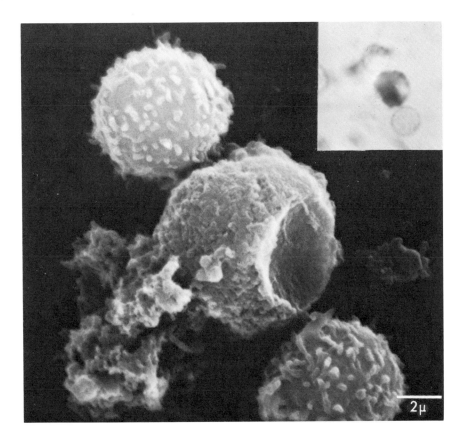

Figure 23. Combined light and SEM of the effector EL-4
tumor cell interaction. The insert shows the light
micrograph of the corresponding SEM interaction shown
in the figure.

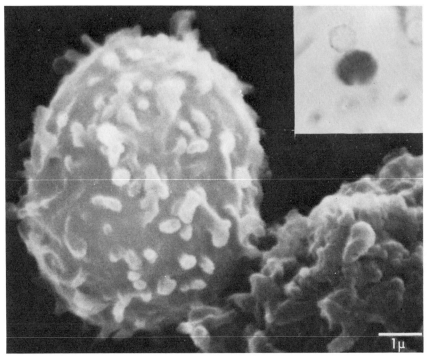

Figure 24. A second combined light (insert) and SEM of the effector cell-EL 4 tumor cell interaction.

The corresponding SEM photographs in Figures 23 and 24 show the cytotoxic lymphocytes to be villous. This further supports our finding that the so called T-cell line of lymphocytes are villous. Figure 23 shows an effector cell completely shearing off the cytoplasm of the EL 4 cell revealing the nucleus, while Figure 24 shows that the interaction between the effector cell and tumor cell is apparently mediated by the microvilli.

Even though effector cell-target cell interactions were quiet readily found by alcian blue staining, the quantitative enumeration of this interaction was impossible, because the EL 4 cells would clump together during incubation. To eliminate this problem, the mastocytoma cell line was utilized as the target. These cells did not aggregate after a three hour incubation but remained in a homogeneous monolayer as shown in Figures 25 and 26. The surface architecture of these cells was quite different from the EL 4 , since the mastocytoma cells were extremely villous (Figures 27 and 28).

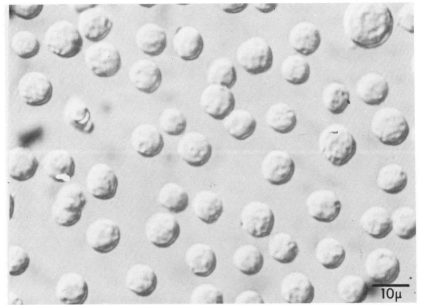

Figure 25. Nomarski photomicrograph of a homogeneous, viable (alcian blue negative) lawn of mastocytoma cells after a three hour incubation at 37°C.

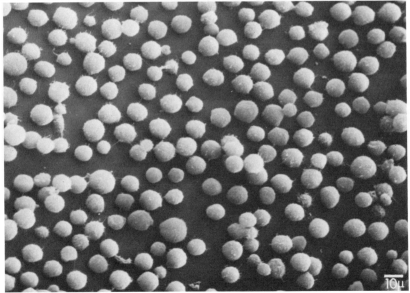

Figure 26. Corresponding SEM photomicrograph of a lawn of mastocytoma cells three hours after incubation at 37°C.

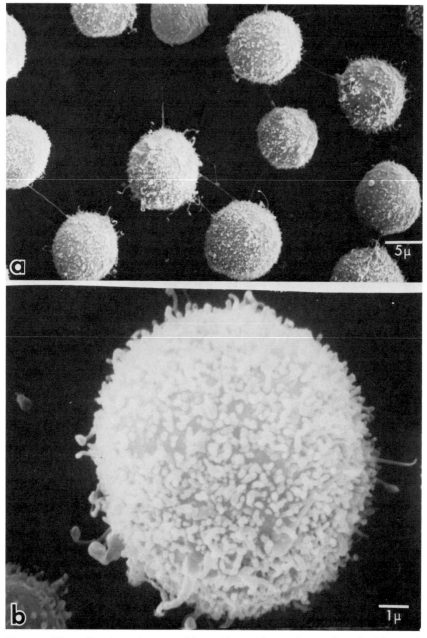

Figure 27. Mastocytoma cells after three hour incubation at 37ºC (a) magnification showing interconnecting microvilli between the cells (b) typical villous mastocytoma cell.

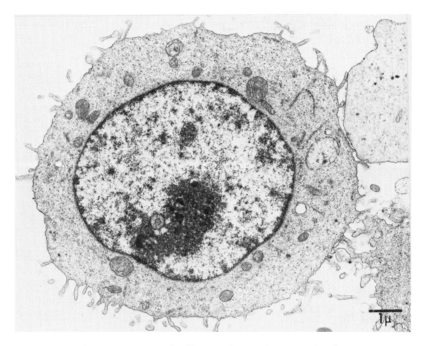

Figure 28. *En face* TEM section of a typical mastocytoma cell.

The effector cell-mastocytoma cell interactions could easily be observed on the microscope slides by the alcian blue stain as demonstrated in Figure 29. This type of destruction was T-cell mediated, since it was seen after the B-cell population was removed by passage through Leukopak columns (Trizo and Cudkowicz, 1974). Tumor cell destruction could also be observed after the action of the effector cell when 0.2% BSA was utilized instead of fetal calf serum (FCS). Such results eliminate the possibility of nonspecific antibody in the FCS causing the tumor cell destruction.

The cytotoxic activity of ILNC against mastocytoma cells was seen even without alcian blue staining, because spherules of debris could easily be observed around the destroyed tumor cells (Figure 30).

Approximately 4-6% of the ILNC cells were judged to be effector cells since they destroy the tumor cells as shown by the alcian blue stain. Uropod extensions of ILNC appeared rarely in the rosette interactions. Almost all of the tumor cells that were destroyed had the effector ILNC binding to them. This suggests that once the rosettes are formed and centrifuged on to the slide, the ILNC and tumor cells stay in contact throughout the 2-3 hour incubation if the buckets are

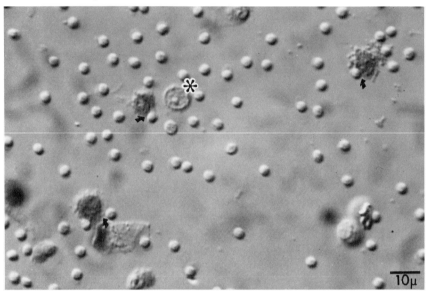

Figure 29. Effector ILNC and mastocytoma cells (30:1) incubated for 2 hours at 37°C. An arrow indicates cell interactions, asterisk-viable mastocytoma cell. Alcian blue stained.

not rocked. Tumor cell damage could be seen after a 30 min. incubation; however, longer incubation times (2-3 hrs) were utilized to assure a more complete tumor destruction.

Figure 31a and b shows a typical effector ILNC-mastocytoma interaction as seen by SEM. The villous cytotoxic lymphocytes appear to be destroying the mastocytoma cell by a process which causes damage to the tumor cell membrane as shown by the formation of spherical debris.

If the ILNC-tumor cell rosettes are incubated on Thermanox slides as shown in the first part of this chapter, these cells can then be prepared for TEM. Briefly, the glutaraldehyde-fixed cells on Thermanox slides are stained with 1% O_sO_4 for 15 min. followed by the alcian blue stain for 5 min. The slides are then dehydrated through a graded acetone series and embedded with Spurr from 100% acetone. Selected rosettes (Fig. 29) were circled and sectioned *en face* for TEM.

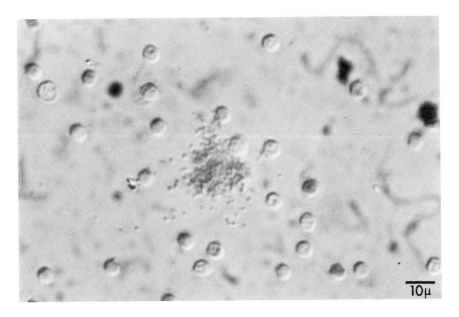

Figure 30. Nomarski photograph showing the cytotoxic effect of the effector ILNC against a target mastocytoma cell after three hours incubation at 37°C.

Figure 28 shows a typical mastocytoma cell by TEM. However, when these tumor cells are incubated to form rosettes with effector ILNC, severe damage to the mastocytoma cytoplasm results as shown in Figures 32 and 33.

Non-immunized LNC also can kill either the EL 4 or mastocytoma cells after rosette formation and incubation. These non-immunized LNC are lymphocytes which are lipase and acid phosphatase negative. This "background" killing by normal LNC has caused problems in utilizing this assay technique for the enumeration of cytotoxic effector cells in immunized mice, since the percentage of cytotoxic lymphocytes in the non-sensitized cell population in most cases has been only a few per cent below the sensitized cell population (e.g., 4% vs 6% for the ILNC). We are currently varying the method of rosette formation and lessening the incubation time in order to obtain a significant amount of killing above the non-immunized controls. However, it must be reemphasized that this "granulated" destruction of the tumor cells is not

145

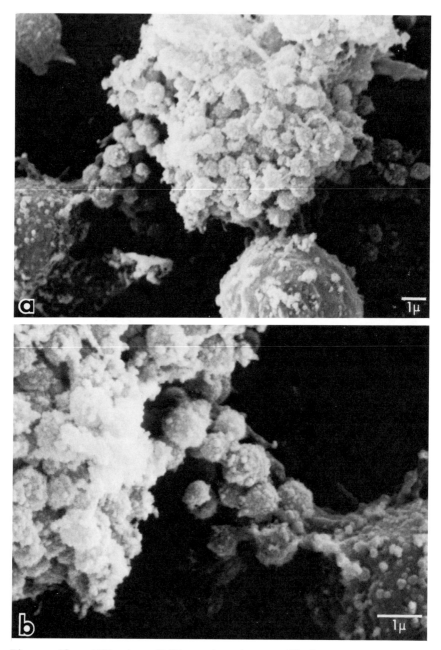

Figure 31. Effector ILNC-mastocytoma cell interaction by SEM. (a) and (b) binding effector cells cause granulation of the mastocytoma cell.

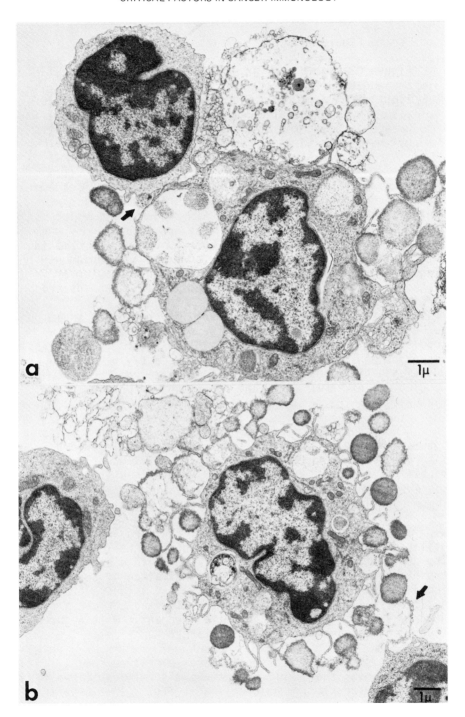

(Caption to Figures 32a and b on previous page)

Figure 32a and b. *En face* TEM of a mastocytoma cell
being destroyed by effector ILNC. The corresponding
light microscope (Figs. 29 and 30) and SEM (Fig. 31),
also show a granulation of the mastocytoma cell membranes as being the mode of destruction of these cells
by the cytotoxic ILNC.Arrows-effector cell interaction.

---

seen in either the pure populations of tumor or LNC [except
for the ILNC which in some cases are contaminated with a
small percentage (<5%) of tumor cells because of the localized subcutaneous injections] when they are incubated by themselves. Only in the presence of both tumor and LNC does the
tumor cell destruction occur. The complement independent
plaque-forming cell described earlier in this chapter is
another example of a cytotoxic lymphocyte which can destroy
foreign cells (SRBC) without prior immunization. The killing
that is being observed quite possibly may represent an immunosurveillance process. It should be stressed that the low
levels of cytotoxicity observed with the Plaque Cytogram Assay
cannot be detected with the ^{51}Cr release assay because of the
relatively high background release of ^{51}Cr from the pure
populations of tumor cells and non-immunized LNC-tumor cell
mixtures.

A non-specific, autodestruction of the EL 4 and mastocytoma tumor cells by simple contact with an allogenic LNC
was ruled out, because rosettes were found frequently between
viable LNC and viable tumor cells. However, as shown above
there is a small but significant population of LNC in the
immune population which can form dead tumor cell rosettes.

In conclusion, light microscopy, SEM, and TEM have been
utilized to describe the effector ILNC-tumor cell interaction.
The destruction of the tumor cells results in disruption of
the plasma membrane with concomitant formation of spherical
debris. The effector cells are lipase and acid phosphatase
negative, villous lymphocytes. Non-immunized LNC can also
destroy the tumor cells by a similar mechanism with apparently identical destruction of the target tumor cell.

This assay technique should have several technical
advantages over the ^{51}Cr method currently being utilized for
measuring cytotoxic lymphoid cell activity. It affords the

advantage of actually being able to enumerate and study these cells on a cellular level. By using both classical morphological and other cellular descriptors, it may be possible to differentiate various subpopulations of effector cells.

Note: There is an abstract listed in this Symposium by Springer et al. which shows the effector cell action by villous, human T-cells against target mammary carcinoma cells.

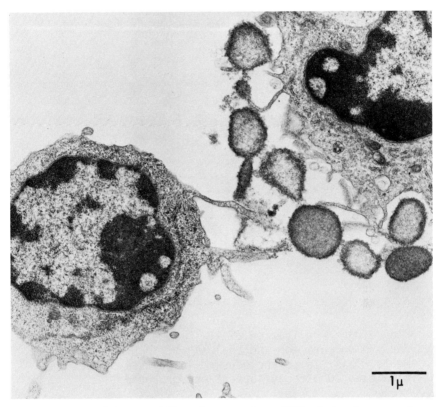

Figure 33. High magnification *en face* TEM photomicrograph showing the interaction between the villous effector LNC and grannulated mastocytoma cell.

CONCLUSION

Cellular assays for several types of immune responses have been described in this chapter. The application of the Plaque Cytogram assay for the enumeration and analysis of IgM antibody-producing cells, spontaneous RFC, complement independent PFC and sensitized and non-sensitized effector cells has been presented. Figure 34 presents a summary of the application of Plaque Cytogram Assay for the study of immunocompetent cells.

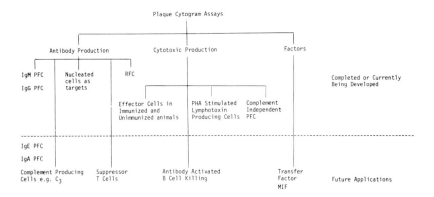

Figure 34. Application of the Plaque Cytogram Assay for the enumeration and analysis of immunocompetent cells. This figure includes cellular assays that are completed, under development and proposed.

REFERENCES

N. Abramson, A.F. Lo Buglio, J.H. Jandl, and R.S. Cotran, J. Exp. Med., 132:1191, 1970.

H.D. Adolphs, Med. Microbiol. Immunol., 158:171, 1973.

L.C. Andersson, S. Nordling, and P. Häyry, Cell. Immunol. 1:315, 1971.

H. Ansley, and L. Ornstein, Technicon Hemalog Advances in Automated Analysis, Vol. 1, p. 5, 1970.

J.F. Bach, G. Biozzi, M.F. Greaves, I. McConnell, H.S. Micklem, E. Moller, and O.B. Zaalberg, Transplant. Proc., 4:335, 1972.

J.F. Bach and M. Dardenne, Cell. Immunol., 3:1, 1972.

A.E. Bussard and J.L. Binet, Nature, 205: 675, 1965.

T.K. Chio, D.R. Sleight, and A. Nisonoff, Fed. Proceed. Abst. No. 3357, (Atlantic City, N.J., 1974).

A.J. Claflin, and O. Smithies, Science, 157:1561, 1967.

A.J. Cunningham, Nature, 207:1106, 1965.

J.J. Cutts, Cell Separation Methods in Hematology, New York:Academic Press, 1970.

N. Donnelly and D.H. Sussdorf, Proc. Soc. Exp. Biol. Med., 142:351, 1973.

F.W. Fitch, D.A. Rowley, and S. Coulthard, Nature, 207:994, 1965.

M.J. Fulwyler, Automated Cell Identification and Cell Sorting (G.L. Wied and G.F. Bahr, Eds.) p. 97, Academic Press: New York, 1970.

F.R. Galey, J.T. Prchal, G.D. Amromin, and Y. Thurani, N. Engl. J. Med. 290:640, 1974.

R.M. Gorczynski, R.G. Miller, and P.A. Phillips, Immunology, 19:817, 1970.

H.G. Gratzner, P. Ahmad, and R.C. Leif, In vitro 9: 373, 1974, abstract.

F.G. Gudat, T.N. Harris, S. Harris, and K. Hummeler, J. Exp. Med., 132:448, 1970.

F.G. Gudat and W. Villiger, J. Exp. Med., 137:483, 1973.

T.N. Harris, K. Hummeler, and S. Harris, J. Exp. Med. 123: 161, 1966.

K. Hannig, Modern Separation Methods of Macromolecules and Particles, Wiley: New York, (T. Gerritsen, Ed.) 1969.

J.S. Haskill, D.G. Legge, and K. Shortman, J. Immunol., 102:703, 1969.

K.E. Hellstrom, and S. Hellstrom, Advances in Cancer Research, Vol. 12, p. 167, Academic Press, New York, 1969.

H.R. Hulett, W.A. Bonner, R.G. Sweet, and L.A. Herzenberg, Clin. Chem. 19: 813, 1973.

K. Hummeler, T.N. Harris, S. Harris, and M.B. Farber, J. Exp. Med., 135:491, 1972.

J.S. Ingraham, and A.E. Bussard, J. Exp. Med., 119:667, 1964.

N.K. Jerne, and A.A. Nordin, Science, 140:405, 1963.

M.M.Kay, B. Belohradsky, K. Yee, J. Vogel, D. Butcher, J. Wybran, and H.H. Fudenberg. Clin. Immunol. Immunopathol. 2:301, 1974.

R.C. Leif, and J. Vinograd, Proc. Natl. Acad, Sci., 51,:520, 1964.

M.M. Kay, B. Belohradsky, K. Yee, J. Vogel, D. Butcher, J. Wybran, and H.H. Fudenberg. Clin. Immunol. Immuno pathol. 2:301, 1974.

W.H. Lay, N.F. Mendes, C. Bianco, and V. Nussenzweig, Nature 230:531, 1973.

R.C. Leif, and J. Vinograd, Proc. Natl, Acad., Sci., 51: 520, 1964.

R.C. Leif, in Automated Cell Identification and Cell Sorting, Edited by G.L. Weid and G.F. Bahr, p. 21, Academic Press, New York, 1970.

R.C. Leif, H.N. Easter, R.L. Warters, R.A. Thomas, L.A. Dunlap, and M.F. Austin, J. Histochem. Cytochem., 19:203, 1971.

R.C. Leif, S. Smith , R.L. Warters, L.A. Dunlap, and S.B. Leif, Submitted for publication, 1975.

S.B. Leif, B.F. Cameron, and R.C. Leif, J. Retoendothel Soc. (Abst. Ed.), 92:390, 1973.

P.S. Lin, A.G. Cooper, and H.H. Wortis, N. Engl J. Med., 289:548, 1973.

R.G. Miller, and R.A. Phillips, J. Cell. Physiol. 73:191, 1969. J. Minowade, T. Ohnuma, and G.E. Moore, J. Nat. Cancer Inst., 49:891, 1972.

P.F. Mullaney, J. Sheinkamp, H.A. Crissman, L.S. Cram, and D.M. Holm, Laser Applications in Medicine and Biology (M.L. Wolbarsht, Ed.) Plenum Press: New York, 1975, in press.

G.N. Papanicolaou, Atlas of Exfoliative Cytology, Harvard University Press, Cambridge, Mass., 1954.

A. Polliack, N. Lampen, B.D. Clarkson, and E. de Harven, J. Exp. Med., 138:607, 1973.

T.G. Pretlow II, E.E. Weir, and J.G. Zettergren, Vol 14 of the International Review of Experimental Pathology, Acadamic Press, 1975.

F. Ruch, Introduction to Quantitative Cytochemistry, Edited by G.L. Weid and G.F. Bahr, Vol. 2, p. 300, Academic Press, New York, 1970.

K. Shortman, Aust. J. Exp. Biol. Med. Sci., 46:375, 1968.

K. Shortman, in Modern Separation Methods of Macromolecules and Particles, Edited by T. Gerritsen, Vol. 2, p. 167, Wiley, New York, 1969.

K. Shortman, E. Diener, P. Russell, and W.D.J. Armstrong, Exp. Med., 131:461, 1970.

K. Shortman, Ann. Rev. Biophys. Bioeng., 1:93, 1972.

J.T. Thornthwaite and R.C. Leif, J. Immunol. 113:1897, 1974.

J.T. Thornthwaite, B.N. Thornthwaite, M.A. Hart, M.L. Cayer and R.C. Leif, Scanning Electron Microscopy/1975 edited by O. Johari and I. Corvin IIT Research Institute:Chicago, 1975a.

J.T. Thornthwaite and R.C. Leif, submitted for publiction, 1975b.

J.T. Thornthwaite and R.C. Leif, J. Immunol., 114:1023, 1975c.

D. Trizo and G. Cudkowicz, J. Immunol., 113:1093, 1974.

H. Walter, Modern Separation Methods of Macromolecules and Particles (T. Gerritsen, Ed.) Vol. 2, p. 121, Wiley: New York, 1969.

H. Walter, R. Tung, L.J. Jackson, and G.V.F. Seaman, Biochem. Biophys. Res. Comm. 48;565, 1972,

G.L. Weid, G.F. Bahr, and P.H. Bartels, Automated Cell Identification and Cell Sorting, Edited by G.L. Weid and G.F. Bahr, p. 195, Academic Press, New York, 1970.

B. Wetzel, G.B. Cannon, E.L. Alexander, B.W. Erickson, Jr., and E.W. Westbrook, Scanning Electron Microscopy/1974, Edited by O. Johari and I. Corvin, p. 581, IIT Research Institute, Chicago, 1974.

N. Williams, N. Kraft, and K. Shortman, Immunology, 22; 885, 1972a.

N. Williams, and K. Shortman, Aust. J. Biol. Med. Sci., 50:133, 1972b.

J. Wybran and H. H. Fudenberg, J. Clin. Invest. 52:1026, 1973.

D.K. Yip, and N. Auersperg, In Vitro 7:323, 1972.

K. Zeiller, G. Pascher, and K. Hannig, H.-S.Z. Physiol. Chem. 351:435, 1970.

K. Zeiller, H.G. Liebich, and K. Hannig, European J. Immunol. 1:315, 1971.

K. Zeiller, E. Holzberg, G. Pascher, and K. Hannig, H.-S.Z. Physiol. Chem. 353:105, 1972a.

K. Zeiller, G. Pascher, and K. Hannig, Prep. Biochem. 2:21, 1972b.

ACKNOWLEDGEMENTS

We are thankful to the Editor of the Journal of Immunology for permission to allow us to reproduce in this chapter Figures 1, 2, 3, 8 and Tables 1, 2, 3 from Thornthwaite and Leif 1974, and Figures 4, 5, 6, 7 and Tables 4, 5 from Thornthwaite and Leif 1975c. We thank Dr. B.D. Watson for proofreading the manuscript and A. Pollack for his work on the Complement Independent PFC. We thank M. Fuentes, D. Prudhomme and P. Fiorentino for making the tissue culture medium and injecting the animals. We thank Dr. D. Marszalek and W. Charm for assistance in the SEM work and M.A. Hart for the TEM work on the EL 4 and SRFC. We thank Drs. T.S. Johnson and C.W. Song for the mastocytoma cells. Finally, we thank the medical illustration service at the Veteran's Hospital for printing the figures. This work was supported by Damon Runyan-Walter Winchell Grant DRG-1232, General Support Grant SOl-RR-05691 and NIH Grant 5-ROl-CA-13441-03.

DISCUSSION

H. Fudenberg, University of California: Two questions.
I'd like to ask. Number one, on the cells which form
plaques, your system would not pick up IgG plaque formers?

R.C. Leif, Papanicolaou Cancer Research Institute:
Right.

H. Fudenberg: Can you distinguish between those and
the macrophages on the same slide?

R.C. Leif: If one accepts lipase activity as a specific descriptor for macrophages, then there is no problem,
one employs the Ornstein Ansley staining procedure. One
could also stain for lipase and then subsequently easily
observe the cells by the combined light and SEM procedure.

H. Fudenberg: Second question. Have you tried to com-
pare the populations obtained with your method with those
obtained by Zeiller with Hannig's electrophoresis system, in
terms of subpopulation.

R.C. Leif: No, we would love to obtain one of Hannig's
apparatus, but no one has donated one yet, and in fact we
have proposed to build our own. Zeiller by the way has a
set of Centrifugal Cytology Buckets.

E.L. Springer, University of California: I have just
three questions. Number one: I noticed that on your protocol for your experiment you used a high concentration of
gluteraldehyde of 4%, could you please tell me exactly how
many milliosmoles this represented in a final concentration?

R.C. Leif: Well, I'm going to tell you a story about
gluteraldehyde and milliosmoles. One, it doesn't mean anything, since the glutaraldehyde is partially polymerized.
Some of the gluteraldehyde immediately penetrates the cells.
The glutaraldehyde which immediately penetrates would have
to be subtracted from the remaining extracellular glataral-
dehyde. The only thing we were ever able to do intelligent-
ly, and I'm not so sure that was too intelligent, was des-

cribed in the first Centrifugal Cytology paper. The diameters of cells fixed in various gluteraldehyde concentrations were measured and compared with the unfixed cells.
Four percent was the optimum concentration. We are now
beginning a study with the AMAC II high resolution electronic volume spectrometer with Dr. Cameron, Mr. Thomas, Mr.
Thornthwaite, Mr. Lopez and Mr. Yopp to find out what is the
optimum fixative and at that point I will start believing
that we are free of fixation artifacts. At present in the
case of Centrifugal Cytology, I always recommend to people
who are using it to obtain a bottle of the fixative from
your present electron microscopist. It's the safest thing
to do. At least the artifacts are consistant.

E.L. Springer: I then take it you have not read Dr.
Hyatt's comments on glutaraldehyde fixation in his recent
two volume series on electron microscopy techniques?

R.C. Leif: I, if I remember rightly I have, and so has
Mr. Thornthwaite, but at present as I said, the real test of
glutaraldehyde fixation will be if the volume of the cells
remains constant. The only way to obtain this information
is with a high resolution electronic cell volume spectrometer such as the AMAC II. Until these tests are completed,
fixation artifacts are possible; although, significant
artifacts are improbable. It unfortunately is the case in
our own research that if we ran all possible preliminary
tests, we would never do the biology which is the reason we
invented all this equipment.

E.L. Springer: Third question. I noticed that you
said you heated your cells at 37^0 and have a diminution of
microvilli. How long did you allow those cells to remain on
the substrate as compared to those cells that were at a
lower temperature?

R.C. Leif: They were on for a half hour, at 37^0, the
other ones were kept in the cold and didn't loose any hair
from the storage. Is that correct Jerry?

*J.T. Thornthwaite, Papanicolaou Cancer Research Inst-
itute:* Yes.

R.C. Leif: Yes. So its really a thermal effect. Now
concerning the substrate, it really isn't glass. The substrate is albumin. Because the glass, the way we prepare

it, is ultraclean and immediately binds albumin. So when one looks at the SEMs every once in a while one can see a scratch and one can really see that the cells are sitting on albumin which is a natural material for cells to be in contact with.

E.L. Springer: All right.

THE CONTRIBUTION OF IMMUNOLOGICAL FACTORS TO THE CONTROL OF METASTATIC SPREAD OF SARCOMATA IN RATS

PETER ALEXANDER and SUZANNE A. ECCLES
Chester Beatty Research Institute
Belmont, Sutton, Surrey,
England.

INTRODUCTION

The concept that the occurrence of malignant cells is much more frequent than that of clinically observable tumours is supported, but not proven, by a number of observations. The hypothesis that the "excess" of cells with malignant potential is eradicated by an immunological process akin to the rejection of allografts and requiring the participation of T-lymphocytes at the afferent and or efferent level, has attracted much attention and some of its proponents have even claimed that specific cell-mediated immunity evolved to provide a means of coping with malignant cells. Unfortunately, this idea has not withstood the test of experiment and there are several studies which show that experimental animals which are depleted of T-cells and which do not reject allografts are not significantly more susceptible to either spontaneous or carcinogen-induced malignancies (e.g. (1) (2)). While some viruses are only oncogenic in immune suppressed hosts such as new-born rodents or adults deprived of T-cells, the "immune surveillance" in this situation is directed against the virus and not the transformed cell. Whether there is no in vivo control over malignant cells or whether they are surveilled by processes not

involving the lymphoid machinery is a challenging
problem which deserves investigation.

The failure to detect T-cell mediated
surveillance at the level of cancer induction does
not, however, mean that the well established
reaction of the host against the tumour-specific
transplantation-type antigens (TSTAs) plays no
role in the natural history of these tumours.
The first indication that immune factors may
influence the dissemination of cancer in vivo came
from experiments (3,4) which showed that tumours
transplanted into rodents exposed to whole-body
irradiation or to anti-lymphocyte serum metastasized more readily than in normal recipients (3,4).
Such studies were not decisive since the procedures which facilitated spread were not only
immunosuppressive but also impaired bone-marrow
function (e.g. availability of monocytes) and
blood clotting which are known to be important in
tumour spread (5).. Indeed, in our laboratory
work on a possible effect of immunity on metastasis was started by a Swedish surgeon,
C-M. Rudenstam, who during a sabbatical leave was
concerned to find out if effects he had ascribed
to clotting defects might in part be mediated by
interference with immune mechanisms. This led
him to the finding (quoted in (6)) that primary
chemically-induced sarcomata in rats which only
rarely metastasized did so if the tumour-bearing
rats were subjected to prolonged draining of
thoracic duct lymph. This initial observation
led us to investigate systematically the effect of
immune parameters on dissemination and metastasis.
While the studies which will be described below
demonstrate that specific immune processes
requiring T-cells exert a controlling effect they
are surely not the only, and very possibly not
even the principal factor, in the development of
metastasis - this, like many other aspects of
malignancy, is a multi-factorial phenomenon.

Grafting tumours into T-cell deprived recipients

Rats were shown (7) to be depleted of T-lymphocytes without a detectable deficiency of bone-marrow function following 1) Six days of continuous drainage of thoracic duct lymph, or 2) Adult thymectomy followed by three sub-lethal doses of whole-body X-irradiation and a period of recovery. Syngeneic rat sarcomata were transplanted into hind legs and 14 days later the legs were amputated - a procedure which removed both the tumour and the draining node - and the rats were then kept for periods up to 60 weeks. Table 1 shows that the incidence of metastasis was greatly increased in such T-cell deprived rats.

TABLE 1

METASTASIS FOLLOWING SURGICAL REMOVAL OF A
GRAFTED SYNGENEIC SARCOMA

Number of animals

Treatment	Surviving at 60 weeks	Dead with no tumour	Dead with lung tumour[+]	Dead with only lymph node tumour
None	$^{50}/_{60}$	2	4	4
Thoracic duct lymph drainage	$^{8}/_{40}$	11*	11	10
Sham cannulation	$^{16}/_{20}$	1	2	1
Thymectomy and irradiation	$^{3}/_{20}$	3	9	5
Sham thymectomy	$^{15}/_{20}$	1	3	1

* All the deaths occurred soon after prolonged draining which is very traumatic.

+ Many of these rats also had lymph node metastases.

Draining of thoracic duct lymph from tumour-bearing rats

Reference has already been made to the finding (6) that if, following the induction of a primary sarcoma by a carcinogenic hydrocarbon and before surgical removal of this tumour, the rats are subjected to prolonged thoracic duct lymph drainage, the rate of "cure" is greatly decreased and the majority of rats die of metastases. This is a complicated situation since removal of thoracic duct lymphocytes while preventing a primary response does not abrogate an already established cell-mediated immune reaction (9). We were also puzzled by the finding that rats bearing primary sarcomata were unable to reject a challenge with the same tumour cells inoculated subcutaneously (10) but yet did not, in general, develop spontaneous metastasis (unless immunosuppressed) although it is to be anticipated that tumour cells are continually shed into the circulation. This conflict was resolved by the finding (6) that the capacity of a tumour-bearing rat to reject an inoculum of the same tumour (i.e. the extent of concomitant immunity) depended on the challenge site, being high for i.v. and low for s.c. or i.m. injected tumour cells. Table 2 shows the resistance of rats with different primary autochthonous tumours to i.v. challenge with autologous tumour cells and very similar findings have also been made for syngeneic transplanted sarcomata (11) where the powerful manifestation of concomitant immunity to i.v. administered cells was shown to be specific, i.e. directed against the TSTAs of the tumour cells.

The metastasis promoting effect of thoracic duct lymph drainage of tumour-bearers and the powerful expression of concomitant

TABLE 2

Capacity of rats bearing primary benzypyrene-induced sarcomata to reject an i.v. challenge consisting of 10^5 tumour cells obtained from the primary tumour by biopsy.

Primary tumour	Number of lung tumour nodules in	
	Autochthonous host	Syngeneic normal rat
A	0	0
B	0	100
C	1	100
D	0	12
E	1	72
F	14	0
G	200	500
H	3	40
I	0	0
J	0	0
K	20	200

immunity to i.v. challenge could be explained if blood- and lymph-borne spread was controlled by an immunologically specific humoral factor which, however, was relatively ineffective - possibly for reasons of physical inaccessibility - against tumour cells at s.c. or i.m. sites. Direct support for this hypothesis came from experiments (12) which showed (see Table 3) that the promotion of metastases by thoracic duct lymph draining could not be prevented by returning the lymphocytes (these were shown to rejoin the re-circulating population) but could be reversed by giving back serum from tumour-bearing rats.

TABLE 3

EFFECT OF REMOVING THORACIC DUCT LYMPH ON
SPONTANEOUS LUNG METASTASES DERIVED FROM
SYNGENEIC SARCOMA IMPLANTED INTO LEG

Day: 1	15 - 20	21	66
tumour implanted	thoracic duct lymph drained	tumour amputated	rats killed lungs examined

Treatment	Lung tumours	
	Incidence	Average weight of lung tumours
None	$^0/_9$	
Sham operation	$^2/_9$	0.15g
Lymph drained	$^9/_9$	3.9 g
Lymph drained; lymphocytes returned	$^9/_9$	2.4 g
Lymph drained + serum from tumour-bearing rats	$^1/_8$	0.1 g
Lymph drained + serum from normal rats	$^8/_8$	2.9 g

Serum rather than lymph plasma was returned since
more than 100ml of lymph plasma was drained daily
and giving this amount of fluid back created
severe physiological problems.

Further support (12) for the concept
that blood-borne spread can be prevented in an
immunologically specific manner by a humoral
factor circulating in tumour-bearing animals came
from studies in which administration of the serum
or lymph plasma of tumour-bearing rats specifically protected against a subsequent challenge of
tumour when given i.v. but not when given s.c.
or i.m.   This experiment is similar to earlier

findings that passage transfer of immunity by antibody can be obtained much more readily if the subsequent challenge is by the i.v. than by the s.c. route. However, in lymph and blood of rats with sarcomata studied in these experiments free antibody could not be detected and there was compelling data to show that while antibody to the TSTA was formed, it was neutralized by TSTA released in a soluble form from the growing tumour (13). We are currently attempting to establish the nature of this specifically protective substance found in blood and lymph of tumour-bearers. It may be a soluble antigen-antibody complex which when combined with monocytes or macrophages renders these specific-ally cytotoxic to the tumour. This would constit-ute an economy in the use of antibody which might come into play twice; initially by direct inter-action with the tumour and secondarily as a complex. That the protective substance is produced by immune lymphocytes is indicated by the fact that immunity to i.v. challenge can be transferred with lymphocytes from tumour-bearers (12).

Control of latent metastases by immune factors

The various immunological manoeuvres which affect the development of metastases arising from a "primary" tumour (either induced, i.e. autoch-thonous, or transplanted) have, in our experiments, had no detectable effect on the growth of this primary. All the data presented so far are, therefore, consistent with the hypothesis that immune factors have the capacity to inhibit individual malignant cells in transit but that their effect on established s.c. or i.m. tumour cells is less pronounced.

Recent experiments which are still incomplete indicate that this may be an over-

simplified view.   We found (see Table 4) that
immunosuppressive treatment following surgical
removal of a grafted s.c. tumour resulted in the
appearance of metastases.   The available data

TABLE 4

EFFECTS OF IMMUNOSUPPRESSION FOLLOWING SURGICAL REMOVAL OF
I.M. TUMOUR ON THE SUBSEQUENT APPEARANCE OF METASTASES
(A SYNGENEIC SARCOMA WAS TRANSPLANTED I.M. IN THE HIND LEGS
OF RATS AND REMOVED BY AMPUTATION OF THE WHOLE LIMB 14 DAYS LATER)

Treatment after surgical removal of tumour	Time after surgical removal of tumour	Deaths from lymph node or lung metastases per group of twenty rats			
		Day 30	Day 50	Day 70	Day 100
None		0	0	1 (5%)	2 (10%)
500 rads X-rays to whole body	1 day	3 (15%)	9 (45%)	11 (55%)	11 (55%)
	1 month	0	5 (25%)	7 (35%)	7 (35%)
Thoracic duct lymph drainage begun	1 day	1 (5%)	3 (15%)	9 (45%)	9 (45%)
	1 month	0	1 (5%)	6 (30%)	6 (30%)

suggest that sarcoma cells are shed from the
original tumour, and in normal animals remain
latent in lymph nodes and in the lung for long
periods - some of them do not manifest within the
ordinary life span of the animal - but following
immune suppression may grow and kill.   As yet,
we do not know if these latent metastases consist
of single cells or of clusters, and if they are
clusters, whether their latency is due to an
equilibrium between immune destruction by the host
and proliferation, or if their growth is limited
because they have not become vascularized.   In
addition to these problems of tumour biology, the

experiment shown in Table 4 poses an important
practical question for the management of
clinically localized cancer.   Attempts to treat
suspected micro-metastasis by cytotoxic chemotherapy following removal of all clinically
evident disease by surgery or radiotherapy is a
line of attack now being investigated widely and
one which appears to have proved valuable in
osteosarcoma.   However, the possibility that
such microfoci of tumour may, in fact, be restrained by the body's immune defences indicates a need
for caution.

Why do some tumours metastasize in an immunologically normal host?

So far I have described experiments with
sarcomas which in immunologically normal animals
metastasize only rarely and which are essentially
"curable" by the equivalent of radical surgery
(i.e. removal of the primary and draining nodes).
Such tumours do not constitute the major problem
of cancer which is concerned with the control of
disseminated disease;   in general primary tumours
and strictly local spread can be successfully
treated.   There are experimental tumours which
disseminate spontaneously and we have compared the
biological properties of a number of rat sarcoma
which vary widely in their metastatic behaviour.

Tumours are made up of both normal and
malignant cells and the mistake must not be made
of equating "cells in a tumour" with "tumour cells"
Evans (14) showed that the content of normal
macrophages varies widely between different tumours
and that the total macrophage content cannot be
estimated by ordinary histological techniques but
requires physiological tests made on cell
suspensions derived from the tumour.   Table 5
shows that there is an inverse correlation between
the number of macrophages in a series of sarcomata

and their capacity to metastasize (8).   Since
macrophages are capable of killing tumour cells
it seems very likely that the macrophages exert a
restraining influence on the tumour.   However,
the influx of host monocytes and macrophages into
tumours requires an active T-cell response and
tumours in T-cell deprived rats - like those used
in the experiments shown in Table 1 - have a very
much lower macrophage content (8).

An attractive hypothesis is to link both
macrophage content and metastatic behaviour to
the magnitude of the immune response to the tumour
and the data shown in Table 5 provide an impressive relation between "immunogenicity" and
metastasis for a series of sarcomata.   These

TABLE 5

Tumour	Macrophage content %		Incidence of metastasis +	Immunogenicity*
	Mean	Range		
MC-3	8	2 - 12	100	$< 10^3$
HSH	12	10 - 15	100	10^4
ASBP-1	22	18 - 26	52	10^5
MC-1(M)	38	36 - 42	25	10^6
HSN	40	34 - 44	32	5×10^6
HSBPA	54	42 - 63	11	5×10^7

+ Following amputation of tumour-bearing limb.

* Number of cells needed to induce a tumour in rats immunized
by excision of i.m. tumour.

findings must, however, be interpreted cautiously
because immunogenicity is measured in these
experiments by the number of tumour cells which
an immunized recipient is able to reject.   This

is not a simple parameter but a complex measurement which involves both the extent of the host
reaction (i.e. the number of cytotoxic cells and
antibody molecules produced) and the effectiveness
with which the tumour cells are able to avoid
destruction by the immune processes of the host.

We are accumulating evidence that for
some tumours at least immunogenicity, as defined
above, is low not because the host response is
limited but because they are able to "escape"
effectively. Thus immunologically specific
cytotoxicity of the cells present in the draining
nodes is the same for rats bearing the highly
"immunogenic" and non-metastasizing MC-1 sarcoma
as for rats with the MC-3 tumour which is
essentially "non-immunogenic" and which has close
to a 100% incidence of distant metastases (15).
However, we have found (15) from tests in tissue
culture that the spontaneous release by living
tumour cells of their TSTAs in a soluble form is
much greater for the MC-3 than the MC-1 sarcoma.
Soluble TSTAs bind to specifically immunized
mononuclear cells and thereby render them
incapable of killing their target. The
inhibition of at least some of the arms of the
specific cytotoxic cell-mediated immune response
of the host by soluble tumour-specific antigens
may make an important contribution to "escape".
We have speculated (10) that the rate of
spontaneous shedding of tumour antigens is one of
the factors which determine whether a disseminated
tumour is destroyed by the immune reaction of the
host. Table 6 summarizes a model, which is
certainly an over-simplification, according to
which escape of a tumour mass is determined by the
concentration of soluble TSTAs in the environment
which intercept the cytotoxic effector processes
of the host. From geometrical considerations it
is obvious that for a given rate of shedding the
concentration of TSTAs will be higher around a

TABLE 6

RELATION BETWEEN ANTIGEN SHEDDING AND METASTASIS

Rate of spontaneous shedding of tumour antigens by tumour cells:	Concentration of soluble antigen surrounding:	
	Macroscopic primary tumour	Microfoci of disseminated tumour
Low (Non-metastatic)	Sufficient to permit escape	Insufficient to avoid destruction by effector processes
High (Metastatic)	Sufficient to permit escape	Sufficient to permit escape

large tumour mass than around a micro-foci. Accordingly, for a tumour with a low rate of shedding such as MC-1, the concentration of soluble TSTAs may be sufficient to protect the primary tumour but not the disseminated cell – hence no metastasis. If the rate of release of TSTAs is high then the disseminated tumour cell may escape.

The capacity of irradiated cells to immunize may also be related to the metastatic capacity. While for non-metastasizing tumours the degree of immunity obtainable with irradiated cells is almost as great as that which can be obtained by excision of a growing tumour this does not apply to the metastasizing tumours studied by us (11), where irradiated cells frequently do not evoke a detectable host response. This is not, however, due to the fact that the tumour cells are not antigenic and living

tumour gives rise to cell-mediated immunity which
is detectable _in vitro_ (15).   When irradiated
cells do not immunize this may be due to rapid
shedding of TSTAs from the membranes.   There is
good evidence that TSTAs have to be presented
within the cell membrane if they are to evoke
a host response.   In a soluble form the TSTAs
can inhibit the effector arms but cannot induce
immunity.   Irradiation with the doses used to
render cells incapable of growing may inhibit
the synthesis by cells of proteins and
consequently TSTAs which are shed from the membrane will not be replaced.   It is, therefore,
conceivable that cells which shed TSTAs spontaneously at a high rate do not after irradiation
evoke a host response.

These investigations were supported by
grants from the Medical Research Council and the
Cancer Research Campaign.

REFERENCES

(1) B.M. Stanford, H.I. Kohn, J.J. Daly and S.F. Soo.   J. Immunol. 110 (1973) 1437.

(2) O. Stutman.   Science, 183 (1974) 534.

(3) B. Fisher, O. Soliman and E.R. Fisher. Proc. Soc. Exp. Biol. Med. 131 (1969) 16.

(4) R.K. Gershon, R.L. Carter and K. Kondo. Nature, 213 (1967) 674.

(5) A.S. Ketcham, H. Wexler and J. Minton. J. A. M. A. 198 (1966) 157.

   C-M. Rudenstam.   Acta Chir. Scand. Suppl. 391 (1968).

(6) P. Alexander and J.G. Hall.   Advances in Cancer Res. 13 (1970) 1.

(7) S.A. Eccles and P. Alexander.   Brit. J. Cancer, 30 (1974) 42.

(8) S.A. Eccles and P. Alexander.   Nature, 250 (1974) 667.

(9) D.D. McGregor and J.L. Gowans.   Lancet (i) (1964) 629.

(10) Z.B. Mikulska, C. Smith and P. Alexander. J. Natl. Cancer Inst. 36 (1966) 29.

(11) J.W. Proctor, C-M. Rudenstam and P. Alexander. J. Natl. Cancer Inst. 53 (1974) 1671-1676.

(12) J.W. Proctor, C-M. Rudenstam and P. Alexander. Nature, 242 (1973) 29.

(13) D.M.P. Thomson, K. Steele and P. Alexander.
     Brit. J. Cancer, 27 (1973) 27.

     D.M.P. Thomson, S. Eccles and P. Alexander.
     Brit. J. Cancer, 28 (1973) 6.

(14) R. Evans.   Transplantation, 14 (1972) 468.

(15) G.A. Currie and P. Alexander.   Brit. J.
     Cancer, 29 (1973) 72.

(16) P. Alexander.   Cancer Res. 34 (1974) 2077.

DISCUSSION

T. Pretlow, University of Alabama Medical Center: In the studies of macrophage frequency, what physiological test did you use, and was it in vitro? Secondly, did you attempt to quantitate the frequency of lymphocytes in the tumors?

P. Alexander, Chester Beatty Research Institute: The methods used for measuring the macrophages in tumors were those developed by Dr. Robert Evans, (J. Natl. Cancer Inst. 1973, 50:277), which consists of making a cell suspension of the tumor, and then culturing in the presence of trypsin. Macrophages stick to the bottom of Petri dishes, even in the presence of trypsin, whereas sarcoma cells do not. Evans showed that this simple test provided a true measure of the macrophage content of tumours in a series of tests in which macrophages were identified by other in vitro tests. We have not yet determined the lymphocyte content of different tumors.

T. Pretlow: In working with several tumors in the same strain of mice we find an enormous difference in the proportion of macrophages as assessed by cytomorphometric studies, and the number that we can obtain in suspension, using a variety of techniques. I wonder if this might not be a significant variable in your experiment?

P. Alexander: Do you mean that you find a variation in macrophages content in different specimens of the same transplanted tumours or in different tumours?

T. Pretlow: No, not for different types of tumors, but in the same strain of mouse, we find a considerable difference in the proportion of macrophages that we are able to recover in suspension, and it seems as though this is an important variable.

P. Alexander: I fully agree -- that was the point I tried to make. Different tumors within the same strains of rats have different macrophage contents and the macrophage contents reflects their biological behavior.

174

T. Pretlow: What I'm saying is that there is not a one to one correlation between the number of macrophages which we find in the solid tumor and the number which we are able to obtain in suspension. In fact, there is an enormous variation.

P. Alexander: I agree.

B. Cameron, Papanicolaou Cancer Research Institute: On the fractionation of serum factors, do you think that the fractionation procedure destroys the activity or, for example, can you re-combine the fractions and recover activity?

P. Alexander: Possibly, though I do not know the reason; aggregation may occur during fractionation. All I know is that we have lost the specific anti-tumour activity of tumor bearing serum when we have attempted separation.

M.R. Schinitsky, Eli Lilly & Company: Can you name either a benign or malignant human tumor which does, or does not metastasize on the basis of tissue macrophages?

P. Alexander: We do not as yet have this data, but we find that the macrophage content of human tumors is very variable and are currently following the patients to see if the macrophage content of tumors is of prognostic significance. But it will take several years before we know the answer.

Z. Brada, Papanicolaou Cancer Research Institute: Have you studied the mechanism of the action that you describe? Is there any relationship between the metastasis formation of your tumors, and for instance, between the number of viable cells in circulation and release of the cells from the primary tumor, and the amount of the critical mass of the cells in the target organ in your case, lung?

P. Alexander: We've tried to measure the number of malignant cells in circulation or rats bearing different sarcomas but have been unsuccessful in getting consistent data. We assume that on several grounds cells are being shed all the time from these tumors but can't prove it.

Z. Brada: And, are you sure that not other factors which are called as soil factors, e.g., coagulation factors, are not involved in the observation?

P. Alexander: As far as we can tell there are no cogula-
tion defects in rats which have been deprived of T cells by
the two procedures used by us. But I must emphasis that the
factors of the type you mentioned are involved in metastasis
and that immunity is only one of many factors involved in
determining the degree of metastasis.

A. Ghaffar, University of Edinburgh: In the model where
you have shown that the immunity can be transferred by serum,
have you looked if it is antibody, and if it is antibody,
could you comment on the mechanism of this immunity?

P. Alexander: These sera have no antibody activity.
There is antibody there, but it is the form of antigen antibody complexes. Whether the immunologically specific protective factor is a circulating antigen antibody complex, or
something else, we do not know because as I told you on fractionation experiments, activity is lost.

A. Ghaffar: What methods then of detecting antibodies
did you use? Was it complement fixation, i.e., complement
mediated cytotoxity or some other method?

P. Alexander: The test used was the mixed cell application procedure which was developed by Dr. Eva Klein.

A. Ghaffar: Well, we find essentially the same thing
by a radio-labeling technique.

E.G. Elias, State University of New York: I have a
question and a comment for Dr. Alexander. The first is the
comment. There is a lot of evidence that the cytotoxic
agents administered as adjuvant to surgery in the clinical
studies could be more harmful than good. Let me point out
that the Swiss Cooperative Group, using the Cytoxan as adjuvant to surgery in lung carcinoma found out that these patients developed early metastasis and died earlier in the
treated group. Recently, the Veteran Administration Group
here in the United States reported that 5-Fu as adjuvant did
not add any advantage in patients with colon carcinoma. We
haven't published our data on Imidazol carboxamide used as
adjuvant to surgical treatment of melonoma which showed no
increase in the survival or delay of metastasis. All these
randomized studies indicates that cytotoxic agents may do
more harm than good as adjuvant to surgery. The osteosarcoma
tumor group that are studying chemotherapy are not randomiz-
ing the patients but are using historical control. The

question I would like to ask you, Dr. Alexander, is, did it make any difference when you collected the serum from the animal-bearing tumors, in other words, did it make any difference whether these animals were having the primary or metastasis before you collected the serum to block the tumor growth in the recipients?

P. Alexander: I do not know the answer because we collected the serum by killing the animals 14 days after tumor transplantation at which time we have no idea whether the animals have distant metastasis. I would like to comment on your comment because we must not overemphasise the role of immunological factors in metastasis. The data does not mean that we should abandon prophylactic chemotherapy after surgery as its effect in reducing residual tumor cells may outweigh any harm done by immunosuppression.

D.M. Lopez, University of Miami Medical School: I would like to comment on the sham surgery that you showed in the first slide, where you have shown that 4 animals out of 9 and later you changed and said there were 2 out of 9, that have had some relief by this method. In connection with this, we have experiences in which by doing sham surgery on animals bearing a chemically induced mouse mammary tumor we have found that you can actually decrease the size of eventual tumor just by this sham surgery, where the tumor burden is not disturbed and we can relieve the immunological anergy that ensues at the very end, when the tumor gets very large. So this might be clarifying the point of your slides.

P. Alexander: Yes thank you very much. I suspect, as you point out, that surgery is itself a minor immunosuppressive procedure. I again don't think it is a terribly severe stress.

D.M. Lopez: On the contrary, I'm saying that it is an immunopotentiator because the tumor gets smaller if you relieve the immunological anergy that ensues in large tumors as measured by lymphocyte stimulation; so what I'm saying is that maybe hormonal effects are at play or some other non-immunologic effect.

ARE AUTOIMMUNE DISEASES AND MALIGNANCY DUE TO SELECTIVE T-CELL DEFICIENCIES?

H. H. FUDENBERG, M.D.
Basic and Clinical Immunology and Microbiology
Medical University of South Carolina

INTRODUCTION

Before proceeding to data directly relevant to the title of this presentation, some introductory comments appear mandatory. Figure 1 illustrates (a) what was known of mammalian cellular immunology in 1970, (b) how much we have learned since then, and (c) how much is still unknown.

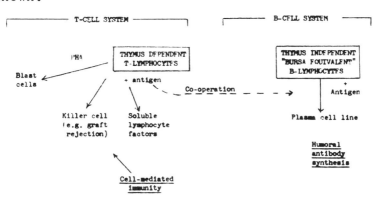

Figure 1. Cellular basis of the immune response (1970 version)

This figure, revised from a paper published by the World Health Organization's Expert Committee on Immunology is based on a consensus arrived at during a week-long meeting in 1970.[1] As shown, the consensus of these "experts" listed only two immunologically important cells: the "T" (or thymus derived) cells, and the "B" lymphocytes. Note that probably the most immunologically important cell system; namely, the macrophage-monocyte system, was not listed, nor were stem cells listed. The figure demonstrates that immunologically virgin "B" cells after encountering an antigenic stimulus, acquire receptors (immunoglobulin molecules), discussed elsewhere in this volume,[2] and upon further exposure to antigen differentiate into the plasma cells, which export into the serum the classical antibodies, (IgG, A, M, D, and E). In 1970, these serum antibodies all were thought to confer protection. I, myself, at present, cannot yet visualize the protective mechanism of serum IgE, nor of Serum IgA, (I believe the latter has no protective effect, in contrast to the IgA on secretory surfaces)[3]

In 1969, though our laboratory had good evidence for suppressor "T" cells, only helper "T" cells[4] were accepted by the "experts," and therefore, only helper, but not suppressor functions are shown for T cells. T cell function was measured in vitro at that time by (a) incorporation of tritiated thymidine into DNA, and no longer by morphologic criteria, ("blast" transformation), although these are not necessarily parallel in abnormal individuals,[5] (b) by release of a number of soluble lymphocyte factors, termed "mediators of cellular" immunity, (c) by rejection of foreign tissue grafts, and (d) "by immune surveillance" i.e. killing of tumor cells in vitro (and, too, I agree with Dr. Alexander's views expressed elsewhere in this volume[6] that T cells are primarily important in monitoring the growth of already established tumors, rather than preventing initiation of tumors). In any event, the Expert Committee at that time felt that there was just one kind of T cell possessing all these functions; we had good evidence that there were at least several subpopulations. For example, one which makes soluble lymphocyte factors differs from that responsible for DNA synthesis in response to antigen;[7] we and others now have evidence that those T cells which possess cytotoxic activity, at least in humans, against tumor cells differ from those producing one or another mediators of cellular immunity.[8,9] (not only T cells, but also B cells, can make at least some of these products, and indeed some can be produced by fibroblasts; hence, I urge that the alternative designation, "lymphokines" be dropped).

Before presenting data relevant to the title of this presentation, "Are Auto-immune Diseases and Certain Forms of Malignancy Due to "T" Cell Deficiencies?", some discussion of the Burnetian clonal selection dogma, very prominent in this symposium, is mandatory. Burnet used three points to butresss his argument for clonal selection.[10] The first point was that cells once committed, were committed not only to antigen, but also to class and subclass and could not switch; as you know, a switch mechanism for IgM to IgG, exists.[11] The immunologically competent cells would rather "switch than fight.

Does clonal selection in a strict sense really exist, i.e. is each virgin immunocyte originally genetically unipotent? Or is each immunocyte unipotent? After exposure to an antigen 1/2 of 1% (approximately) of lymphocyte can combine with two antigens, at least in vitro.[12] By analogy (perhaps not valid) a sea urchin egg, or a mammalian ovum, has the potentiality of giving rise to 10,000 different products, presumably, but once hit by a sperm, the ovum differentiates, and produces only one product. If two sperm hit one ovum within 1 micro-second, (or perhaps 1/10 of a

micro-second) non-identical twins result.* Is it
conceivable, perhaps, that the mammalian lymphocyte is really totipotential, that when hit by
one antigen changes in surface properties immediately shut off its potential to respond to all
other antigens? (Unless a second antigen hits
within a microsecond, in which case the very small
percentage of double producers results.) Another
tenet of the Burnetian concept, directly relevant
to autoimmune disease, is that autoantibodies
arise as a result of formation of forbidden
clones, so that a normal inidvidual does not make
autoantibodies, and autoimmune disease occurs only
in situations when "forbidden clones" arise.[10]
In 1960, and subsequently, we showed that most
normal individuals have small amounts of autoanitbodies in their sera. My own concept is that
these autoantibodies are present in small amounts
in all normal individuals to eradicate aged or
damaged tissue,[13-17] and that the level of B
cells producing autoantibodies is kept in check by
T-suppressor cells.[14,16,17] With the diminution
of T cell immunity, the level of T cells suppressing autoantibody-producing B cell (and also
suppressor T cells destroying "autoantigens" by
cell mediated mechanisms) "autoimmune" cells
increase markedly, resulting in autoimmune
disease.[13-17] This hypothesis, of course,
differs markedly from the "forbidden clone"
concept. (See "note added in proof")

IMMUNOLOGIC DEFICIENCY AND "AUTOIMMUNE DISEASE
a. Animal observations: T cell deficiency and
viruses
        Kidneys taken from patients with lupus
nephritis have "lumpy-bumby" deposits of IgG and
complement as demonstrated by immunofluorescence.
The Fl offspring of New Zealand Black mice have a
genetic predisposition to the same sort of renal
disease, and their kidneys bind IgG and complement
in the same patterns. Figure 2 (page 5), is
representative of results obtained on immuno-
flourescent straining of kidneys of a strain of
mice, (RF/Un) which does not develop renal disease

*About once in 200 pregnancies

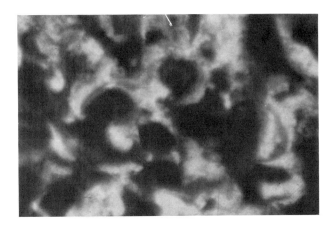

normally, but after neonatal thymectomy developed renal disease with these "lumpy-bumpy" deposits.[18] When we administered interferon (which presumably interferes with viral replication) to neonatally thymectomized (RF/Un) mice, the renal disease and IgG and complement deposits in the kidney did not occur.[19] Therefore, we concluded that the apparent "autoimmunity" was due to a T-cell defect and also that a virus was somehow involved in the pathogenesis of the disease.

b. Selective deficiency of T cell sub-populations

As you know, T cells, especially, secrete a whole host of mediators of cellular immunity, e.g. macrophage, activating factor, differing chemotactic factors for various types of leucocytes, cytotoxic factors destroying foreign antigens (for example, tumor cells); growth inhibiting factors, permeability factors, mitogenic factors, interferon (Table 1 page 6). It is quite conceivable that many of these factors, none of which have been purified, are the same; however, there is evidence that many do indeed differ from one another. Is it then conceivable that a selective T-cell deficiency can exist in which only one population, making only one of these mediators of cellular immunity, is deficient? So far, no one knows whether one type

Table 1

Mediators of Cellular Immunity Elaborated by Sensitized Lymphocyte after Addition of Antigen.

1. Skin Permeability Factor.
2. Chemotactic factors for macrophages.
3. Macrophage migration inhibitory factor (MIF).
4. Macrophage activating factor (same as MIF?).
5. Chemotactic factors for other leukocytes; neutrophils, eosinophils, basophils, lymphocytes.
6. Granulocytic migration inhibitory factor (LIF)
7. Growth inhibitory factors; clonal inhibitory factor, proliferation inhibitory factor.
8. Lymphocytotoxin (toxic for all cells other than lymphocytes).
9. Osteoclast activating factor.
10. Collagen synthesizing factor.
11. Interferon.
12. Mitogenic factor(s) for lymphocytes.

of lymphocyte makes all of these, or whether each chemically distinct mediator is produced by a different T cell. (I personally believe each mediator is produced by a different subpopulation.)[20] In terms of tumor growth, the clonal inhibiting factors, and the cytotoxic factors would, of course, be extremely important, and a selective deficiency of cells producing these selective T-cell deficiencies for antigens present in an oncogenic virus could be critical.

THE GENETIC NATURE OF SUCH IMMUNE DEFECTS.

a. Human Family Studies:
Figure 3 (page 7) shows a family with immune deficiency and autoimmune disease, studied initially in 1958. The proband (indicated by the arrow) was a 35-year-old female who had agammaglobulinemia since age 19, with recurrent pneumonias. Her sister had increased immunoglobulins and rheumatoid factor, and her mother had increased immunoglobulins, rheumatoid factor, and arthritis. One uncle had died of polyarteritis, a related disease, another uncle

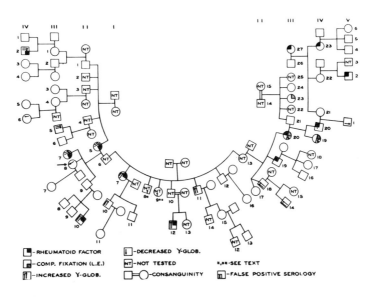

Figure 3. Family tree of patient with idiopathic acquired agammaglobulinemia.

had died in infancy of recurrent infection, (suggesting immune deficiency). Scattered through the family are individuals with rheumatoid factor, lupus factor, and/or increased immunoglobulin (due to deficiency in suppressor T cells?) i.e. individuals with marked qualitative and quantitative abberations of immunoglobulins.(21) Although these individuals were all from one family, the observed phenomena could be environmental rather than genetic. However, in generation II, two brothers who owned a store on Park Avenue quarrelled, and dissolved their partnership. One brother eventually wound up living on Park Avenue, the other in Bedford-Stuyvesant Town. Their offspring had never talked with, or even seen each other; yet, the offspring of both brothers, down to grandchildren (generation IV) had a high incidence of abnormalities. (In terms of environmental controls, I´m told that Park Avenue versus Bedford-Stuyvesant Town is as good as one can do.)+ Furthermore, some of these people were scattered from Wisconsin to Berkeley,

+Kurt Hirschhorn, M.D. - personal communications

185

to Virginia, and so forth. Studies of a dozen
families of patients with "acquired" ("adult
onset") agammaglobulinemia disclosed that each
proband had at least one first degree relative
(that is, a parent or a sib) with a quantitative
or qualitative abberation of immunoglobulins.[21]

Figure 4 shows a family from Sacramento,
California with various autoimmune phenomena.

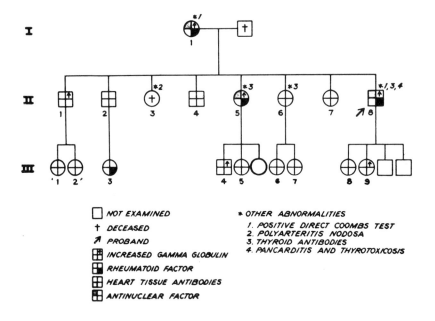

Figure 4.   Family   with   multiple   autoantibodies
(See text)

The proband had a positive direct Coomb's test
(and hemolytic anemia), antibodies to heart (and
myocarditis) to thyroid, (and thyrotoxicosis) and
also had rheumatoid factor, and antinuclear
antibodies, although he had no clinical evidence
of lupus or of rheumatoid arthritis. His mother
had positive Coombs' test and mild anemia; she had
antinuclear factor and rheumatoid factor. His
sibs and their children had a high incidence of
increased immunoglobulins rheumatoid factor, lupus
factor, and of antibody to colon.[22]   One of
these individuals (II$_5$), asymptomatic at the time,
but with thyroid antibodies, two years later

developed thyrotoxicosis; one who had antibodies
to colon (III_6) four years later developed
ulcerative colitis. [23] One sib had previously
died with what looked like polyarteritis; hence it
seems that these serologic abnormalities, with or
without disease occur in families. An unusually
high incidence of lymphoreticullar malignancy has
also been observed in such families (e.g. 24).
Presumably a genetic predisposition results in
suseptibility to clinical symptoms of immunodeficiency (recurrent infection), of autoimmune
disease, and of immunoproliferative disorders.
Although most of the malignancies in these
individuals are lymphoreticular malignancies,
other types do occur.
    Which of the three events, namely, immuno-
deficiency, autoimmune disease or malignancy is
the primary event? (Fig. 5)

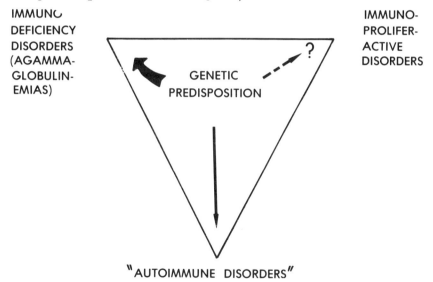

IMMUNO-
DEFICIENCY
DISORDERS
(AGAMMA-
GLOBULIN-
EMIAS)

GENETIC
PREDISPOSITION

IMMUNO-
PROLIFER-
ACTIVE
DISORDERS

"AUTOIMMUNE DISORDERS"

Figure 5. Which comes first?

In patients with "adult onset" agammaglobulinemia,
i.e. deficient humoral immunity, cellular immunity
eventually declines. Why individuals with
"acquired agammaglobulinemia" lose cellular immune
function, after about 10 years of disease, is
unknown, but such individuals do not develop
autoimmune disease, (e.g. rheumatoid arthritis)

until after many years of recurrent infections,
(rheumatoid arthritis), i.e. about 10 to 15 years
after the onset of the symptoms of agammaglobulinemia.(25) We postulated that preferential
loss of suppressor T cells was responsible for the
autoimmune phenomena.(16,17)#

Why is there a higher incidence of lymphocytic malignancies in immune deficiency as
composed to normals? Normals presumably devleop
mutant lymphocyte cell clones; if the mutants are
antigenically positive relative to the normal
cell, the mutants will be eradicated; a few
mutants presumable antigenically negative,
relative to the host will persist, and perhaps
become a lymphoma. In the agammaglobulinemic
patient, who has lost cellular immunity, the
antigenically negative mutant clones presumably
persist to the same extent as in normals, but in
addition, the antigenically positive mutants
cannot be eradicated because of deficiencies in
cellular immunity. Presumably, in immune deficiency, lymphocytes divide more frequently to try
to compensate for the immunologic defect. Each
division produces some chance of chromosomal abberation; hence the additional mechanism could
account for the incidence of lymphomas in far
higher than that of other tumors, in immune
deficiency whether genetic(25) or acquired. (due
to "immuno suppressant drugs").(28)

b. Animal Studies: "Selective" defects

In animal studies, inbred strains of mice were
immunized with synthetic polypeptide antigens, one
composed of a polylysine backbone, and polyalanine
polyglutamine, and a tyrosine tip, (T,G)-A-L,
another with the same polypeptide with histidine
tip, (H,G)-A-L, (Figure 6 page 11) (let's term
the two antigens antigen 1 and antigen 2). CBA
mice responded very poorly to antigen one, whereas
C57 mice responded well; the F_1 hybrids gave an
intermediate response. (Figure 7 page 12)

#Indeed, it seems not unlikely that an abnormal
increase suppressor T-cell number or function is
present initially, and that this is the cause of
the marked increase in immnoglobulins.(26)

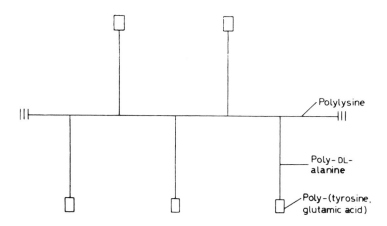

Figure 6. A structural diagram of (T,G)-A--L

In contrast, after injection of antigen 2, CBA
mice responded well and CB7 poorly, and F_1 hybrids
again gave intermediate results.[29] These data
document that the inability to respond to a simple
antigen is based on genetic differences. (The
strains were termed "responders" and "non-
responders" to one or the other antigen.) The
genes responsible for the differences in immune
response of various mouse strains (Ir genes) to
these and other antigens have been shown to be
closely linked to the histocompatibility
genes.[30]

The differences in immune response in inbred
animals to one or another antigen are well
documented, but other interpretations of the cause
of these differences have been obscured by seman-
tics. "Responders" and "non-responders" in
reality are "high responders" and "low responders." In view of linkage of the Ir genes to H-2
locus, and since the differences cited in (29)
appear to exert their effects in T cells, McDevitt
postulated a difference in helper T-cell configuration at the membrane level as the explanation for
differences in response.[31] (I would prefer to
attribute such genetic difference in height of
response to the possibility that high responders,
on a genetic basis, have a low number or low activity of "specific" suppressor T cells, whereas
low responders have a high number thereof.) Gen-

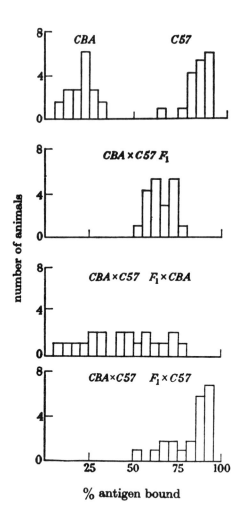

Figure 7. Response of CBA and C57 mice, their F_1 offspring and the F_1 by parental backcrosses to (T,G)-A-L.

etically determined differences in ability of T cell to kill tumor cells of one type, but not another, have also recently been demonstrated in inbred mice[32], and we have inferential evidence

for similar differences in humans.[33] We have
shown that humans may also have specific defects
restricted to a single antigen, namely staphyl-
ococcus; such individuals have severe recurrent
staphylococcal infection all their lives, but
handle every other organism well.[34] In any
event, these animal and human data indicate that
deficient immune responses can involve deficiencies not only of products of a whole class of
cells, like T cells, or B cells (e.g.
agammaglobulinemia) or of subclasses thereof, but
also deficiencies in response against one given
antigen, (i.e. selective deficiencies).

To test whether the high incidence of autoimmune phenomenon and malignancy in patients with
acquired agammaglobulinemia and their first degree
relatives already alluded to is due to a genetic
defect having as its primary effect immunologic
impairment, we studied individuals with "acquired
agammaglobulinemia" (onset of symptoms after 15
years of age). Dr. Tormey, then in our laboratory, devised a system to test lymphocytes placed
under maximum metabolic stress;[35] analogous to
making a diagnosis of diabetes by measuring not
the fasting blood sugar, nor even by performing a
glucose tolerance test, but rather by doing a
cortisone-glucose tolerance test. (As you know,
immunology is a "backwards" science; when the
immunocyte is stimulated, the sequence of biosyn-
thetic events is not DNA, then RNA, then protein;
but the stimulated immunocyte instead synthesizes
proteins, then RNA then lastly DNA.) Maximal DNA
synthesis occurs about 70 hours after exposure to
the mitogen, Phytohemagglutinin (PHA); RNA synthesis is maximal 24 hours after exposure to
mitogen.[36] For DNA synthesis in our assay the
cells are planted at time 0, PHA is added immediately, aminopterin added 24 hours later to create
a metabolic block (of thymidylate kinase) and the
block then bypassed at 64 hours by adding an
excess of thymidine (labelled with isotope) and
the cells harvested after the period of maximum
incorporation, (64-70 after PHA is added) and DNA
synthesis measured. RNA synthesis was measured by
allowing the endogenous system to decline to a
baseline level; since RNA synthesis is maximal 24
hours after PHA stimulation, the PHA was added at

191

42 hours, labelled RNA precursor added at 66 hours, and the cells harvested at 68 hours after PHA addition (Fig. 8) so that amount of labelled precursor incorporated into DNA and RNA could be measured simultaneously.[37]

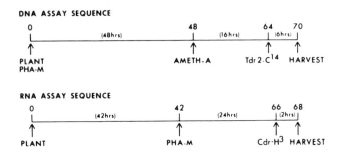

Figure 8. Schematic representation of assay systems for incorporation of labeled precursors into leucocyte DNA and RNA in phytohemagglutinin-stimulated leucocytes in *in vitro* culture. Tdr-2-C¹⁴=thymidine-2-C¹⁴; Cdr-H³=tritiated cytidine; AMETH-A=amethopterin plus adenosine; PHA-M=phytohemagglutinin.

Figure 9. (page 15) shows a summary of the early results. The range of both DNA and RNA synthesis normals (in counts per minute, per ten to the sixth lymphocytes) is great. (DNA synthesis on the left, RNA on the right in the figure shown.) In the patients with "acquired" agammaglobulinemia, DNA and RNA synthesis were very low, lower than any normal.[37] More important, their asymtomatic parents (who had normal levels of immunoglobulins) were all markedly below normal in the assay cited.[38] (Figure 10 page 16) (Protein synthesis was also subnormal) We have studied many more patients than shown in this early figure; whenever it has been possible to obtain two parents of one patient, they both show the defect, suggesting that acquired agammaglobulinemia is a genetically determined (autosomal recessive) disorder.

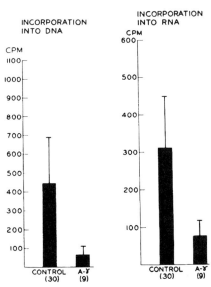

Figure 9 • Incorporation of labeled precursor into DNA and RNA of leukocytes from thirty control subjects and nine patients with "acquired" agammaglobulinemia. Incorporation of labeled precursor is indicated along the ordinate in counts per minute; the height of each bar indicates the mean incorporation value for each group, and the brackets enclose ± one standard deviation.

SUPPRESSOR T CELLS

Although the concept that suppressor T cells exist was highly controversial five years ago, most immunologists now accept the existence of such cells. (I might mention that when we first suggested the concept of suppressor T-cells in 1966, the experts denounced in scatologic terms;[27] the concept that a deficiency thereof might be responsible for auto-immune disease and at least some types of malignancies were greeted by universal shouts of derision.)[27] Nonetheless, it still takes a certain amount of courage to state that suppressor-T cells are a different population than the helper T cells. Dr. Gershon[39] interpreted his data as evidence for helper and suppressor functions occurring in the same cell depending on the magnitude of the signal and the amount of antigen, and on allosteric or other effects. The next several tables are taken from data obtained by Dr. Roberta Kamin in my lab-

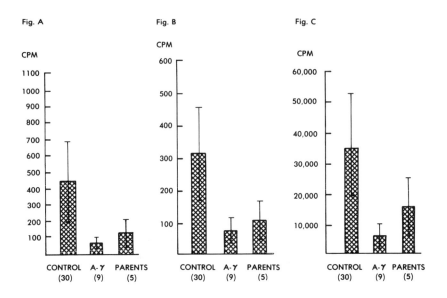

Figure 1∅.   (A) Incorporation of thymidine-2-C^{14}
into   DNA   of   lymphocytes   from   patients   with
"acquired" agammaglobulinemia, their parents, and
control subjects.   (B) Incorporation of uridine-5-
H^3 into RNA by lymphocytes from subjects depicted
in (A).   (C) Incorporation of DL-Leucine-1-C^{14}
into   protein   (TCA-precipitable   material)   in   the
culture medium during in vitro lymphocyte culture
in   phytohemagglutinin-stimulated   lymphocytes.
Incorporation of labeled precursor is indicated
along the ordinate in counts per minute.

oratory(4∅); they indicate that, in the rabbit, T
cells with suppressor function differ in localization from T cells with helper functions.   In
these studies we measured the response of lymphoid
cells from spleen cells of an immunized rabbit (by
Jerne plaque formation) to sheep red cells, to
keyhole   limpet   hemocyanin,   or   to   a   hapten.
Lymphocytes from various organs were tested for
ability   to   suppress   plaques   by   animals   using
varying numbers of spleen lymphocytes and varying
number of lymphocytes isolated from various other
organs.   Table 2 (page 17) is a summary of a
whole vast array of experiments using different

numbers of spleen lymphocytes.

TABLE 2

Suppression of Secondary *in vitro* SRC Response of Spleen Cells
by Normal Lymphoid Cell Populations

Numbers indicate PFC/Culture

Expt.	Spleen Cells		Control	Supplemental Cell Added (3 x 10^7)			
				Normal Spleen	Normal Peyer's patch	Normal Appendix	Autologous Appendix
1	5.0×10^6	IgM:	33,000	3,200	3,900	3,475	3,215
		IgG:	39,000	2,000	1,900	1,665	305
	2.5×10^6	IgM:	8,560	2,344	1,320	1,225	2,000
		IgG:	15,000	655	280	0	0
	1.25×10^5	IgM:	950	1.165	470	310	953
		IgG:	715	435	22	0	0
2	5.0×10^6	IgM:	24,000	4,300		5,650	1,872
		IgG:	24,000	0		4,350	3,000
	2.5×10^6	IgM:	6,000	5,100		2,450	1,475
		IgG:	13,000	0		0	0
	1.25×10^6	IgM:	1,825	2,850		1.450	670
		IgG:	760	0		0	0

As shown, suppression of response to S-RBC were
produced by lymphocytes from Peyers Patches and
appendix, but not by thymus cells (or lymph node
cells). Same results were obtained using as
antigen, a hapten (lac) as with sheep red blood
cells (Table 3).

TABLE 3

Suppression of Secondary in vitro Lac Response by Normal Cell Population

Numbers indicate PFC/Culture

	Controls		Supplemental Cell Added (3 x 10^7)					
	No. Ag	Ag	Lac Appendix	Normal Appendix	Normal Spleen	Normal Peyer's	Normal Thymus	Lac Thymus
IgM:	16	480	229	256	139	72	555	36
IgG:	177	12,562	2,120	4,536	1,500	1,554	9,525	35,300

Therefore, at least by geographic distribution, suppressor T cells differ from helper cells.

This was true for both primary response and secondary response, and for both IgG and IgM response. Maximal suppressor effects were observed at 24 hours after initiation of culture (Table 4).

TABLE 4

Suppression of Secondary in vitro SRC Response of Spleen Cells by Appendix Cells: Effect of Adding Appendix Cells at 24-48 hrs. after Culture Initiation.

Numbers indicate PFC/Culture

| Expt. | | Control | Supplemental Cells: Appendix (1.5×10^7 Viable) | | |
			0 hr.	24 hr.	48 hrs.
1	IgM:	15,750	2,800	2,196	7,300
	IgG:	3,550	0	0	0
2	IgM:	160,000	27,000	14,300	42,500
3	IgM:	30,400	4,250	592	
	IgG:	6,900	1,080	0	

Autologous cells from appendix of an immunized animal suppressed spleen lymphoctyes to the same extent as cells from normal appendix (Table 3). Similar responses were obtained with S-RBC and with the lac antigen. These suppressor cells from appendix are indeed T-cells as shown by the fact that the suppressor effect was markedly diminished, by treatment with anti-thymocyte serum and complement. Nylon fiber depleted cell populations (i.e. B cell depleted populations) gave similar results as whole appendix lymphocytes,[40] again showing that the suppressor cells are T cells.

One of the interesting observations in clinical immunology is that patients with IgA deficiency have a high incidence of various types of autoantibodies.[41] Since IgA cells predominate in the Peyer Patches, and since suppressor cells also predominate there, this is another link for the absence of suppressor cells and auto-immunity.

In terms of malignancy, we have found that the newborn rabbit does have T suppressor cells in his thymus.[42] (The newborn mouse has larger numbers, but the newborn mouse is much more immature than the rabbit). As the rabbits age, the number of T suppressor cells in Peyer Patches declines.[42] As you know, most forms of malignancy increase with aging. Have we indirect additional (though poor) evidence that a decline in T suppressor cells, associated with aging, is associated with increased incidence of malignancy? We have shown that what we call the "active T-cell" population[43] (not the total T cells) decrease in aging in man.[44] The high incidence of autoantibodies in human malignancies[45] is also compatible with deficiency of suppressor T cells.

THEORETICAL CONCEPTS

At least two kinds of suppressor T cells conceivably exist, and a deficiency of either could result in auto-immune disease. Defects in one type, "antigen-specific" suppressor T cells, should theoretically produce organ specific auto-immunity, (e.g. thyroiditis, adrenalitis, antibody hemolytic anemia). Defects of, "non-specific" T cells, lead to autoimmune conditions associated with non-organ specific "autoantibodies," as in lupus, rheumatoid arthritis, and chronic active hepatitis.

Figure 11 (page 20), illustrates our recent concepts of suppressor T cells. (As shown, they could come from several organs. We now know that the primary site of suppressor T-cell activity is the appendix and Peyer Patches; they are absent in thymus, present in only small numbers in lymph nodes). Could it be that T-suppressor cells, each act on a different clone of "autoimmune" cells, e.g. one set of suppressor T-cells monitors clone #1, making autoantibodies to kidney cells, another set monitors clone #2, making autoantibodies to gastric parietal cells, another set clone #3, making autoantibodies to thyroid, another clone #4, making autoanitbodies to red cells? If so, diminution in one or another "set" of suppressor T cells would cause, for instance, pernicious anemia, adrenalitis, thyroiditis, etc. (Fig. 11a) On the other hand, could it be that the suppressor

197

T cells lack specificity and react randomly
against all these autoimmune clones? (Fig. 11b)
As yet, we really do not know the answer.

Figure 11.   T-Suppressor Cells Hypothesis

T- SUPPRESSOR CELLS

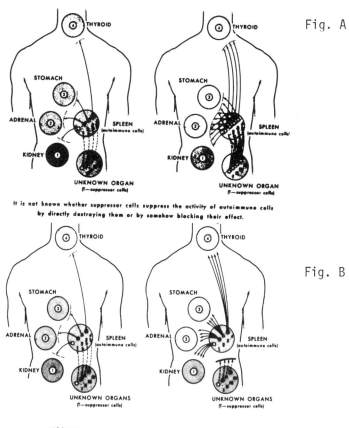

Fig. A

It is not known whether suppressor cells suppress the activity of autoimmune cells
by directly destroying them or by somehow blocking their effect.

Fig. B

NORMAL   T—CELL IMMUNE DEFICIENCY

The information generated thus far in our
laboratory is limited to only non-specific T cell
suppressor effects; it should be pointed out in
this context that in non-organ specific autoimmune
diseases in man (e.g. rhumatoid arthritis, lupus,
chronic active hepatitis) and mouse (NZB

auto-immune syndrome) immunoglobulin levels rise;
if the T suppressor cells were specific we would
not expect all immunoglobulin levels to rise,
because any one antibody wouldn't account for more
than, at most, one percent of the total
immunoglobulin. (And indeed, Ig levels are not
elevated in adrenalitis, thyroiditis, etc.)
However, it is likely that both kinds of T
suppressor cells exist. Furthermore, we don't
know whether suppressor cells suppress the
activity of autoimmune cells, (both autoimmune T
cells and autoimmune B cells) by direct
destruction of these cells or by somehow blocking
their effect perhaps by elaboration of soluble
factors. I prefer the latter interpretation, but
our data just isn't firm enough to state this as
anything other than hypothesis.

SUMMARY

To recapitulate, the T suppressor cells,
presumably coming from the appendix and Peyer
Patches of normal man, presumably modulate the
level of autoimmune cells in lymph nodes, spleen
and other organs to modulate the levels of both
autoantibodies and cellular autoimmunity to
various body organs and tissue. In T-cell immune
deficiency, T suppressor cells may be dispro-
portionately diminished either in number or in
function; (we can't discriminate between these as
yet) so that the autoimmune clones increase and
cause disease.

In terms of malignancy, selective defects
genetically determined that may predispose are:
1. diminution in number or function of
   suppressor T cell
2. diminution in number or function of a T
   cell subpopulation responsible for
   production of "cytotoxic factor," "clonal
   proliferation factor," or some other
   mediator of cellular immunity
3. A selecive immunologic defect to antigenic determinants on one or another
   oncogenic virus.

These possibilities are not mutually
exlusive; such postulated defects are probably a

necessary, but not sufficient, cause for appearance of neoplasia.

Note added in proof:
Recent observations of other suggest most, if not all, non-inbred organisms possess potentially self-reactive (i.e. "autoimmune") clones of lymphocytes. Gebhardt, B.M., et.al., J. Exp. Med., No. 2: 370-382, 1974.

(1)   Fudenberg, H. H., Good, R. A., Hitzig, W. H. et al: Primary Immune Deficiencies: Report of A WHO Committee.   Bulletin, WHO Committee, 45: 125-142, 1971.

(2)   Roelants, G.E., Recognition of Antigen By T Lymphocytes, this volume.

(3)   Fudenberg, H.H.: Immunoglobulins: Structure, Function and Genetic Control. (Johnson & Johnson Symp.) in IMMUNOLOGIC INCOMPETENCE. Year Book Publishers, E.R. Stiehm and B.M. Kagan (Editors) pp. 17-37, 1971.

(4)   Mitchell, G. F., and Miller, J.F. A. P. (1968). Proc. Nat. Acad. Sci., U.S., 59, 296.

(5)   Douglas, S. D., Fudenberg, H. H.: Med. Clin. N.Amer. 53: 903-922, July, 1969.

(6)   Alexander, P., Role of Immunity In Dissemination and Metastasis, this volume.

(7)   Spitler, L. E., Benjamini, E., Young, J. D., Kaplan, H. and Fudenberg, H. H.: J. Exp. Med., 131: 133-148, January 1970.

(8)   Dennart, G. and Lennox, E.S., J. of Immunology, 13:1553-61, 1974.

(9)   Fudenberg, H.H. and Haskill, J.S., in preparation

(10)   Burnet FM: The Clonal Selection Theory of Acquired Immunity, Nashville, Tenn., Vanderbilt University Press, 1959.

(11)   Fudenberg, H.H., Wang, A.C., Pink, J.R.L. and Leven, A.S.: Ann. N.Y. Acad. Sci., in press.

(12)   Decker, J. M., Clarke, J., Bradley, L. M., Miller, A., and Sercarz, E. E., J. of Immunology, 113:1823-33, 1974.

(13)   Fudenberg, H.H.: Immunologic deficiency, autoimmune disease and lymphoma: Observations, impications, and speculations, Arthritis Rheum. 9:464-472, 1966 (Invited review).

(14)   Fudenberg, H.H.: Genetically Determined Immunologic Deficiency: Facts and Fancies. In IMMUNOLOGIC DEFICIENCY Diseases in Man, R.A. Good (Ed.) IV: (1) 340-348, February 1968.

(15)   Fudenberg, H.H.: Are Autoimmune Diseases Immunologic Deficiency States? Hospital Practice, 3: 43-53, January 1968.

(16)   Fudenberg, H.H.: Genetically determined abnormalities in antigen-antibody interaction, In Proceedings of Third International Congress of HUMAN GENETICS, Neel, J.V., and Crow, J.F.,

Editors, The Johns Hopkins Press, Baltimore, 1967. pp. 233-246.

(17) Fudenberg, H.H.: (Editorial) Amer. J. Med., 51: 295-298, September 1971.

(18) Guttman, PLH., Wuepper, K.D., and Fudenberg, H.H.: Vox Sang. 12:329-339, 1967.

(19) Guttman, P.H., Davis W.C., Fudenberg, H.H. and Merigan, T.C.: Vox Sang., 17: 278-288, 1969.

(20) Fudenberg, H.H., in "Lymphokines," NIH task force Nov. 14,15, 1974 (Bethesda, Md.) Natl. Cancer Inst., Monographs, in press.

(21) Fudenberg, H.H., German, J.L., III and Kunkel, H.G.: Arthritis Rheum, 5:565-588, 1962.

(22) Fiaklow, P.J., Fudenberg, H.H. and Epstein, W.V.: Amer. J. Med. 36:188-199, 1964.

(23) Fudenberg, H.H. and Franklin, E.C.: N.Y. Acad. Sci. 124:884-895, 1965 (Invited Review).

(24) Gatti, R. A., and Good, R. A.: Cancer 28:89-98, 1971

(25) Douglas S.D., Goldberg L.S., Fudenberg H.H.: Amer. J. Med. 48:48, 1970.

(26) Waldmann, T. A., ct. al, Lancet - p. 609, 1974.

(27) Workshop on myelonic proteins, homogeneous antibody, and autoimmunity, Nat. Inst. Rheum. Arth., Bethesda, Md., J. Immunology, 107, 1971.

(28) McKhann, C. F.: Primary malignancy in patients undergoing immunosuppression for renal transplantation. Transplantation 8:209-212, 1969.

(29) McDevitt, H.O., Sela M: J. Exp. Med. 122:517, 1965.

(30) Benacerraf, B. and McDevitt, H. O., The histcompatbility linked immune response genes. Science (Wash., D.C.). 175:273, 1972.

(31) Hammerling, G. J., Masuda, T. and McDevitt, H.O., J. Exper. Med., 1180-1200, 1973.

(32) Vachek, H. and Kolsch, E.: The Genetic Control of T Cell-meditated Immunity, 27,507, 1974.

(33) Fudenberg, H.H., Byers, V.S. and Levin, A.S.: Viral Etiology of Human Osteosarcoma: Evidence Based on Response to Tumor-Specific Transfer Factor and on Immuno-Epidemiologic Studies, in FUNDAMENTAL ASPECTS OF NEOPLASIA. Springer-Verlag, N.Y., in press.

(34) Davis, W.W., Douglas, S.D., Fudenberg, H.H.: Intern. Med. 69:1237, 1968.

(35) Tormey, D.C. and Mecller, G.C.: Blood,

26:569, 1968.
(36)   Mueller,   G.C.   and LeMahiev,   M.,   Biochem.
Biophys. Acta., 114, 100, 1968
(37)   Tormey, D.C., Kamin, R.M. and Fudenberg,
H.H.: J. Exp. Med. 125:863-872, 1967.
(38)   Kamin, R.M., Fudenberg, H.H. and Douglas,
S.D.: Proc. Nat. Acad. Sci., 60:881, 1968.
(39) Gershon, R., this volume.
(40)   Kamin, R.M., Henry, C. and Fudenberg, H.H.,
J. Immunol., 113:1151-1161, 1974.
(41) Wells, J.V., Michaeli, D. and Fudenber, H.H.:
Auto-Immunity   in   Selective   IgA   Deficiency.   in
PRIMARY IMMUNODEFICIENCY DISEASES IN MAN., NATL.
FOUNDATION, in press.
(42)   Kamin,   R.M.,   and Fudenberg,   H.H.,   in
preparation.
(43)   Fudenberg, H.H., Wybran, J. and Robbins, D:
T-Rosette-Forming   Cells,   Cellular   Immunity   and
Cancer, N. Engl. J. Med., Vol. 292, p. 475, 1975.
(44)   Fudenberg,   H.H.   and   Robbins,   D.,   in
preparation.
(45)   MacKay, I.R., Wells, J.V. and Fudenberg,
H.H.:   Clin.   Immunol.   and   Immunopathol.,   in
preparation.

ACKNOWLEDGMENTS

Original   work   reported   herein   was   sponsored   by
grants   from   the   N.I.H.   (AM-163213,   HD-05894,
AI-09145).

We are indebted to the following publishers for
permission to reproduce various figures.   Fig. 3,
Karger Press, Basel Switzerland (Guttman, et.al.,
VOX SANG., 12, 1967.) Fig. 4, Grune and Stratton
(Fudenberg, et.al., ARTHRITIS RHEM., 5, 1962.)
Fig. 5, N.Y. Academy of Science Press (Fudenberg,
et.al., ANN. N.Y. ACAD. SCI. 124, 1965.)   Fig. 7,
The Rockefeller University Press (McDevitt and
Sela, J. EXP. MED., 122, 1965.)   Fig. 9, The
Rockefeller University Press (Tormey, et.al., J.
EXP. MED., 125, 1967.) Fig. 10, National Academy
of Science (Kamin, et.al., PROC. NATL. ACAD. SCI.,
60, 1968.)

The following figures and tables are modifications. Fig. 1, Fudenberg, et.al., BUL. WHO, Vol. 2, 45. Fig. 8, Fudenberg, HOSP. PRACT. 1968. Fig. 11, Fudenberg, et.al. NOBEL SYMPOSIUM 3, 1967. Tables 2 through 4 from Kamin, et.al., J. IMMUNOLOGY, 1974.

DISCUSSION

M. Teodorescu, University of Illinois: I would like to make a short comment and ask a question regarding the suppressor T cells. We have some evidence that actually in the rabbit, the cells that are able to suppress are the B cells, immunoglobulin bearing cells. We showed this regarding mitogen stimulation. I wonder whether in your experiments you have some hard evidence that the cells that perform suppression are T-cells in the rabbit. And whether, in the human, is like in the rabbit or like in the mouse.

H.H. Fudenberg, University of California: I'm sorry if I didn't make this point clear. In the rabbit, we show these were T cells because the effect was eradicated by anti-rabbit T cell antiserum plus compliment and the same effect was obtained by T cells but not B cells isolated by nylon column.

M. Teodorescu: In the rabbit?

H.H. Fudenberg: In the rabbit.

H.H. Fudenberg: These were rabbit cells. Now we have deliberately not studied the effect on mitogen activation, which to us is an artificial system. Many people were playing with suppressors of mitogen-induced effects. In contrast, we are looking at response to antigen. I'm sorry if I didn't make this clear. We studied a response to sheep red cells, to keyhole limpet hemocyaninm and to a lac hapten, and found suppression to all of these antigens. Mitogen studies are nice and they give very good quantitative figures, but I remain unconvinced of their significance in relation to biologic activities. Everytime we get into an arguement regarding significance of mitogen I remember that the only effect of mitogens in respect to the human species I know of is one case reported of a child that ingested poke weed and developed a syndrome resembling infectious mononucleosis, with blast cells in his peripheral blood. We don't know what mitogens do in terms of normal function. Perhaps we don't know how antigens act but they at least have some known biological relevance.

M. Teodorescu: So these are suppressor T cells in the rabbit not B cells?

H.H. Fudenberg: These are rabbit T cells.

R. Hard, Medical College of Virginia: In most experimental systems in mice, hypergammaglobulinemia develops. How do you square these findings with the hypogammaglobulinemia patients which you suspect have T cell deficiency?

H.H. Fudenberg: That is a very good question. We have studied the T cell deficiency in the "acquired" agammaglobulinemia not in the original. The T cell difficiency appears only after about 10 years of their disease. We tried to find suppressor activity in agamma patients about 10 years ago and couldn't. I guess we looked at the wrong patients. Most of the patients we had were of long duration. But Dr. Waldman at the NIH has reported several months ago some but not all of these patients with acquired agammaglobulinemia, (I don't know how he selected them. My own impression is that he selected the new ones). Some of these patients had T cell suppression of immonoglobulin (Ig) synthesis. In otherwords, if he got rid of their T cells and put their own B cells alone in culture, they make immunoglobulin as normals would. The mixture would not. Agamma T cells added to normal B cells would suppress Ig synthesis. In a paper published by us in 1962, we showed that as the disease progress as in patients with acquired agammaglobulinemia their Ig levels would gradually rise, perhaps by 50%. This doesn't mean very much if the patient had 10% of normal Ig to begin with, a 50% rise would give him 15% instead of 10%. Here we didn't really know what to make of these findings. But based on the hypothesis, that this was due to a suppressor effect we actually treated these patients with corticosteroids, since T cells presumably are more steroid sensitive than B cells. We used this therapy even though the infectious disease expert said it was dangerous. Their Ig levels rose and they got better, as gauged by fewer infections.

M.M. Sigel, University of Miami Medical School:
I think suppressor cells are a family of cells or even a universe of cells, and until we really get to understand their functions, (whether cell to cell contact is required or soluble mediators are involved) it is premature to sort them out at this stage. The thing I would like to indicate,

however, is in line with your ontogenetic data, the early appearance of suppressor function. We find early appearance of suppressor function phylogenetically, lower fishes, the sharks, possess suppressor cells even though they may be deficient in certain T functions.

H.H. Fudenberg: The data fits with out theories of the work we've been doing on evolution of immune response in the human feti. The current ban on fetal research is going to delay our work on suppressor cell and fetuses.

C. Bell, University of Illinois: I have observed a similar negative feedback regulation or suppression by immunoglobulin negative, (Ig$^-$) lymphocytes (LC) on the Ig$^+$ LC in the rabbit. I have some data which partly agrees with yours in regard to the suppression. In my experiments the suppression was affectuated by rabbit lymphocytes lacking membrane immunoglobulin (Ig$^-$LC or T-LC) and assayed for immunoregulation on rabbit lymphocytes showing membrane-Ig (Ig$^+$LC or B-LC). However, I noted that educated Ig$^-$LC (T-LC) supernatant cell free fluids under defined conditions (as presented in my poster session) can actually exert a positive immunoregulatory effect on Ig$^+$LC (B-LC) facilitating the responses of Ig$^+$LC to SRBC. Have you noticed any positive feedback immunoregulation in your system?

H.H. Fudenberg: We really haven't tried the supernatants yet, they are stored away until we find the optimal age of rabbits for maximal suppressor function in absence of helper phenomena, but your observations are fascinating.

C. Bell: Thank you.

R. Citrobaum, University of California: I don't think anybody denies that you can see suppressor activity in some systems in some way in all animals. Your hyopthesis though is based on the absence of suppressor activity in old animals, I didn't see any data to support that.

H.H. Fudenberg: The hypothesis of patients with agammaglobulinemia is based mainly on the wearing out of cellular immunity in agammaglobulinemias after they've had no humoral antibody for some time and this development of autoimmune phenomena only in those individuals only when cellular immunity declines, as well as, the fact that autoimmune stigmita without disease are present in high

207

incidence in family members, of such patients. As I've said, this talk was in large part going to be "immunophilosphy", and I would show some data which would support but not prove the hypothesis. I don't claim that they proved anything here.

R. Citrobaum: Just to take a lymph node from an old rabbit and add it to your system and show that you don't get suppression would be very simple and very to the point.

H.H. Fudenberg: We're looking right now at various organs from rabbits of different ages in this system. Right now I can tell you that the appendix and Peyer's patch of a 3 month old rabbit have more suppressor activity than that of a new born rabbit and less suppressor activity than that of a year old rabbit. Thats all I can tell you now. I can also give you some hypothesis to why nude mice don't develop autoimmune diseases and contact NZB but I don't think you'd believe that.

M. Cohn, Salk Institute: I was trying to think during your talk if there is any one question I could ask you to show you how confused your concept is. I just want to have a yes or no answer to it. Do you have a reason to distinguish between autoimmunity destroying the T cell function that you are measuring and the distrupted T cell function being responsible for the autoimmunity. Can you distinguish between autoimmunity leading to a loss of a "suppressor function" or a loss of a suppressor function creating autoimmunity? Do you know which is cause and which is effect?

H.H. Fudenberg: If I have to answer it in one word, "no".

M. Cohn: No.

H.H. Fudenberg: However, many autoantibodies appear 5 years before subsequent disease. So if you're going to say which comes first, I would say the disease comes later.

M. Cohn: You giving an explanation, but you do not have a reason.

H.H. Fudenberg: All right, that all.

A.L. Goldstein, University of Texas: I would like to report the results of recent studies with the NZB mouse which suggest that a decrease in thymosin levels and loss of suppressor T cells may result in the onset of autoimmune disease. Recent studies of Mike Dauphinee and Norman Talal, and Jean-Francois Bach and Mireille Dardenne in NZB mice indicate that the sequence of events preceeding the onset of an autoimmune disease in the NZB mouse is as follows: Thymosin levels in the blood decrease in the first weeks of life; this is followed by decline in spontaneous rosette-forming cells in the spleen and by the eighth week of life, there is a loss of suppressor T cells. Cell-mediated immunity falls and several months later, the mouse develops an autoimmune disease similar in many respects to systemic lupus. So at least with regard to the possible etiology of the disease, there is now evidence that would suggest a defect at the level of the endocrine thymus. Most recently, Scheinberg and Cathcart at Boston University have found that the peripheral blood lymphocytes of patients with active systemic lupus but not inactive systemic lupus respond to thymosin in vitro. This later observation would also suggest a possible role for thymosin in the etiology and perhaps treatment of autoimmune diseases like systemic lupus.

H.H. Fudenberg: Mel Steinberg at the NIH also has evidence that the decline in suppressor T cell functions preceeds appearance of autoantibodies and subsequent auto-immune disease in the NZB strains.

M. Cohn: Yes, but you know this is all a question of assay and sensitivity and we're too big a group to get into this. But, let me just make the point about the origin because you're not actually discussing the origin of suppressor cells and how distintion of specificity are made. All that is being put aside and its confused and part of the philosphy is to clarify that. All right now if in the case of the NZB mouse, a noncytopathogenic virus appears on the surface of a cooperating T cell. Now we don't use the word T cell, we have to talk about the function of this on the surface of cooperating T cell and this was now recognized as a foreign surface determinent. Then you would end up with abnormal induction or in this sense an analogue of allogenic induction. This system would now sabotage the immune system and cascade into generalized autoimmunity, which is the case in the NZB mouse. Now what target organ finally gets effected and how good your assays are is another question, but what you do do is you direct your immune system now against self components and against foreign components and its not very effective, which is what you are measuring when you are measuring your suppressor activity. And as Dixon showed a long time ago, surprisingly enough in the old NZB mouse, they respond very well to things like gammaglobulin and serum albumin, but respond very poorly to KLH which is very foreign. So the question I asked was essentially the origin of it and it is quite clear that you could sabotage a suppressor activity by a prior immunological defect.

C. Chang, Tufts University: I would like to hear your comment on the prospect of trying to experimentally suppress T cell immunity selectively, and thereby enhance the auto-immunity. Have you ever done anything along this line, or are you planning to?

H.H. Fudenberg: As I understand your question, how would one try to selectively suppress T cells and thereby increase autoimmune disease? We are trying to devise methods for separating subpopulations of T cells now. Until this can be done I think its impossible to delete any one specific subpopulation and Dr. Haskill in our group from Charleston is attempting to separate these cells. When we can do this then I think we will be able to selectively remove the suppressor T cells from animals. We now have chromic thoracic duct drainage with return of lymph and removal of lymphocytes. When we can separate these cells then hopefully we will be able to do just what you said.

THE ROLE OF BLOCKING SERUM FACTORS IN IMMUNITY TO EMBRYONIC
TUMOR ANTIGENS

K. HELLSTRÖM and I. HELLSTRÖM
Departments of Pathology and Microbiology
University of Washington Medical School

Abstract: Many tumors appear to share antigens with
     normal embryonic cells, in addition to the more specific
     transplantation antigens, which they also possess. Data
     have been summarized indicating that embryonic anti-
     gens, often complexed with antibodies, are circulating
     not only in tumor-bearing but also in certain tumor-
     (or embryo-) immunized hosts, and can block lymphocyte
     mediated immune reactions to such antigens present on
     tumor cells. This is compatible with the hypothesis
     that the poor ability of embryonic antigens to evoke
     a tumor specific transplantation resistance is due t
     their great capacity to form, and to act, as blocking
     factors,abrogating lymphocyte mediated, cytotoxic
     reactions.

INTRODUCTION
     Several lines of evidence indicate that cells from many
neoplasms have antigens which are also present on normal,
syngeneic embryonic cells and which can, therefore, be referred to as phase specific or embryonic tumor antigens (1,2).

     Brawn described in 1970 that lymph node cells (LNC)
from multiparous mice can be cytotoxic to cells from various syngeneic methylcholanthrene induced sarcomas, as measured by the microcytotoxicity assay (3), and he postulated
that the cytotoxic reactions were directed against embryonic
antigen(s) present on the neoplastic cells. Dierlam et al
(4), as well as Baldwin et al (5), confirmed these findings
and showed, in addition, that the cytoxic lymphocyte effect
can be blocked by serum from pregnant mice. Although the
antigens in these reactions are generally referred to as embryonic, there is no absolute proof that they are, indeed,
embryonic. They might, for example, be viral antigens pre-

211

sent on fetal cells and neoplastic cells alike and immunizing during a normal pregnancy. This reservation holds true also for the work described in this paper.

The fact that cytotoxic reactions to embryonic tumor antigens can be detected in vitro by studying LNC from multiparous mice, has led to fairly extensive experiments to test whether similar reactions can lead to tumor destruction in vivo. Baldwin et al (6) tried to adoptively transfer tumor immunity by giving LNC from multiparous mice, but did not succeed in conferring any resistance to transplanted tumor cells. This failure reminded of findings of Ting et al (7), who used embryonic cells in an attempt to immunize mice against tumor transplants. There is thus a dilemma: embryonic tumor antigens appear, on the one hand, to be good targets for a cytotoxic immune response in vitro, while they do not, on the other hand, seem to function as targets for tumor rejection in vivo.

One may speculate about alternative explanations for this discrepancy (8). One possibility is that the density of the embryonic antigens at the tumor cell surface is insufficient for them to function as targets for tumor rejection. Alternatively, the embryonic antigens may be too loosely associated with the cell surface to be targets for a cytotoxic response, except under very special in vitro conditions, or they may very easily modulate (9) upon exposure to antibodies. Still another possibility is that the embryonic antigens, alone or complexed with antibodies, are highly capable of blocking lymphocyte mediated cytotoxic reactions and that their presence in animals immune to embryonic antigens will effectively prevent tumor cells from destruction by reactive lymphocytes.

We will now discuss a series of experiments performed to search for blocking factors to embryonic tumor antigens, to characterize such factors to some extent, and to investigate their role in vivo. Part of our data has been published recently (8,10); experimental details (not included here) are given in the published papers.

RESULTS AND DISCUSSION

A. Reactivity of LNC from pregnant mice on syngeneic tumors. Our first step was to establish a system in which LNC mediated cytotoxic reactions to embryonic tumor antigens could be regularly detected. Cells from two transplanted BALB/c methylcholanthrene induced sarcomas (1315 and 1321), as well as from BALB/c 3T3 lines transformed to neoplasia in vitro, were exposed in standard microcytotoxicity assays to LNC from multiparous BALB/c mice or from age matched, virgin female controls.

TABLE 1

Summary of tests on cytotoxicity of lymph node cell (LNC) from multiparous versus virgin (control) BALB/c mice on syngeneic target cells.

Target cells	Neoplastic and/or transformed	% Reduction of target cells per well w/ 1.5×10^5 LNC M±SE *
1315	+	36.5 ± 2.5
1321	+	32.9 ± 4.2
3T3-MSV	+	41.6 ± 4.3
3T3-SV40	+	27.0 ± 4.1
3T12	+	20.8 ± 3.2
3T3	−	-10.0 ± 4.1
Skin Fibroblasts	−	- 5.3 ± 3.9

* Reduction in % of the number of target cells/well remaining attached. Mean percentage reduction (± SE) for all experiments performed (a minimum of 8 per group) is indicated.

As summarized in Table 1, both chemically induced sarcomas tested, one 3T3 line transformed by the SV40 virus in vitro, one 3T3 line transformed by the Moloney sarcoma virus, and a spontaneously transformed 3T3 line, were all sensitive to exposure to LNC from multiparous BALB/c mice. The sensitivity of the different lines vary, however. Fibroblasts from adult skin and non-transformed 3T3 cells were not affected by exposure to LNC from pregnant, as compared to control, mice.

A cytotoxic effect was commonly seen with LNC harvested already during the first pregnancy, and with LNC obtained after a completed pregnancy; it was most regularly detected, however, using LNC from multiparous mice, taken during pregnancy.

The effector cells appeared to have the θ marker, or to be dependent on the function of a cell having that marker, since incubation of effector cell populations with anti-θ serum and complement abolished most of the cytotoxicity seen against tumor target cells (8).

B. Blocking of the tumor cell cytotoxic effect of LNC from multiparous mice by serum from pregnant or tumor-bearing mice. Dierlam et al (4), Baldwin et al (5,6) and others have found that sera from multiparous mice can block the cytotoxic reaction of LNC from such mice on cultivated tumor cells.

TABLE 2

Blocking of the cytotoxic effect of LNC from syngeneic multiparous mice by serum from multiparous as compared to virgin mice. Cells from tumor 1315 used as targets.

Serum dilution	Mean % blocking serum activity
1:10	82
1:20	95
1:40	48
1:80	2

Table 2 summarizes a large number of experiments performed to confirm and extend these observations. As is apparent from the table, sera from multiparous mice were found to inhibit the cytotoxic effect of LNC from pregnant mice, and this was generally seen up to a serum dilution of 1:40. Sera taken during the latter part of the first pregnancy were also blocking, as were sera taken 30 days after a completed pregnancy (sera taken later were not tested).

TABLE 3

Blocking of the cytotoxic effect of LNC from syngeneic multiparous mice by serum from tumor-bearing mice. Same sera tested against both target cells

Target cells	% Blocking activity of serum from		
	1315 tu. bear.	1321 tu. bear.	Multipara
1315	214	32	107
	116	65	98
	65	12	NT
	168	105	66
1321	37	129	87
	14	90	97
	32	56	NT
	24	70	167

NT= not tested

Table 3 summarizes data obtained with sera from tumor-bearing mice. These sera could also block the cytoxic effect of LNC from multiparous mice. It was, unexpectedly, found that their ability to do so was greatest when the sera were harvested from mice carrying the respective target tumor under study.

The blocking effect of serum could be removed by absorption with tumor cells or with normal embryonic cells, as summarized in Tables 4-5. Absorption with the same amount of adult, normal cells did not remove it. The cells used for absorption could be either derived from culture or taken directly from the animals; the latter finding suggests that at least some of the antigens involved in these reactions are expressed in vivo.

TABLE 4

Absorption of the blocking activity of serum from multiparous mice with cultivated tumor cells.

Target cells	% blocking activity after absorption with				
	1315	3T3–MSV	1321	Fibroblasts	3T3
1315	5	NT	NT	>100	NT
	NT	21	NT	NT	>100
	NT	15	NT	NT	65
	-17	NT	33	92	NT
	-174	NT	100	>100	NT
3T3–MSV	27	NT	NT	79	NT
	NT	3	NT	NT	29
	NT	-3	NT	NT	73
1321	40	NT	21	>100	NT

TABLE 5

Absorption of the blocking activity of serum from multiparous mice with cells taken directly from mice (without culturing).

Target cells	% Blocking activity after absorption with		
	1315	Embryo	Adult kidney
1315	NT	13	>100
	2	17	36
3T3-MSV	NT	-3	>100
	NT	5	67
	-50	35	69

Attempts were then made to raise antisera with "un-blocking" properties (11) by immunizing rabbits with BALB/c mouse embryos, following a protocol described by Bansal and Sjögren (12). As shown in Table 6, it was possible, following immunization of rabbits with embryos and repeated absorptions of their sera in vitro and in vivo, to obtain antisera which, when mixed with sera from multiparous mice, could cancel the blocking effect of the latter. An unblocking effect was often seen also when the rabbit serum was diluted ten times more than the blocking serum.

TABLE 6

Exp No.	Unblocking serum pool No.	Dilution	Target cells	Percent blocking activity with multiparous mouse serum and: Unblock. rabbit sera	Control rabbit sera
1	I	1:10	3T3-MSV	-26.5	27.2
		1:50		-33.3	23.8
2	I	1:25	1315	-52.5	73.4
3	I	1:10	1315	-21.2	60.9
		1:25		- 7.2	37.5
		1:50		10.5	110.5
		1:100		- 3.0	93.2
4	II	1:10	1315	12.4	94.2
		1:25		0	106.1
		1:50		17.5	74.5
		1:100		50.4	61.4

218

C. Preliminary studies on the nature of the blocking and
unblocking serum factors. The blocking activity of serum from
multiparous mice was removable by passage through columns
removing either IgG2a or IgG2b immunoglobulins, and it couldbe
recovered in eluates from such columns. Passage of serum
through columns removing IgM or IgA did not abrogate its
blocking activity, while passage through columns removing
IgG1 occasionally decreased it. These data, which will be
presented in detail by Tamerius et al elsewhere, are summarized in Table 7.

TABLE 7

Removal of blocking activity of multiparous serum by passage
through immunoabsorbent columns removing IgG2a and IgG2b
immunoglobulins. Data from 3 experiments summarized.

		Mean % blocking
IgG1	effluent	66
	eluate	29
IgG2a	effluent	0
	eluate	91
IgG2b	effluent	0
	eluate	86
IgM	effluent	71
	eluate	0
IgA	effluent	119
	eluate	0

Removal of immunoglobulins from an unblocking rabbit serum removed its unblocking activity, which was then recovered again in the eluate (Table 8). This indicates that the factors responsible for the unblocking effect are, at least partially, antibodies.

TABLE 8

Removal of unblocking activity from rabbit antiserum by passage through column removing immunoglobulins.

Serum	CI% *	Blocking %
BALB/c contr.	29.8	C
BALB/c multip.	-10.6	135.6
BALB/c multip. + Rabbit contr.	0.5	98.3
+ Rabbit contr. (Ig abs.)	-4.3	114.4
+ Rabbit contr. (Ig eluate)	11.7	60.7
BALB/c multi. + Rabbit unbl.	38.6	-29.5
+ Rabbit unbl. (Ig abs.)	2.1	93.0
+ Rabbit unbl. (Ig eluate)	22.9	23.1

When blocking sera from multiparous mice were passed through columns to which unblocking (as compared to control) rabbit sera had been bound, the blocking activity was lost (Table 9). These findings suggest that the blocking effect may, at least partially, be mediated by antigens binding to the rabbit antibodies. The findings presented in Tables 7 and 9 are thus compatible with the hypothesis that the blocker is often an antigen-antibody complex.

CI* = The cytoxic index, the 15 percentage reduction of target cell numbers per well with immune is compared to control lymphocyte.

TABLE 9

Removal of blocking activity from multipara serum by passage through immunoabsorbent containing rabbit antibodies to mouse embryo cells.

Serum from pregnant BALB/c passed through column loaded with:		Mean % blocking activity
Rabbit anti-moust embryo serum	effluent	0
(absorbed w. adult mouse cells)	eluate	83
Rabbit control serum (from same	effluent	55
rabbit (absorbed w. adult mouse c)	eluate	0

D. Searches for factors blocking reactivity to embryonic tumor antigens in mice immunized with either neoplastic or embryonic cells. One possible explanation why common putatively embryonic, tumor antigens can be more easily detected in vitro than in vivo might be that they are so capable of blocking the immune response that they cannot induce a reaction leading to tumor rejection.

Experiments summarized in Table 10 are compatible with this view, even if they do not prove that it has to be correct. The table shows that sera from mice immunized against the tumor specific antigens of either of two chemically induced sarcomas (1315 and 1321), and showing specific transplantation resistance against the respective tumors, could block the cytotoxic effect of LNC from multiparous mice. Sera from the same mice did not, on the other hand, block the cytotoxic effect of LNC immune to the tumor specific transplantation antigens of the same neoplasms.

TABLE 10

Blocking activity of sera from mice immunized with tumor cells. Cells from tumor 1315 used as targets.

LNC donor	% blocking activity of sera from				
	1315 tu. bearing	1315 tu. removed	1315 tu. removed, chall. 1315	1321 tu. bearing	1315 tu. removed
Multipara	53	NT	48	NT	NT
	127	107	56	NT	NT
	NT	37	30	NT	45
Immune to 1315	106	-20	5	20	NT
	31	-41	-1	-4	NT

Mice immunized with BALB/c embryos were studied as well. Their LNC were cytotoxic to plated tumor cells, and their sera blocked this cytotoxic effect, as well as that of LNC from multiparous mice; the latter finding is not included in Table 10. The embryo immunized mice did not have any detectable transplantation immunity against the two chemically induced sarcomas used for the tests.

A correlation thus existed between the in vitro and the in vivo observations, if the combined effect of LNC and serum from the immune donors was taken into account, since sera blocked immune reactions against common, embryonic antigens also when they were taken from animals with transplantation immunity against the unique antigens but not against any common ones.

E. Preliminary attempts to manipulate the immune response to embryonic tumor antigens in vivo. The finding that unblocking sera to embryonic tumor antigens can be raised led us to test whether inoculation of such sera to mice immunized with tumor or embryonic cells could influence the take of a small tumor transplant of chemically induced sarcomas (1315 or 1321). Table 11 summarizes preliminary experiments performed to study this.

TABLE 11

Studies on the effect of combined immunization of BALB/c mice with embryonic cells and inoculation with unblocking serum, followed by inoculation with 1315 tumor cells.

Immunization	No. mice w. tumor 12 d. after inocul.	No. mice with tumor 14 d. after inocul. (mean tu. diam. in parenthesis)	No. mice dead of tumor 20 d. after inocul.
# 1315 + control serum	4/10	5/10 (2.4)	7/10
+ unblock. serum	0/9	6/9 (2.9)	4/9
Embryo + control serum	6/10	7/10 (4.5)	3/10
+ unblock. serum	1/10	3/10 (2.2)	0/10
Adult kidney + control serum	6/10	6/10 (4.7)	4/20
+ unblock. serum	2/10	7/10 (4.6)	2/9
Total. Control serum	16/30	18/30 (4.2)	14/30
Unblock. serum	3/29	16/29 (3.6)	6/28

223

As shown in Table 11, the immunization of BALB/c mice with syngeneic embryos or with tumor 1315, combined with inoculation of unblocking rabbit serum, slightly, but significantly, prolonged the latency period before transplanted 1321 tumors were palpable, as well as the life span of the inoculated mice. No such difference was observed when, on the other hand, the mice were challenged with sarcoma 1315.

These findings may have alternative interpretations. They are, however, compatible with the notion that the inoculated antisera depressed tumor growth because they either acted as "unblockers", or contained lymphocyte dependent antibodies against common embryonic antigens, or were cytotoxic to cell carrying embryonic antigens. If any of these alternative interpretations is correct, certain possibilities may open for manipulation of the immune response to embryonic tumor antigens in a prophylactically or therapeutically useful way.

F. Evidence for reactivity to embryonic (?) antigen in mice undergoing liver regeneration. Table 12 gives data from two recent experiments, in which we investigated whether any LNC reactivity similar to that seen in pregnant mice could be detected in adult mice undergoing liver regeneration following partial hepatectomy; the control LNC donors were sham operated litter mates of the hepatectomized animals.

TABLE 12

Cytotoxic effect of LNC from hepatectomized mice on cultivated neoplastic cells.

Exp. #	Days between Hep. ect. and test	Number of effector cells/wells x 10³	% Reduction of target cells/well			
			#1315 tumor cells	3T3-MSV tumor cells	BALB/c fibroblasts	3T3
1	10	150	28.8	20.6	15.9	14.0
		75	37.0			
	34	150	33.9	15.8	7.0	11.5
		75	35.2			
2	10	150	43.2	40.2	-30.5	26.7
	20	150	42.5	13.4	-18.4	1.3
	22	150	28.1	32.0	-9.1	-6.7
	81	150	32.1	38.9	-3.6	9.2

It appears that LNC mediated cytotoxicity was detected on
1315 and 3T3-MSV target tumor cells, but not on the two types
of control cells used, following hepatectomy. This cytotoxic
effect, as well as that of LNC from multiparous mice, could
be blocked by serum taken from mice undergoing hepatectomy
(Table 13). The blocking activity was removed from such
serum by absorption with cells from regenerating liver or
from tumor 1315. These findings are presented in more detail
elsewhere (13).

TABLE 13

Blocking of the cytotoxic effect LNC from multiparous
or hepatectomized mice on tumor cells by serum from
hepatectomized mice. 1315 target tumor cells used.

Exp. #	Days between hep.ect.and bleed.	% CI contr.ser.	% Block. by 1:10 dil. hep. ect.ser.
1	7	48.7	53.8
	7-10		67.8
	21		80.1
	80		-7.8
2	8-22 abs.contr. liver	21.0	62.5
	abs.regener. liver		-20.7
	abs. 1315 tumor		-100
3	8-22 abs.contr. liver	46.1	96.0
	abs.regener. liver		-41.6
	abs. 1315 tumor		14.2
	unabsorbed		100.0

If further work will confirm and further extend these
data, they will have an important implication in demonstrating reactivity to antigens shared by tumor cells under certain conditions (beyond pregnancy) when neoplasia is not
involved. The role in vivo of this latter reactivity is, as
yet, unknown.

REFERENCES

(1) Proceedings of the First Conference and Workshop on
     Embryonic and Fetal Antigens in Cancer, N.G. Anderson
     and J.H. Coggin, Jr., eds. Oak Ridge National Laboratory
     (1971).

(2) Third Conference on Embryonic and Fetal Antigens in
     Cancer, N.G. Anderson and J.H. Coggin, Jr., co-chair-
     men, Cancer Res. 34, (1974) 2021.

(3) R.J. Brawn, Int. J. Cancer, 6 (1970) 245.

(4) P. Dierlam, N.G. Anderson, and J.H. Coggin, Jr., in
     Ref. 1, p. 303.

(5) R.W. Baldwin, Advanc. Cancer Res., 18 (1973) 1.

(6) J.R. Baldwin, and M.J. Embleton, Int. J. Cancer,
     13 (1974) 433.

(7) C.C. Ting, D.H. Lavrin, G. Shieu, and R.B. Herberman,in
     Ref. 1, p. 223.

(8) K.E. Hellstrøm, and I. Hellstrøm, Int. J. Cancer,
     (1975a, in press).

(9) L.J. Old, and E. Boyse, Ann. Rev. Med., 15 (1964) 167.

(10) K.E. Hellstrøm, and I. Hellstrøm, Int. J. Cancer,
     (1975b, in press).

(11) K.E. Hellstrøm, and I. Hellstrøm, Adv. Immunol.,
     18 (1974) 209.

(12) S.C. Bansal, and H.O. Sjøgren, Int. J. Cancer, 9
     (1972) 490.

(13) I. Hellstrøm, K.E. Hellstrøm, and M. Nishioka,
     Nature (1975), in press.

     This investigation was supported by grants CA 10188 and
CA 10189 from the National Institutes of Health, by grant
IC-56D from the American Cancer Society, by contract
NIH-NCI-71-2171 within the Virus Cancer Program of the
National Institutes of Health and by contract NO1 CB 23887
from the National Cancer Institute.

DISCUSSION

E.W. Lamon, University of Alabama: Dr. Hellstrom, I noticed that in some of your unblocking experiments you showed a negative blocking effect. Do you think this is conceivably the same phenomenon as antibody dependent lympho- cyte cytotoxity?

K.E. Hellstrom, University of Washington: I didn't have too much time to go into the antibody dependent lymphocyte toxicity, but as you know from your own work with Eva Klein and from the work of Pollack in our laboratory that one does indeed see lymphocyte dependent antibodies in these systems. Whether the negative unblocking is expected there, I don't know for sure, but I believe that it is most likely that.

V. Jansons, College of Medicine and Dentistry of New Jersey: In your lymphocyte cytotoxicity test, where you found differences, for instance, in the transformed cell versus the normal, (SV40-3T3 versus 3T3) did you use trypsin- ized normal cells also?

K.E. Hellstrom: In those cases we trypsinize the cells with the weakest trypsin dose that we can use and still get them..., free cells, that we can plate. And we plate them on day zero. We added the lymphocytes on day one.

H. Whitten, University of Alabama: Dr. Hellstrom, your blocking studies have led to a better comprehension of hypo- responsiveness at the effector level. However, don't you think that an analysis of antigen mediated (tolerizing) or antibody mediated (enhancing) events that are operative in the primary response in allowing early tumor growth are more important ultimately?

E. Klein, Karolinska Institute: I'm sorry, but Dr. Hellstrom says that he doesn't get your question, so maybe you can look for him after...

H. Whitten: Right.

(Editor's note) The following discussion concerns material verbally presented at the meeting but not contained in the manuscript.

E.L. Lloyd, Argonne National Laboratory: In one of your slides you showed the number of patients with recurrence of disease within one year and the frequency of blocking in those patients. I think you showed that 3 out of 23 did not block within this period, I wonder if you would care to comment on what the nature of these tumors was? Was it different from those that did show blocking activity?

K.E. Hellstrom: Those where it did not block... we have been studying it primarily in very large groups of melanoma patients and where we did not see blocking, the difference, the selection of a patient was to try to select patients that were as clinically similar as possible, and then to do in vitro test of sera from such patients for blocking, some of the sera blocked, some did not block, the question we asked was "Did these have any predictive value as to the probability of tumor recurrence within a year?". The data that came out was that if few of the patients whose sera did not block had recurrence within a year. A much larger number of patients whose sera did block, did have recurrency within a year.

E.L. Lloyd: But they were all malignant melonoma cases?

K.E. Hellstrom: Yes.

E. KLein: Thank you very much Dr. Hellstrom.

CURRENT STATUS OF SELECTED APPROACHES TO IMMUNOTHERAPY

WILLIAM D. TERRY, M.D.
Immunology Branch
National Cancer Institute
National Institutes of Health

INTRODUCTION

The concept of manipulating the immune system as part of
the treatment of patients with cancer is an historically
venerable one and there are reports in the literature that go
back to the 1890's describing attempts at clinical immunotherapy (1). This presentation consists of a brief review of
the status of some of the more recent efforts to study immunotherapy in animals and to use immunotherapy as an experimental treatment for patients with malignant disease. Only
a limited spectrum of the manipulations currently being investigated will be reviewed.

The basic premise of immunotherapy is that tumor cells
contain specific antigens that differentiate them from their
normal tissue counterparts, and that the immune system of a
tumor bearing patient recognizes these antigens and makes an
effective immune response against them, leading to the death
of a significant number of tumor cells. All approaches to
specific immunotherapy, whether active or adoptive, require
that there be tumor associated antigens. Other immunotherapies are based on the premise that even if one cannot develop an immune response directed specifically against the
tumor, the evocation of an irrelevant immune response in the
immediate vicinity of tumor cells will lead to the destruction of tumor cells as "innocent bystanders". Such "non-
specific" immunotherapies require that a strong delayed hypersensitivity reaction be initiated within the tumor site
and depend upon the fact that non-specific cytolytic cells
and factors are generated and the assumption that these cells
and factors can kill tumor cells.

Evidence for the idea that experimentally derived tumors

do indeed have antigens on their cell surfaces against which syngeneic animals can respond was first convincingly produced by Ludwig Gross who demonstrated that immunization of mice with a syngeneic tumor increases resistance to subsequent challenge with the same tumor, but not resistance to challenge with immunologically unrelated tumors (2). A large body of work has been performed utilizing this type of challenge-protection experiment and there is no question that most experimentally induced tumors do indeed have tumor associated antigens. The evidence that spontaneous animal tumors also have tumor associated antigens is considerably weaker, but a full discussion of this topic is beyond the scope of this review.

The analogous experiments designed to determine whether human tumors have tumor associated antigens cannot be performed. It is impossible to do challenge protection experiments, both because it would be ethically impermissible and because there are no inbred strains of human beings. Evidence that human tumors have tumor associated antigens and that the immune system of a tumor bearing patient recognizes these antigens depends therefore on indirect analyses, most of which are carried out in vitro. Indirect studies are always much less powerful than the direct biologic demonstration of a tumor associated antigen and at the present time it is probably fair to say that while there is suggestive evidence that tumor associated antigens are present on some types of human tumors, the strength of the evidence varies and in many cases, is subject to real question.

The driving force behind the development of clinical immunotherapy has been the 200 year long history of anecdotal clinical observations that the development of a severe infection in a patient with a malignant tumor might lead to regression, or even disappearance, of the tumor. These observations led Coley and others to study the effects of intentionally induced bacterial infections, or application of bacterial toxins, on the growth of established human malignancies. Unexpected regressions were seen and reported (reviewed in 3). Retrospective studies of patients having surgery for lung cancer have also shown that those patients who developed post-operative empyema had improved survival relative to those who had an uncomplicated postoperative course (4).

A review of these clinical observations leads to the reasonable hypothesis that infection or bacterial products released by infectious organisms stimulates the immune system in such a way that there is better reactivity against tumors. There are a large class of substances known as immunoadjuvants or immunopotentiators which have the capacity to increase immune system reactivity. One major approach to modern immunotherapy, therefore, has been to explore the usefulness of immunoadjuvants in the treatment of established cancer, and what follows is a description of some of the animal studies and clinical trials that have been carried out.

I. The use of adjuvants or delayed hypersensitivity agents at the tumor site.

A. Animal models.

1. Drs. Rapp, Zbar and their colleagues have developed a model in which a transplantable chemically induced guinea pig hepatoma is injected into the skin of syngeneic strain 2 guinea pigs (5). One week later, when intradermal tumor nodules are approximately 1 cm in diameter, and when tumor cells have already metastasized to regional lymph nodes, BCG, an attenuated strain of Mycobacterium bovis developed by Calmette and Guerin and used as a vaccine against tuberculosis, is injected directly into the tumor. If sufficient numbers of viable BCG organisms are injected, a high proportion of the tumors regress and these animals are rendered resistant to subsequent challenge with the same tumor. Verification and amplification of this model have been provided by Baldwin and his colleagues with rat tumors (6).

a. Elements of this model. i) The animals must be capable of making an immune response to the BCG; ii) it is possible that the animals must also be capable of making an immune response to the tumor; iii) the BCG must be injected directly into the tumor; iv) the BCG must be living and an adequate number of organisms used.

b. Limits of this model. i) The tumor must not be too big. If one waits much past seven days, the effectiveness of injecting BCG is decreased; ii) intratumoral injection of BCG is much less effective if the tumor is subcutaneous or intramuscular; iii) the tumor was chemically induced and is maintained by transplantation; it is not a spontaneous tumor.

c. Mechanisms. While there is considerable information about what BCG does when it is injected into an

233

immunocompetent animal (7), there is as yet no definitive answer to the question of how the intratumoral injection of BCG causes the regression of tumor and the elimination of metastases.

i) One possibility is that the development of a long lasting delayed hypersensitivity and chronic inflammatory reaction in the vicinity of the tumor as well as in the draining lymph nodes, leads to the "passive" killing of tumor cells by activated macrophages and lymphoid cells, as well as by the release of cytotoxic lymphokines. Tumor cells would be destroyed as "innocent bystanders" by these various processes.

ii) Speculation about mechanisms in this model is complicated by recent evidence that this guinea pig tumor shares surface antigens with BCG organisms (8,9), raising the possibility that animals become immunized to the BCG and react against the tumor by virtue of antigenic cross reactivity. BCG should therefore be more effective against those tumors sharing antigens with BCG, and this should be experimentally verifiable.

B. Clinical models.

1. The first modern clinical attempts to intentionally establish delayed hypersensitivity reactions in the region of a tumor were carried out by Edmund Klein (10). This clinical work antedated the experimental work in animals and, as is so often the case in medicine, was initiated because of observations in the clinic by an astute clinician. Klein noted that a topical chemotherapeutic agent used in the treatment of skin cancer was much more effective when the patient had an "allergic" reaction to the drug. Based on these observations, he began to sensitize patients to a good inducer of delayed hypersensitivity, dinitrochlorobenzene (DNCB). Once the patient had been sensitized, DNCB was then applied to the tumor in the absence of chemotherapeutic agents. Klein found that with at least certain types of tumors (eg, basal cell carcinomas), he could induce the complete disappearance of the local lesions. Other investigators have repeated Klein's studies and have verified the essential parts of his findings (11).

a. Elements of this model. i) The patient must make an immune response to DNCB. ii) DNCB must be applied directly to the tumor.

b. <u>Limits of this model</u>. i) The effectiveness of the treatment is dependent upon the histology of the tumor; it is considerably more effective on superficial spreading basal cell carcinomas then it is on nodular basal cell carcinomas, and it is essentially ineffective against melanoma nodules. ii) This is a relatively ineffective way to treat large tumors. iii) Almost without exception, if the treated tumor does regress, other untreated tumors do not; the effect is local and there is no evidence of a systemic effect.

c. <u>Mechanisms</u>. i) The destruction of tumor cells is presumably through the mechanism of the innocent bystander (as was described for I.A.1.c.i).

2. Another clinical model, more directly comparable to the guinea pig model, is the intralesional injection of BCG into intradermal malignant melanoma nodules. Morton and other investigators have used this approach in patients with metastatic melanoma limited to skin and have found that in a majority of such patients, 90% of injected nodules disappear (12). In addition, uninjected nodules also disappear in about 5 to 10% of the cases. Frequently these nodules are physically quite close to the injected nodules.

a. <u>Elements of this model</u>. i) The patient must be immunocompetent and must be capable of making an immune reaction against BCG. ii) BCG must be injected intralesion-ally. iii) There is a low frequency of regression of unin-jected nodules.

b. <u>Limits of this model</u>. i) This approach ap-pears to be of little value if melanoma deposits are subcu-taneous or if there is visceral disease.

c. <u>Mechanisms</u>. i) Again, the innocent bystander effect is the most likely mechanism. ii) Bucana and Hanna have, however, provided recent evidence that at least some human melanoma cells share surface antigens with BCG (9). It is therefore possible that immunization with BCG leads to crossreactive immune responses against melanoma tumor cells. iii) Speculations about the causes of regression of uninjec-ted nodules include a number of possibilities. Intravascular dissemination of BCG from the intratumoral injection site could lead to localization of BCG in uninjected melanoma nodules. In this case, mechanisms would be similar to those for the intratumoral injection. Another possibility is that during the course of the destruction of the injected nodules, there may be more effective immunization against tumor associated antigens, leading to specific immune rejection of uninjected tumor nodules. Finally, immunity against BCG could lead to crossreactive immunity against tumor cells in uninjected nodules.

d. Hazards. Intralesional injection of BCG causes frequent morbidity, including fever, an influenza-like syndrome, hepatic dysfunction and granulomatis hepatitis (13). Several deaths have been reported (14). The nature of the lethal event is not   clear, but may include allergic reactions to BCG, and induction of coagulation disorders.

II. The systemic use of adjuvants.

A second major approach to immunotherapy involves the stimulation of delayed hypersensitivity systemically, as opposed to locally at the site of the tumor. The impetus for this approach comes primarily from immunoprophylaxis experiments in animals in which it was shown that immunoadjuvants administered prior to tumor transplantation led to either a decrease in the number of successful tumor transplants and/or a prolongation of survival (15). This approach was extended by treating animals with BCG and other adjuvants after they had been transplanted with a tumor.

A. Animal models.

1. In the murine L1210 leukemia model Mathé demonstrated that BCG given intraperitoneally to animals 24 hours after a tumor graft caused retardation of tumor growth and reduction in mortality (16). Several other models have been studied in which systemic BCG with chemotherapy (17,18), surgery (19) or hormonal therapy (20) caused cure of some tumors.

B. Human models.

1. Studies of systemic adjuvants in man were carried out by Dr. Mathé and his colleagues in patients with acute lymphoblastic leukemia (21). Subsequent to remission induction, patients were randomized to receive either no further therapy or one of three forms of immunotherapy; a) Pasteur BCG applied by scarification; b) allogeneic tumor cells given subcutaneously; or c) the administration of both allogeneic tumor cells and BCG. The duration of complete

remission of patients in the immunotherapy group (all three types of treatment grouped together) was significantly prolonged relative to the control group. Because of the multiple forms of treatment used, the study is not easy to evaluate. No additional clinical trials confirming the usefulness of this form of immunotherapy in acute lymphoblastic leukemia have been published, and several trials of BCG alone, using different substrains of BCG and different routes of administration, have reported no significant effect (22, 23).

2. The next major trial published also used a combination of BCG with tumor cells, but in patients with acute myelogenous leukemia (AML). Powles et al. induced remission with chemotherapy and then randomized patients to maintenance chemotherapy, or maintenance with a combination of chemotherapy and immunotherapy (24). The immunotherapy consisted of Glaxo BCG, administered with a multipuncture Heaf Gun, and allogeneic AML blast cells that had previously been harvested by performing leukapheresis on patients with acute leukemia. Each week the patient received BCG in one limb and approximately 10^9 irradiated tumor cells injected intradermally and subcutaneously in the other three limbs.

Results of this trial (recently updated; personal communication, R. Powles) have shown an increased median survival for patients receiving immunotherapy and chemotherapy (estimated median survival of 74 weeks) as compared to patients receiving chemotherapy alone (estimated median survival of 39 weeks). The p value for significance of difference of death rates is less than 0.01 (Table 1). In addition, survival following first relapse and duration of first remission is reported as being longer in the immunotherapy plus chemotherapy group than in the patients receiving chemotherapy.

a. Elements of this model. i) The tumor load is first reduced with chemotherapy; chemotherapy is continued during maintenance with immunotherapy. ii) This is a randomized trial, with simultaneous controls. iii) Glaxo BCG is given intradermally by Heaf Gun, and is not in proximity to tumor cells. iv) Allogeneic irradiated tumor cells are administered intradermally and subcutaneously. v) Immunotherapy is continuous until relapse.

b. Limits of this model. i) Positive effects are significant but no apparent long term survivors (ie,

cures). ii) There is no way to tell whether the positive
effects are due to BCG alone, cells alone, or require both.

c. <u>Mechanism</u>. i) If these effects are mediated
by an immunologic mechanism they could be due to stimulation
of either nonspecific or specific immunity. Nonspecific
effects could involve activation of macrophages or other immune cells that kill tumor cells without specificity. Specific effects could be due to increased magnitude of the pre-
existing specific anti-tumor response. ii) Powles has raised
the alternative possibility that nonimmunologic effects might
be involved. For example, BCG might stimulate an increased
production of normal bone marrow stem cells, thereby increasing protection against the effects of cytotoxic chemotherapy
with resultant better resistance to terminal marrow failure
or to infection.

TABLE 1

Immunotherapy in Acute Myelogenous Leukemia

		Powles	Vogler	Gutterman
No. of patients	C + I	30	18	14
	C	22	23	21
Estimated median	C + I	44	39.4[*]	>72[**]
Remission duration	C	27	26[*]	60[**]
Estimated median	C + I	74[†]	84.2[††]	Too
Survival	C	39[†]	70.4[††]	Early

[*] p = 0.002; [**] p = 0.04; [†] p = 0.01; [††] p = 0.005
   C = chemotherapy   I = immunotherapy

3. Another study of systemic BCG in acute myelo-
blastic leukemia has been carried out by the Southeastern
Cancer Study Group. Vogler and Chan, writing for this group,
reported on a study in which chemotherapy was used to induce
remission and patients were then randomized to receive either
a short course of BCG followed by chemotherapy, or chemotherapy alone (25). BCG of the Tice strain was given intradermally by multiple puncture in all four extremities each week

for four weeks. Median duration of remission for the immunotherapy group was 39.4 weeks as compared to 26 weeks for the
chemotherapy group (p=0.002). More recent information on
this trial indicates that the immunochemotherapy group has an
estimated median survival of 84.2 weeks, while the estimated
median survival of the chemotherapy group is 70.4 weeks
(p=0.025) (Table 1).

        a. Elements of this model. i) The tumor load
is reduced with chemotherapy prior to the use of the immunotherapy; chemotherapy is continued during maintenance. ii)
This is a randomized trial, with simultaneous controls. iii)
Tice BCG is given intradermally and is administered by multiple puncture (Tine method). iv) BCG is administered only
during the 4 weeks after consolidation.

        b. Limits of this model. i) Preliminary eval-
uation indicates that although the use of BCG has led to increased survival, there will be no long term survivors.

        c. Mechanism. Probably as described for
II.B.2.i.

        4. The most recently reported trial of the use of
BCG in patients with adult acute leukemia also shows some
positive effects in the subset of patients with acute myelogenous leukemia. Gutterman et al. studied a consecutive
series of 14 AML patients who received BCG in addition to
chemotherapy following remission induction and consolidation
(26). Clinical results were compared to a previous consecutive series of 21 patients with AML who had similar but not
identical induction chemotherapy, and identical maintenance
chemotherapy but without BCG. BCG used was fresh liquid
Pasteur strain and it was applied by scarification three
weeks out of four, with chemotherapy given on the fourth
week. The results show a prolongation of estimated remission
duration with a median of greater than 72 weeks for the immunochemotherapy group versus an estimated median remission
duration of 60 weeks for the chemotherapy group (p=0.04)
(Table 1). This study has been in progress for a period of
time too short to permit evaluation of survival data. It is
of some interest that the reported estimated median remission
duration for the Powles and Southeastern studies are 27 and
26 weeks respectively for the groups receiving chemotherapy
alone, while the comparable value for the Gutterman study is
60 weeks. The nature of this discrepancy will have to be determined before comparative evaluation of the results of

these different studies can be carried out.

    a. <u>Elements of this model</u>. i) Tumor load is reduced with chemotherapy prior to the use of immunotherapy; immunotherapy and chemotherapy are continued during maintenance. ii) This is a non-randomized trial with historical controls. iii) Liquid Pasteur BCG is used by scarification.

    b. <u>Limits of this model</u>. i) It is too early to permit full evaluation. ii) Two-thirds of the control patients had different remission induction and consolidation chemotherapy than did the treated patients. It is not clear how this might effect duration of remission and/or survival.

    c. <u>Mechanism</u>. Probably as described for II.B.2.i.

General Comments.

  None of these three studies is finally evaluated, since patients are still being followed. Even though conclusions concerning the effect of this form of immunotherapy will have to be deferred for several years, some comments can be made. The three studies will never be directly comparable because of differences in chemotherapy, in method, frequency of administration, and strain of BCG, and the additional use of allogeneic cells in one trial. Despite all of these differences, it is clear that the use of BCG, with or without allogeneic cells, increases the duration of remission and probably will increase the survival of patients with AML. There is no evidence that the use of allogeneic cells adds an additional therapeutic effect. A randomized study in which patients are treated with BCG plus allogeneic cells would be required to establish this point.

  It is also clear that there is no compelling evidence that the therapeutic effect of BCG is an immunologic one. Powles has made suggestions of some nonimmunologic mechanism that might account for the prolongation of survival and remission duration and other suggestions could be envisioned. Careful study of this point will be important in further evaluating the role of immunoadjuvants in the treatment of AML.

    5. BCG has also been used as a systemic immunostimulant in patients with disseminated malignant melanoma. Gutterman <u>et al</u>. have reported a trial in which 101

consecutive patients with unresectable metastatic melanoma
received repeated courses of chemotherapy (with dimethyl
triazeno imidazole carboxamide (DTIC)) and immunotherapy
(with liquid Pasteur strain BCG applied by scarification)
(27). Clinical results were compared with results in a previous consecutive series of 111 patients treated with DTIC
alone.

Estimated median durations of survival, remission, and disease stability were essentially the same for
both groups. If instead of the median data, the 0.25 percen-
tile data are evaluated, there appear to be significant differences favoring the immunochemotherapy group for each parameter.

a. Elements of this trial. i) A large and variable amount of tumor is present when immunotherapy is initiated; chemotherapy and immunotherapy are continued until
patient has significant progression. ii) This is a nonrandomized trial with historical controls. iii) Liquid Pasteur
BCG is used by scarification.

b. Limits of this trial. i) Probably will be
no long-term survivors.

c. Mechanisms. i) Probably as described for
II.B.2.c.ii. ii) There is the additional possibility of antigenic crossreactivity between BCG organisms and melanoma
cells (see I.B.2.c.ii.).

6. A study of patients with Stage III or Stage II
malignant melanoma has been reported by Morton (12). Tumor
burden was reduced in Stage III melanoma by resecting large
visceral and subcutaneous metastases. Postoperatively, Tice-
strain BCG was given intradermally alone by the Tine technique, or mixed with irradiated autologous or allogeneic tissue
culture melanoma cells. Stage II patients were treated with
BCG alone (Tice-strain intradermally by Tine technique) or
with BCG given the same way and with either autologous or
tissue culture irradiated melanoma cells injected at a separate site. Results were compared with historical controls
from the same or other institutions.

Recurrence rate and survival of 39 Stage III
patients given immunotherapy appear to be improved relative
to historical controls from other institutions. Similarly,
67 patients with Stage II disease given immunotherapy appear

to have a decreased recurrence rate relative to 34 simultaneous but nonrandomized control patients from the same institution.

      a. Elements of this trial. i) Stage III--surgically remove as much tumor tissue as possible before immunotherapy. ii) Stage III--nonrandomized with surgically noncomparable historical controls from other institutions. Stage II--nonrandomized but simultaneous controls from same institution. iii) Tice BCG given intradermally by Tine technique, either alone or with autologous or allogeneic irradiated melanoma cells at a separate site (Stage II) or Tice BCG mixed with tumor cells (Stage III).

      b. Limits of this trial. i) Apparent positive effects are not statistically evaluable (preliminary, nonrandomized trial). ii) Therapies are varied and Stage III historical controls are surgically noncomparable so that evaluation is difficult.

III. The last immunotherapeutic approach that will be discussed is one in which tumor cell surfaces are altered by enzymatic treatment. There are a number of ways to do this, but the discussion will be limited to the use of neuraminidase, an enzyme which releases neuraminic acid (sialic acid) from polysaccharide chains. Immunoprophylaxis experiments showed that neuraminidase treated tumor cells yielded fewer metastases, and increased tumor transplantation resistance in allogeneic and syngeneic hosts (28,29). Subsequent experiments explored the usefulness of neuraminidase in the treatment of established tumors.

    A. Animal models.

      1. In the model developed by Simmons, a tumor is transplanted subcutaneously into syngeneic mice and allowed to grow until it is from 0.3 to 1 cm. in diameter (30). Control animals, not given further treatment, all die with progressively growing tumor. Other animals are treated with injections of the same tumor, preincubated with vibrio cholera neuraminidase (VCN), at a site far removed from the growing tumor. VCN treated cells are given alone, or with BCG. Results vary with different tumors and different strains of mice, but from 10% to 60% of treated animals have regression of the tumor and are "cured". The use of BCG appears to increase the number of regressions, at least for some of the tumor models.

a. <u>Elements of this model</u>. i) Animals must
be immunologically competent. ii) Immunotherapy is given at
a site distant from the primary tumor. iii) Release of
sialic acid appears to be critical. Heat inactivated or substrate inhibited VCN preparations are ineffective. iv) No
reduction of tumor mass prior to immunotherapy. v) Syngeneic
transplantable tumor is used.

b. <u>Limits of this model</u>. i) Tumors must be of
relatively small size. Delay of treatment markedly decreases
effectiveness. ii) Tumors studied usually killed without
metastasizing. iii) There are no published reports substan-
tiating the model.

c. <u>Mechanisms</u>. The mechanism is not known. It
is known that the serum of some strains of mice contain a
"natural" IgM antibody that reacts with mouse cells after
they have been treated with VCN (31). It has been hypothe-
sized that VCN-treated tumor cells interact with this antibody, and the consequence might be improved immunogenicity
for a variety of cell surface antigens, including the tumor
associated antigens (32). This could lead to increased
levels of cellular and/or humoral reactivity against the established tumor, and in some animals, to cure.

2. A second animal model utilizes a similar approach in the L-1210 leukemia of DBA/2 mice (33). Animals
are given leukemic cells intraperitoneally. Two days later
they are treated with a chemotherapeutic agent, and four days
after that, VCN treated L-1210 cells are given intraperitoneally with or without BCG or MER. Untreated animals die very
rapidly. Animals receiving chemotherapy alone have improved
survival, but few cures. Animals receiving immunotherapy in
addition to the chemotherapy have the best survival, with as
many as 55% long term survivors (cures). The main elements
of this model have been substantiated by the work of
Kollmorgen <u>et al</u>. (34).

a. <u>Elements of this model</u>. i) Animals must be
immunologically competent. ii) Immunotherapy is given in
same physical location as transplanted tumor (intraperoneal-
ly). iii) Release of sialic acid is critical. iv) Cyto-
reductive therapy is required before immunotherapy. v) Syngeneic transplantable tumor is used.

b. <u>Limits of this model</u>. i) Treatment must be
early. Delay of chemotherapy or immunotherapy reduced

effectiveness.

        c. <u>Mechanism</u>. Presumably as for III.A.1.

  B. <u>Clinical trials</u>.

      At the present time, no clinical trials with enzymatically modified cells are far enough advanced to report any results. Trials are in progress in which 1) patients with a variety of solid tumors are immunized with their own VCN treated tumor cells (Simmons); 2) patients with AML are immunized with allogeneic VCN treated leukemia blasts (Holland); and 3) patients with melanoma are immunized with allogeneic VCN treated melanoma cells that are grown in tissue culture (Terry).

DISCUSSION AND CONCLUSION

      This review has emphasized selected approaches to immunotherapy. Relatively recent more comprehensive reviews of immunotherapy are available (35-37).

      Limited generalizations can be made concerning the animal and human studies discussed in this review. Regardless of the immunotherapeutic approach, more impressive effects are seen when immunotherapy is applied either before a tumor grows very large, or after the tumor mass has been reduced by surgery, chemotherapy or hormonal therapy. This implies that there is a quantitative balance between a tumor and the immune system. The nature of this balance and the elements critical to shifting the balance in either direction are unknown.

      In all systems using "non-specific" local or systemic immunostimulation, positive effects are usually not seen unless the animal or patient is immunocompetent, or can be rendered immunocompetent by the adjuvant being used. It follows from both of the preceding generalizations that the next generation of clinical trials of immunotherapy should be directed toward immunocompetent patients with small amounts of tumor.

      Presently available immunotherapeutic manipulations are quite crude and reflect the limited information available concerning tumor-host interactions. Expanding knowledge in the immunobiology of tumor host relationships should permit more refined and effective immunotherapy for human cancer.

REFERENCES

(1) J. Hericourt and C. Richet, C.r. hébal. Seanc, Acad. Sci., 121 (1895) 567.

(2) L. Gross, Cancer Res, 3 (1943) 326.

(3) H.C. Nauts, New York Cancer Research Institute. (Monogr 8), 1969.

(4) J.C. Ruckdeschel, S.D. Codish, A. Stranahan and M.F. McKneally, NEJM, 287 (1972) 1013.

(5) B. Zbar, I.D. Bernstein, G.L. Bartlett, et al., J. Natl. Cancer Inst., 49 (1972) 119.

(6) R.W. Baldwin and M.V. Pimm, Eur. J. Clin. Biol. Res., 16 (1971) 875.

(7) G.B. Mackaness, P.H. Lagrange and T. Ishibashi, J. of Exp. Med., 139 (1974) 1540.

(8) T. Borsos and H.J. Rapp, J. Natl. Cancer Inst., 51 (1973) 1085.

(9) C. Bucana and M.G. Hanna, J. Natl. Cancer Inst., 53 (1974) 1313.

(10) F. Helm and E. Klein, Arch. Dermatol., 91 (1965) 142.

(11) W.R. Levis, K.H. Kraemer, W.G. Klingler, G.L. Peck and W.D. Terry, Cancer Research, 33 (1973) 3036.

(12) D.L. Morton, F.R. Eilber, E.C. Holmes, J.S. Hunt, A.S. Ketcham, M.J. Silverstein and F.C. Sparks, Ann. Surg., 180 (1974) 635.

(13) F.C. Sparks, M.J. Silverstein, J.S. Hunt, C.M. Haskell, Y.H. Pilch and D.L. Morton, N. E. J. Med., 289 (1973) 827.

(14) C.F. McKhann, C.G. Hendrickson, L.E. Spitler, A. Gunnarsson, D. Banerjee and W.R. Nelson, Cancer, in press.

(15) L.J. Old, D.A. Clarke and B. Benacerraf, Nature, 184 (1959) 291.

(16) G. Mathé, Rev. franc. Et. Clin. Biol., 13 (1968) 13.

(17) J.L. Amiel and M. Berardet, Eur. J. Cancer, 6 (1970) 557.

(18) W.J. Pearson, G.R. Pearson, W.T. Gibson, et al., Cancer Res. 32 (1972) 904.

(19) F.C. Sparks, T.X. O'Connell and Y-TN Lee, Surg. Forum, 24 (1973) 118.

(20) W.F. Piessens, R. Heimann, N. Legros, et al., Eur. J. Cancer, 7 (1971) 377.

(21) C. Mathé, R. Weiner, P. Pouillart, et al., Natl. Cancer Inst. Monogr, 39 (1973) 165.

(22) Leukaemia Committee and the Working Party on Leukaemia in Childhood, Br. Med. J., 4 (1971) 189.

(23) R. Heyn, W. Borges, P. Joo, et al., Proc. Am. Assoc. Cancer Res., 14 (1973) 45.

(24) R.L. Powles, D. Crowther, C.J.T. Bateman, et al., Br. J. Cancer, 28 (1973) 365.

(25) W.R. Vogler and Y. Chan, Lancet, ii (1974) 128.

(26) J.V. Gutterman, E.M. Hersh, V. Rodriguez, K.B. McCredie, et al., Lancet, ii (1974) 1405.

(27) J.V. Gutterman, G. Mavligit, J.A. Gottlieb, M.A. Burgess et al., NEJM, 291 (1974) 592.

(28) G. Gasic and T. Gasic, Proc. Nat. Acad. Sci., 48 (1962) 1172.

(29) B.H. Sanford, Transplantation, 5 (1967) 1273.

(30) _____, Science, 174 (1971) 591.

(31) B.H. Sanford and J.F. Codington, Tissue Antigens, 1 (1971) 153.

(32) S.A. Rosenberg and S. Schwarz, J. Natl. Cancer Inst., 52 (1974) 1151.

(33) J.G. Bekesi, J.P. Roboz, L. Walter and J.F. Holland, Behring Inst. Mitt., 55 (1974) 309.

(34) G.M. Kollmorgen, J.J. Killion, W.A. Sansing and J.C. Bundren, in: The Cell Cycle in Malignancy and Immunity, U.S. Atomic Energy Commission (1974), in press.

(35) G.A. Currie, Brit. J. Cancer, 26 (1972) 141.

(36) R.C. Bast, Jr., B. Zbar, T. Borsos and H.J. Rapp, NEJM, 290 (1974) 1413.

(37) E.M. Hersh, J.U. Gutterman, and G. Mavligit. Immuno-therapy of Cancer in Man (Charles C. Thomas, Springfield, 1973)

DISCUSSION

R. Citronbaum, National Institutes of Health: I just
want to make one comment which perhaps you touched on, but
was not, I think, brought home forcefully enough, and that
is that in humans there have not been demonstrated conclusively tumor specific transplantation antigens; merely tumor
associated substances. Now, these substances probably are
not very specific; that is they are maybe made by all cells.
And I'm sure you are well aware that a presumed antigen,
like carcino-embyinic antigen although made in colon carcinoma, pancreatic and others, is also made, in tiny bits, by
normal liver cells. So if we consider the possibilities -
I don't want you to think that I'm against immune therapy
but I just think that we should consider the possibilities
of what we are doing to the patient. That is, if we try to
immunize against a tumor associated substance which is part
of the normal development of other tissues, the possible
consequences of these acts for instance, with carcinoembryonic antigen, may be disastrous. C.E.A. is expressed
on liver cells and the liver turns over 100% within one
year. We would come to the obvious conclusion that perhaps
immunotherapy would not be very safe.

W.D. Terry, National Cancer Institute: In the first
place, it is important to make a distinction between fetal
antigens, and tumor associated transplantation antigens.
The published work of Baldwin makes it quite clear that
these two categories of antigens may have very different
implications in terms of host immunity to tumors; an immune
response to fetal antigens does not necessarily protect
against subsequent challenge with a tumor. Attempts to
immunize patients with cancer are directed towards immunization against tumor associated antigens, not fetal antigens.
It is possible that in the course of these attempts, patients
may become immunized against fetal or other normal tissue
antigens. This would require breaking the self tolerance
assumed to exist for these antigen systems. If this occurred, some types of autoimmunity might develop. However, in
general, we are dealing with patients who have limited hopes
of survival and under those circumstances the risks of
causing harm in the distant future appear to be worth

taking.

R. Citronbaum: This is why I said that I did not want my comments to be construed that I was against immunotherapy.

W.D. Terry: No, not at all.

R. Citronbaum: However, as we go along in chemotherapy and we find that patients now will live five and ten years; whereas before they were living three months. Then we may start to get into real problems with immunotherapy. I just want to look down the road at some of these.

W.D. Terry: We are so early in the development of immunotherapy that I do not think it is terribly useful to look very far down the road at possible late complications. Our job at the present time is to find immunotherapeutic manipulations that are demonstrably effective in patients with cancer. In attempting to achieve that goal, there are two factors that make clinical immunotherapy exceedingly difficult. One is the ethical consideration that makes one wish to try out new forms of therapy only on patients who have essentially a negligible chance of survival. This usually means patients who have an extensive amount of disease. On the other hand, the available information from animal models suggests that immunotherapy is only effective when a very small tumor load is present. Because of this, the exploration of usefulness of immunotherapeutic approaches must be carried out in individuals with a small tumor load and frequently, this will mean patients with an anticipated survival or moderate duration. The repeated administration of BCG is an example of an approach which has some morbidity, but where this morbidity appears acceptable when compared to the known risks of the diseases in which it is being utilized.

B. Becker, Purdue University: I would suggest that people who are working with BCG would also try other bacterial species; there are quite a few including related Corynebacterium, Thermomonospora and Micropolyspora genera because they have a similar polysaccharide antigen of arabinose, galactose and perhaps mannose. Of the natural products from plants, I would select polysaccharide gums which contain arabinose, galactose and/or other monosaccharides in the polymer.

W.D. Terry: As I indicated previously, my review only

covered certain aspects of work currently in progress. As you know, many other adjuvant like materials are under investigation and, for example, Corynebacterium parvum is being used both in animal studies and in clinical trials. Investigators in this field have to make decisions concerning which of the available materials appear to be most promising for clinical investigation based on prior animal experimentation. My hope is that we will achieve some understanding of the principles involved from the preliminary studies that are being carried out and that then we will be able to proceed on a more rational basis to determine which immunostimulants should receive extensive clinical trials.

B. Becker: I just want to point out the uniqueness of arabinose in these organisms I mentioned, and the polymers and their absence in the mammalian cell. At least, the literature doesn't show arabinose being on the mammalian cell surfaces to a great extent.

G.M. Kollmorgen, Oklahoma Medical Research Foundation: You indicated that one of the requirements for successful immunotherapy was an immunocompetent host. Which in vivo or in vitro tests of immunocompetence correlate best with patient response and prognosis?

W.D. Terry: A number of studies have been performed and somewhat different answers have been reported concerning the correlation between tests of immunocompetence and prognosis. A part of the difference seems to be determined by the particular tumor being studied. In general, tests of existing delayed hypersensitivity and of the capacity to be newly sensitized and give a delayed hypersensitivity reaction appear to be amongst the most useful in providing information that will ultimately correlate with prognosis. Considerably more work will be required in this area.

M. Teodorescu, University of Illinois: In some surveys using automatic thermography that we were doing in Bucharest, Dr. Mogos, and I on 135 cancer patients for 4-5 years; we found that the reaction to skin-reactive factors correlates very well with survival time and tumor evolution. Besides, we found that a unique inocculation inside the tumor of autologous mitogen induced lymphokines, which induced tremendous reactions resulting, in some cases, in tumor rejection. I can say this particularly about one patient who was not treated by any other means. She survived about five years although that patient was, at the moment of treatment, in a very advanced form. So, this correlates very well at the clinical level with the experiments done in the guinea pigs. It is probable that inocculation of lymphokines triggers a strong response inside the tumor, which can bring about longer survival time, due to subsequent establishment of specific antitumor immunity.

IMMUNOLOGICAL ASPECTS OF BURKITT´s
LYMPHOMA AND THE EPSTEIN-BARR VIRUS

EVA KLEIN
Department of Tumor Biology
Karolinska Institutet, Stockholm Sweden

Studies on Burkitt lymphoma initiated a few years ago were motivated by the recognition of the disease as a separate clinical entity occurring in a geographically defined area and by the often dramatic efficiency of even inadequate chemotherapy. These two facts intrigued virologists - an infectious factor was supposed to be involved in the etiology of the tumor - and tumor immunologists - the clinical improvements were regarded to be brought about by host response towards tumor specific antigens. Host response is known to exist in virally induced experimental tumor systems. Looking back on the exciting development of the field one may state that the virologists are probably fully satisfied. Two important facts emerged: The discovery of Epstein Barr virus determined the causative agent for infectious mononucleosis and incriminated herpesviruses with oncogenic potential. On the basis of the EBV studies herpesviruses with oncogenic potential were searched for in animal systems and indeed found (1).

Concerning the immunology of the tumor host relationship in the Burkitt patient, while immunological response to certain viral antigens has shown correlation with the clinical course, much is still to be learned about anti-tumoral response.

The herpesvirus EB, isolated first from a Burkitt lymphoma drives lymphoid cells to proliferate in vitro. It seems to be the factor responsible for establishment of human lymphoblastoid lines (2). Very few of such lines produce infectious virus and the presence of viral genetic information demonstrated either directly by nucleic acid hybridization or by revealing virally determined antigens is the handle by which the virus can be detected in them.

The known EBV determined antigens are - in the order

they appear in the viral cycle: EBNA - nuclear antigen, MA -membrane antigen(s), EA - early antigen(s), VCA - viral capsid antigen(s).

The nuclear antigen EBNA: this was the last one to be discovered as it is assayed now (3). However, it is probably identical (4) with the antigen(s) detected by complement fixation early in the studies on Burkitt lymphoma (5, 6, 7, 8). Most human sera have anti-EBNA activity. Among the EBV determined antigens this is the one present in all cells carrying the EBV genome. Studies on EBNA have led to a series of new findings:

The presence of EBNA has an absolute correlation with the demonstrability of EBV-DNA by nucleic acid hybridization, both in lymphoblastoid cell lines and in biopsy material (3, 9, 10, 11, 12). In nude mouse propagated nasopharyngeal carcinoma, the EBNA test has been instrumental in localizing the genome to the carcinoma cell as from such tumors the infiltrating human lymphocytes are eliminated (13).

In the metaphase plates of EBV-DNA carrying cells, all EBNA appears to be localized to the chromosomes (3). Moreover, it was demonstrated in the chromatin fibrils of the interphase nucleus (14). Thus EBNA is a virally determined or virally changed chromosomal protein. Its regular presence in all genome positive lines makes it perhaps the most interesting among the EBV-determined antigens. As long as the genetic information for EBNA synthesis is present, it appears bound to all chromosomes. Interestingly it is expressed on mouse chromosomes in mouse/human hybrid cells in which the parental mouse cell is genome negative. With the progressive loss of human chromosomes EBNA was found to disappear from the hybrid clones before all human chromosomes were lost (EBV-DNA was also lost) (15). The exact localization of the EBV-DNA to individual human chromosomes is not determined yet.

Twenty-six of 27 African Burkitt lymphomas with histologically confirmed diagnosis were found to contain EBV-DNA (10-101 viral genomes per cell), as determined by nucleic acid hybridization. In 25 of the 26 EBV DNA-positive lymphomas the EBV-determined nuclear antigen was also detected. Technical reasons may have accounted for the apparent EBNA-negativity of one EBV DNA-positive biopsy.

Four African lymphoma biopsies, one with a definite diagnosis and three with a questionable diagnosis of Burkitt's
lymphoma were EBV DNA- and EBNA-negative. The same
was true for a collection of Swedish cases of Hodgkin's disease, lymphocytic lymphoma, chronic lymphatic leukemia
and some other lymphoproliferative malignancies. Thus,
there was excellent agreement between the presence of EBV
DNA and of EBNA in tumor biopsies (9, 11). The EBNA
test appears a relatively simple way for the detection of the
virus genome, provided it is carried out with appropriate
technique. It is of interest that several of the patients with
EBV-genome and EBNA-negative malignant lymphomas had
high serum titers of EBV antibodies. This indicates that the
virus does not readily travel along with malignant lymphomas as a passenger in the seropositive patients. In comparison with other lymphomas, African Burkitt's lymphoma of
the high endemic areas is unique in that the tumors (with
rare exceptions) represent the proliferation of an EBV-genome carrying clone. These findings urges the necessity to
distinguish between EBV-seropositive status and evidence
for EBV-genome-carrying neoplastic cells.

Table I summarizes the tests performed in our and in
other laboratories, concerning the occurrence of EBV-DNA
(detected by nucleic acid hybridization), and the EBV-determined nuclear antigen (EBNA) in biopsies from human lymphoproliferative malignancies. Three main points emerge:
a) Presence of the nuclear antigen is strictly correlated with the presence of the viral genome (9).
b) When present, there are multiple genome copies
per cell. This is true in biopsies and for EBV-carrying
established lines (9, 16, 17).
c) Among the various human tumors tested, only
African Burkitt's lymphoma and nasopharyngeal carcinoma
carry detectable viral genomes (11). As mentioned before
non-African Burkitt-like lymphomas, or non-Burkitt lymphomas from patients with high antibody titers, are devoid
of the viral genome (17, 18).
The EBNA provides also a tool for virus infectivity
assay. The above mentioned transforming characteristic of
EBV is exploited for virus detection (19). EBNA detection
in virus infected lymphocytes turned out to be a useful parameter, reducing the time of the assay (20, 21). Thus the
assay can be read either by looking for antigenic conversion
or establishment of a cell line. It is of interest that a considerably higher proportion of cells become EBNA-positive
in an infected cell population than what eventually grow as a

line. Instead of using blood lymphocytes lymphoblastoid cell lines devoid of EBV (a few such lines exist) can be used as target cells (20). This type of assay, with EBNA detection as method, is technically less cumbersome.

TABLE 1

EBV-DNA and EBNA in lymphoma biopsies

Diagnosis	Geographical origin	EBV-DNA[&] (no. pos/ total)	(mean no. genomes)	EBNA (no. pos/ total)
BL[x]	East Africa	26/27	38	25/27
BL?[xx]	East Africa	0/3	2	0/3
BL	East Africa	23/23	(10^S)	n. t.
BL	East Africa	22/23	38	n. t.
BL	East Africa	n. t.	n. t.	12/12
BL	Europe	n. t.	n. t.	0/3
BL	USA	0/4	neg.	n. t.
Lym-phoma[§]	Sweden	0/6	< 2	0/6
CLL[§§]	Sweden	0/4	< 2	0/4
CLL	Sweden	n. t.	n. t.	0/21
ALL[+]	Sweden	n. t.	n. t.	0/6
H. D.[++]	Sweden	0/7	2	0/7

&) cRNA/DNA hybridization unless otherwise indicated
x) Burkitt´s lymphoma
xx) The diagnosis of Burkitt´s lymphoma was questionable
S) DNA/DNA hybridization
§) Low differentiated solid lymphocytic lymphoma
§§) Chronic lymphatic leukemia
+) Acute lymphatic leukemia
++) Hodgkin´s disease

The function of EBNA is completely unknown. Its regular presence in all virus carrying transformed cells is at least consistent with the possibility that it may play some important role in EBV-induced transformation. Conceivably, it might have some regulatory function, e. g. in restricting the initiation of the viral cycle from integrated viral genomes. Alternatively, it may play some structural role, e. g. in stabilizing the association between the multiple viral genome load and the chromatin of the transformed cells. As a third alternative, EBNA may reflect a purely coincidental change of some chromosomal protein in virus genome carrying cells, or the accidental attachment of a viral product to the chromatin.

Early antigen (EA). This antigen complex was discovered by Henle et al. (22). They observed that certain Burkitt lymphoma, nasopharyngeal carcinoma and infectious mononucleosis sera that stained the cells of a virus producer line (detecting VCA), in addition stained a certain proportion of cells in the EBV superinfected VCA negative Raji cell line. In contrast, most healthy donor sera did not stain these cells. Superinfection induced thus a new antigen(s) in Raji cells against which only some donors, particularly those with an active EBV-related disease, had antibodies. Later it was found (23) that this new antigen, designated EA (early antigen), contained two components with distinct specificity, D (diffuse), present as finely distributed material in both nucleus and cytoplasm and R (restricted), present as large clumps of cytoplasmic material. Both R and D appear within 12-24 hours after superinfection. In addition to antigenic specificity, they also differ with regard to their susceptibility to various solvents, e. g. ethanol.

The appearance of EA signals the entry of the cell into the lytic cycle (24). In EA positive cells RNA, DNA and protein synthesis is inhibited. It is not known whether EA itself is responsible for this inhibition, or is preceeded by the production of an inhibitory protein. In abortively superinfected lines all EA positive cells die and do not continue the viral cycle. In virus producing lines, on the other hand, at least a proportion of the EA positive cells go on to viral DNA synthesis and, subsequently, to the synthesis of late viral antigens and virus particles.

The chemical nature of EA is not known, but some experiments carried out by Ernberg and Brown suggest that it may be a glycoprotein.

Membrane antigen (MA). In contrast to the regular, correlation between EBNA and the EBV-genome, the serologically detectable membrane antigen (MA) is not detected with equal regularity on lymphoid cells. Originally, it was demonstrated in Burkitt lymphoma biopsies (25).

MA is not present on cells of nonvirus-producer lymphoblastoid lines. Numerous virus-producer lines, express it on a variable proportion of the cells (26), depending on the culture conditions (27).

Recent experiments by Ernberg et al. (28) have led to a distinction between early membrane antigen (EMA), present on cells that are not engaged in virus production and uninfluenced by DNA inhibitors, and a late membrane antigen (LMA), found on the surface of virus producing cells and on virus particles. EMA and LMA differ in antigenic specificity.

During an earlier phase of development, prior to the distinction between EMA and LMA, MA was subdivided into three serologically distinct subcomponents (29). It is likely that all three represent the EMA complex.

The close parallellism between neutralizing antibody and anti-MA titers suggests that at least some MA components are also present on the viral envelope (30). This was also shown directly by immunoferritin studies (31). It is also clear, however, that the viral envelope has some specificities of its own, not represented within the MA complex. This evidence comes from a study of the anti-MA titer (measured by the blocking of direct membrane fluorescence) and the virus neutralization titer, measured in three different tests (32), in a variety of Burkitt lymphoma, nasopharyngeal carcinoma, and other EBV-positive sera. There was a good correlation between the three neutralization tests and also between the neutralization titers, on the one hand, and the anti-MA titers, on the other, but the latter correlation was only true for so-called concordant sera, i. e. sera with an anti-MA and anti-VA titer in essentially the same (double high or double low) class. Discordant sera, however, with high anti-VCA (and often anti-EA) but low MA titers showed strong neutralization. These sera came from BL or NPC patients with large tumors. Since the sera had high titers against EA and VCA as well, anomaly was the low anti-MA titer. Thus, according to the present analysis,the viral envelope contains the antigenic components of both the early and the late MA complex but, in addition, it has some further, "private" components of its own.

Viral capsid antigen (VCA). Reactivity of sera from various categories of human population with this antigen provided the information about the widespread of the EB virus (33). Moreover seroconversion to anti-VCA positivity in connection with the disease gave the proof that EBV is the etiological agent of infectious mononucleosis (34, 35).

Antibodies reacting with VCA are thus present in the serum of most healthy individuals (33). Burkitt cases differ in that they have high titers. Eightly percent of Burkitt sera react in dilution over 1:160. Among age matched African controls only 14% showed similarly strong reactivity (36). Patients with nasopharyngeal carcinoma have also regularly high titers (37). Only a proportion of patients with other lymphoid malignancies and non-African Burkitt cases have high titers (38, 39, 40, 41, 42) and as discussed before such tumors were shown later to lack both the viral genome and EBNA.

Antibodies to VCA are detected on acetone fixed preparations by indirect immunofluorescence. Nuclear and cytoplasmic staining can be seen in a low proportion of cells in EBV carrying cultures (33). The antigen positive cells are degenerating and all contain virus particles detected by electron microscopy. Burkitt biopsy cells do not have VCA or particles.

In nonproducer lymphoblastoid lines which carry the EBV genome VCA containing cells cannot be detected. In some of these,superinfection and induction with BudR or IudR leads to expression of viral antigens, occassionally also VCA (43, 44). The nature of the antigen was detected in experiments in which it was shown that positive sera agglutinated unenveloped EBV particles and reacted with viral capsids.

Clinical correlations. The question arises whether EBV-related antibody levels or titer changes correlate to clinical status. African Burkitt patients are without exception MA and VCA seropositive. A high proportion (75%) have antibodies against EA also. High titers, particularly against the R subcomponent of EA, or increasing such titers correlate to a comparatively great risk for recurrence and/ or death (46). Studies on 59 BL patients have shown that the anti-MA or anti-VCA level alone at admission did not have prognostic significance. However, extreme values of the quotient anti-VCA/anti-MA correlated to a significantly poorer prognosis than intermediate quotients. In other words when the two titers were compared, patients with "concordant" i. e. high-high or low-low titers have favorable prognosis. The limits defined were 333 to anti-VCA and 25 to the anti-MA titers (47).

The different survival rates in the serologically "discordant" and "concordant" groups were statistically significant. The biological basis for these findings is presently unknown.

There is evidence from the analysis of Burkitt and nasopharyngeal carcinoma patients´sera that anti-VCA titers reflect the tumor burden, extreme high titers indicating large tumors. In such a patient, strong anti-MA activity might be instrumental in keeping the disease under control. This would explain the relatively better prognosis of the high-high titered patients compared to the high VCA - low MA titered ones, and also the low-low titered patients, indicating less advanced tumor status. However to the explanation for the unfavorable prognosis in the low VCA - high MA titered patients, further assumptions have to be introduced.

In three patients with prolonged remission period, decrease of anti-MA but not of anti-VCA titers occurred before recurrence (46, 47).

Sera of four cases with recurrence later than 1 year after initial admission and at least 6 months of remission before the recurrence were studied horizontally. Three of the patients had a sudden decrease of anti-MA reactivity several months before recurrence while other antibody levels were unaffected. The fourth case had slowly increasing anti-MA titers. This relapse differed from the other three by occurring in the originally affected region, and differed from most BL tumors by being near-tetraploid (48, 50). This tumor may have been immunoresistant that managed to escape the increasing anti-tumor immune response. Findings in animal systems have shown that tetraploid tumors have a growth advantage over genetically related but diploid tumors in the presence of immune response directed against cell surface antigens.

The mechanisms leading to the drop of anti-MA activity was investigated. As such sera were anticomplementary, a search was made for specific antigen-antibody complexes in the serum. When brought to low pH an antibody fraction with high anti-MA reactivity was separated through membrane filtration (49).

Low anti-MA reactive pre-recurrence sera from two other cases with late relapse and by high-reactive sera before the titer drop as well as high-reactive sera from the post-relapse period, when the titers had increased again were analyzed similarly. Only the relatively low-reactive sera close to recurrence increased their anti-MA reactivity significantly by acid treatment (47). This finding indicates the presence of immune complexes with MA specificity in such sera. The antigen part of such complexes has yet to be demonstrated.

When BCG "immunotherapy" was administered to BL patients in remission, increase of anti-MA but not of anti-VCA or anti-EA levels occurred. The significance of the anti-MA increase is further indicated by the fact that non-EBV-associated antibodies showed, only occasionally and when so, small changes during the treatment (52).

Further cases from the Uganda Cancer Institute treated by Drs. Ziegler, Magrath and Olweny were studied also. These patients received during remission Pasteur BCG by dermal scarification with short intervals. The sera of these patients showed anti-MA titer increases between 1 and 4 log steps and it was noticed that patients with a titer increase of more than 3 steps during the first month of treatment relapsed less often. Anti-VCA and anti-EA titers were unaffected. The anti-MA titer increase after the BCG treatment seemed to persist for long time. The data do not prove an effector role of anti-MA antibodies in suppression of tumor growth, neither does the drop of such antibodies before some forms of recurrences, but the findings may suggest this (47, 53).

Cell mediated cytotoxicity has been studied quite extensively. Peripheral lymphocytes of Burkitt remission patients were found to be not cytotoxic to autologous established tumor lines (54). Normal lymphocytes exposed to established, autologous EBV-carrying lines were found to differentiate to blasts and exert cytotoxicity to a variety of cell lines, including EBV genome negative B and T cells (53). Sensitivity to this killing effect appears to be an individual characteristic of each line that can not be related to known antigen specificity. It must be noted, furthermore, that such "autologously educated" lymphocytes do not kill Burkitt lymphoma biopsy cells. The in vivo significance of the phenomenon is therefore questionable.

Recently, Svedmyr and Jondal have made some important findings concerning the atypical cells of the peripheral blood in acute infectious mononucleosis (54, 55, 56, 57). These atypical cells are largely T-cells, since they form SRBC-rosettes. Since EBV can be expected to infect B, not T-cells (56, 58) it was reasonable to assume that they may represent reactive cells, sensitized against EBV-infected cells. Jondal and Svedmyr tested the peripheral lymphocytes of acute IM patients, in comparison with healthy controls, for cytotoxic effect against EBV genome negative or positive lines.

Generally, both IM and normal lymphocytes show a certain non-specific cytotoxicity against both EBV-genome positive and negative cell lines. The cell type responsible to the effect is equipped with complement receptors (59). It was thus possible to remove them after they formed EAC rosettes. Subsequently, the cytotoxicity of the normal lymphocyte population disappeared. In contrast, the cytotoxicity of the IM lymphocytes disappeared towards the EBV negative targets but remained unaltered for the genome positive lines (58, 60). There was no difference between the sensitivity of virus producer lines with and non-producer lines without serologically detectable MA. Sensitivity depended thus on the presence of the viral genome. This suggests that EBV-transformed cells may carry membrane antigens which are not detected in the serological tests as carried out presently, but can nevertheless serve as targets of EBV-determined, lymphocyte mediated rejection reactions. The nature of these ("lymphocyte defined?") antigens will be of great interest for further studies.

In a few Burkitt cases the biopsy cells were found to react with antiserum directed against IgG. This reactivity can be due to surface localized immunoglobulin but this is most often IgM (59). IgG may also represent antibodies coating cell surface antigens (62).

Assuming that the antibody coat may lead to cytotoxicity we provided effector factors. We have exposed 7 biopsies to human or guinea pig complement. Moreover, 8 biopsies to lymphocytes derived from normal blood, also after previous incubation with rabbit anti-human IgG serum. No cytotoxicity was obtained. The failure to prove the presence of antibodies by these functional tests may have been due to methodological factors or to the limited number of biopsies tested. It has to be pointed out that sera of all Burkitt patients contain MA reactive antibodies.

As mentioned before, peripheral lymphocytes of Burkitt patients were not found to be directly cytotoxic to autologous tumor cells established in culture but were induced to synthesize DNA and became subsequently indiscriminative killer cells. On the other hand, in a few cases studied, lymphocytes derived from lymph nodes were cytotoxic (64).

We have studied four Burkitt biopsies for the presence of admixed T-lymphocytes. When the cell suspension was mixed with sheep erythrocytes the proportion of rosette forming cells was in all cases about $1/10^3$. In a recent publication higher proportion (4 - 38%) of rosettes was reported (65). From one biopsy which yielded sufficient amount of material such rosetting cells were enriched by Ficoll Isopaque sedimentation. After removal of the erythrocytes from the rosettes the cell suspension was assayed for cytotoxicity against lymphoblastoid lines with and without EBV and also against the biopsy cells. Cytotoxicity was registered only towards the EBV positive and biopsy target cells (66). This approach will be followed up on other cases.

The significance of the known EBV immunological reactivities in relation to the clinical findings are as follows: Anti-VCA activity in high titers occurs regularly in Burkitt and nasopharyngeal cancer patients. Extreme high titers were found in patients with nasopharyngeal carcinoma with large tumor load. High anti-EA activity is particularly related to the diagnosis of Burkitt lymphoma and during remission to risk of recurrence.

Tentatively one might conclude that antibodies to MA have some role in the control of the disease, as indicated by the drop in titers before recurrence and the rise in titers after BCG treatment.

It is of interest that two children with T cell deficiency were found to have high anti-VCA titers which decreased after thymus grafting (67). Moreover, in a survey of Hodgkin´s patients, a interesting correlation was found:

263

patients with low T cell functional parameters had often
high anti-VCA titers (68). Would these two findings indicate
that EBV carrying cells are suppressed by immunological
surveillance? Our understanding about the antitumor response of the Burkitt and nasopharyngeal carcinoma patients is far from satisfactory. It is most likely that more
refined techniques in the analysis of specific cellular response will give more insight. Clarification of the details
of the host response in infectious mononucleosis seems to
be a promising working direction.

REFERENCES

(1)   Oncogenesis and Herpes Viruses, eds. de Thé and H.
zur Hausen (Nuremberg Symp., Agency for Research
on Cancer, Lyon, in press).

(2)   G. Miller, Yale J. Biol. Med., 43 (1971) 358.

(3)   B. M. Reedman and G. Klein, Int. J. Cancer, 11
(1973) 499.

(4)   G. Klein and V. Vonka, J. Nat. Cancer Inst., in
press.

(5)   D. Armstrong, G. Henle and W. Henle, J. Bact., 91
(1966) 1257.

(6)   J. H. Pope, M. K. Horne and E. J. Wetters, Nature
(London), 222 (1969) 186.

(7)   P. Gerber and D. R. Deal, Proc. Soc. Exp. Biol.
Med., 134 (1970) 748.

(8)   V. Vonka, M. Benyesh-Melnick, R. T. Lewis and
I. Wimberly, Arch. Gesamte Virusforsch., 31 (1970)
113.

(9)   T. Lindahl, G. Klein, B. M. Reedman, B. Johansson
and S. Singh, Int. J. Cancer, 13 (1974) 764.

(10)   B. M. Reedman, G. Klein, J. H. Pope, M. K. Walters,
J. Hilgers, S. Singh and B. Johansson, Int. J. Cancer, 13 (1974) 755.

(11)   G. Klein, Cold Spring Harbor Symp., in press.

(12)   G. Klein, T. Lindahl, M. Jondal, W. Leibold, J.
Menezes, K. Nilsson and C. Sundström, Proc. Nat.
Acad. Sci., in press.

(13)   G. Klein, B. C. Giovanella, T. Lindahl, P. Fialkow,
S. Singh and J. S. Stehlin, Proc. Nat. Acad. Sci., in

press.

(14) G. F. Bahr, U. Mikel and G. Klein, submitted for publication.

(15) G. Klein, F. Wiener, L. Zech, H. zur Hausen and B. Reedman, Int. J. Cancer, 14 (1974) 54.

(16) M. Nonoyama and J. S. Pagano, Nature New Biol., 233 (1971) 103.

(17) H. zur Hausen, Int. Rev. Exp. Path., 11 (1972) 233.

(18) J. S. Pagano, H. H. Chien and P. Levine, New Engl. J. Med., 289 (1973) 1395.

(19) D. J. Moss and J. H. Pope, J. Gen. Virol. 17 (1972) 233.

(20) G. Klein, B. Sugden, W. Leibold and J. Menezes, Intervirology, in press.

(21) W. Leibold, T. D. Flanagan, J. Menezes and G. Klein, J. Nat. Cancer Inst., in press.

(22) W. Henle, G. Henle, B. Zajac, G, Pearson, R. Waubke and M. Scriba, Science, 169 (1970) 188.

(23) G. Henle, W. Henle and G. Klein, Int. J. Cancer, 8 (1971) 272.

(24) L. Gergely, G. Klein and I. Ernberg, Virology, 45 (1971) 22.

(25) G. Klein, P. Clifford, E. Klein and J. Stjernswärd, Proc. Nat. Acad. Sci., 55 (1966) 1628.

(26) G. Klein, G. Pearson, G. Henle, W. Henle, G. Goldstein and P. Clifford, J. Exp. Med., 129 (1969) 697.

(27) J. Yata and G. Klein, Int. J. Cancer, 4 (1969) 767.

(28) I. Ernberg, G. Klein, F. M. Kourilsky and D. Silvestre, J. Nat. Cancer Inst., 53 (1974) 61.

(29) A. Svedmyr, A. Demissie, G. Klein and P. Clifford, J. Nat. Cancer Inst., 44 (1970) 595.

(30) G. Pearson, F. Dewey, G. Klein, G. Henle and W. Henle, J. Nat. Cancer Inst., 45 (1970) 989.

(31) D. Silvestre, F. M. Kourilsky, G. Klein, Y. Yata, C. Neauport-Sautes and J. P. Levy, Int. J. Cancer, 8 (1971) 222.

(32) A. de Schryver, G. Klein, J. Hewetson, G. Rocchi, W. Henle, G. Henle, D. J. Moss and J. H. Pope, Int.

J. Cancer, 13 (1974) 353.

(33) G. Henle and W. Henle, J. Bact., 91 (1966) 1248.

(34) G. Henle, W. Henle and V. Diehl, Proc. Nat. Acad. Sci., 59 (1968) 94.

(35) A.S. Evans, J.C. Niederman and R.W. McCollum, New England J. Med., 279 (1968) 1121.

(36) P. Gunvén, G. Klein, G. Henle, W. Henle and P. Clifford, Nature, 228 (1970) 1053.

(37) A. de Schryver, S. Friberg, Jr., G. Klein, W. Henle, G. Henle, G. de Thé, P. Clifford and H.C. Ho, Clin. Exp. Immunol. 5 (1969) 443.

(38) B. Johansson, G. Klein, W. Henle and G. Henle, Int. J. Cancer, 6 (1970) 450.

(39) P.H. Levine, D.V. Ablashi, C.W. Berard, P.P. Cargone, D.E. Waggoner and L. Malan, Cancer, 27 (1971) 416.

(40) W. Henle and G. Henle, Nat. Cancer Inst. Monogr., 36 (1973) 79.

(41) B. Johansson, G. Klein, W. Henle and G. Henle, Int. J. Cancer 8 (1971) 475.

(42) P.H. Levine, D.A. Merrill, N.C. Bethlenfalvay, L. Dabich, D.A. Stevens and D.E. Waggoner, Blood, 38 (1971) 479.

(43) P. Gerber, Proc. Nat. Acad. Sci. (Wash.), 69 (1972) 83.

(44) G. Klein and L. Dombos, Int. J. Cancer, 11 (1973) 327.

(45) S.D. Mayyasi, G. Schidlousky, L.M. Bulfone and Buscheck, Cancer Res, 27 (1967) 2020.

(46) W. Henle, G. Henle, P. Gunvén, G. Klein, P. Clifford and S. Singh, J. Nat. Cancer Inst., 50 (1973) 1163.

(47) P. Gunvén, Thesis, Karolinska Institutet, Stockholm, Sweden.

(48) G. Klein, P. Clifford, G. Henle, W. Henle, G. Geering and L.J. Old, Int. J. Cancer, 4 (1969) 416.

(49) P. Gunvén, G. Klein, W. Henle, G. Henle, G. Rocchi, J.F. Hewetson, A. Guerra, P. Clifford, S.

Singh, A. Demissie and A. Svedmyr, Int. J. Cancer, 12 (1973) 115.

(50)   P. Clifford, N. Gripenberg, E. Klein, E. M. Fenyö and G. Manolov, Lancet (1969) 517.

(51)   T. Mukojima, P. Gunvén and G. Klein, J. Nat. Cancer Inst., 51 (1973) 1319.

(52)   P. Gunvén, G. Klein, J. Onyango, G. Henle, W. Henle, P. Clifford, S. Singh, A. Demissie and A. Svedmyr. J. Nat. Cancer Inst., 51 (1973) 45.

(53)   Ziegler et al., in preparation.

(54)   S. H. Golub, E. A. J. Svedmyr, J. F. Hewetson, G. Klein and S. Singh , Int. J. Cancer, 10 (1972) 157.

(55)   E. A. Svedmyr, F. Deinhardt and G. Klein, Int. J. Cancer, 13 (1974) 891.

(56)   P. J. Sheldon, E. H. Hemsted, M. Papamichail and E. J. Holborow, Lancet (1973) 1153.

(57)   A. M. Denman and B. K. Pelton, Clin. Exp. Immunol., 18 (1974) 13.

(58)   M. Jondal and G. Klein, J. Exp. Med., 138 (1973) 1365.

(59)   M. Jondal and H. Pross, Int. J. Cancer, in press.

(60)   E. Svedmyr and M. Jondal, to be published.

(61)   P. J. Fialkow, E. Klein, G. Klein, P. Clifford and S. Singh, J. Exp. Med., 138 (1973) 89.

(62)   G. Klein, P. Clifford, G. Henle, W. Henle, L. J. Old and L. Geering, Int. J. Cancer, 5 (1969) 185.

(63)   E. Klein, to be published.

(64)   J. Hewetson, S. H. Golub, G. Klein and S. Singh, Int. J. Cancer, 10 (1972) 142.

(65)   R. L. Gross, C. M. Steel, A. G. Levin, S. Singh and G. Brubaker, Int. J. Cancer, 15 (1975) 139.

(66)   M. Jondal, E. A. Svedmyr and E. Klein, to be published.

(67)   L. Businco, E. Ressa, G. Giunchi and F. Aiuti, Clin. Exp. Immunol., in press.

(68)   B. Johansson, G. Holm, H. Mellstedt, W. Henle, G. Henle, G. Söderberg, G. Klein and D. Killander, Oncogenesis and Herpes Viruses, eds. de Thé and

H. zur Hausen (Nuremberg Symp., Agency for Research on Cancer, Lyon, in press).

DISCUSSION

M.M. Sigel, University of Miami School of Medicine: I think I was able to follow everything you said, except the last part of the last slide, where ordinary lymphocytes are quite cytoxic for your cultures, 110% release of chromium. The very last culture that was resistant to T cells was highly susceptible to something else.

E. Klein, Karolinska Institute: Three EBV positive cell lines were used as targets for assaying cytotoxic effect of T cells separated out from Burkitt's biopsy. As control U562 which is not an EBV positive line was used. This cell line is highly sensitive to cytotoxic effect of lymphocyte carrying complement receptors. After these were eliminated from the normal lymphocyte population U562 cells were not killed. This was used as a control system. This EBV negative cells are not killed by the T cells isolated from the Buskitt biopsy. The other targets, three EBV positive lines and the biopsy were damaged by these T cells.

M.M. Sigel: Okay, now, are presumably T cells present in the normal population that was able to kill?

E. Klein: No.

M.M. Sigel: When you take a non-purified population of lymphocytes and kill your cells.

E. Klein: Yes, but if you remove the EAC positive cells you get no killing.

M.M. Sigel: The thing I want to know is whether these same T cells derived from Burkitt's would be acting as sur-pressor cells when added to your other cells. Could they inhibit the reaction of your lymphocytes?

E. Klein: That I don't know.

P. Alexander, Chester Beatty Research Institute: Is the presence of the nuclear antigen always associated with the presence of viral DNA in the presence of the cell?

E. Klein: Right. A 100% correlation.

P. Alexander: Now, if one takes most of the people here; we take our peripheral white cells, we can establish a lymphoblastoid cell line indicating that some of those cells must have had EBV virus in their genomes. Is that right? So surely you would expect an element of positivity with your nuclear antigen on ordinary buffy coat cells of normal people.

E. Klein: We do not find them.

P. Alexander: Yes.

E. Klein: There is now a discussion going on between my husband and Epstein. Because George Klein likes to think that these EBV positive cells which you release from host response when you establish the cultures are kept down in a normal host by the host's immune response. Accordingly you would expect that you can find them somewhere among the lymphoid population. But nobody has seen them and that is why Epstein thinks that there are no transformed cells that grow out in the culture, but some cells under the culture condition release EBV and transform B cells. Thus according to him there are no transformed cells in vitro.

P. Alexander: But, are all your lymphoblastoid cells lines positive?

E. Klein: Yes, they are all positive. All except now there are three or four which have been established from non-Burkitt's lymphoid tumors.

P. Alexander: Concerning the prechusors for the cells taken from the donor which give rise to those lymphoblastoid cell lines, are there no positive cells among them?

E. Klein: The question is, whether you would find them. Because their frequency might be very low.

P. Alexander: I see. Maybe so. The other question I wanted to ask is when you show that the membrane antigen did appear shortly before clinical recurrence that of course as you pointed out, that would be easy to understand and would be nicely explained by antigen release. The thing which I found puzzling, however, was that it rose again when you had recurrent disease. When surely that should now be vast antigen overload. Yet in every one of your cases, it dipped, or in 3 out of 4 it dipped, before there was clinical evidence. As soon as you had recurrent disease, it rose again.

E. Klein: You can of course give an explanation, but this may not be the mechanism. At a certain time there is antigen excess, thereafter antibody response gets stronger and there will be again free antibody.

L.J. Greenberg, University of Minnesota: I have a question for Dr. Klein, Dr. Terry or anyone else in the audience who uses BCG. I wonder if there is any particular genetic background associated with improvement of the disease state? I'm referring of course to the histocompatibility system.

E. Klein: Well, I know that the T cell had this correlation of the nasopharingeal carcinoma involved in each of the HLA type, but I would not be able to explain to you. For me it's enough to see that he has some correlation with another pharingeal carcinoma and one HLA.

L.J. Greenberg: Is this response to BCG?

E. Klein: I'm sorry, that I don't know.

L.J. Greenberg: Perhaps I'm not being very clear. Can the response observed with BCG be explained on the basis of a particular histocompatibility background?

E. Klein: May I throw back the question. Because this could be done in mice, why do you ask it?

L.J. Greenberg: Well, to begin with, there is suggestive evidence that the tuberculin response is associated with HLA system. If this is indeed the case then one might be able to predict which individuals with cancer would respond favorably to BCG.

E. Klein: I see.

M.M. Sigel: This comment may be related to Dr. Alexander's question, but I was not sure about the response. There is the everpresent question as to the immunologic basis underlying the difference between the infectious mono and Burkitt's; one a self-limiting benign disease; the other a progressive malignancy. Perhaps in infectious mono where you do get cells with integrated genoms and expression of new antigens, there is elimination of these cells by virtue of their being endowed with novel antigens, by the T cells that you describe. Do you find, in people who have recovered from an infectious mono, a dominance of these T cells?

E. Klein: People with infectious mononucleosis are presently being followed by measuring active T cells. We have no results yet.

R. Rovoltella, Central National Research: Dr. Klein, when you mentioned an anti-complementary activity of the sera in these patients, you found a good correlation between the anti-complementary activity and the type of antibodies... do you have any information about the profile of the complement during the time course of the disease?

E. Klein: No.

INTEGRATION OF THE EFFECTS OF THYMOSIN AND OTHER HORMONES IN THE REGULATION OF HOST IMMUNOLOGICAL COMPETENCE

ABRAHAM WHITE

Syntex Research and Department of Biochemistry,
Stanford University School of Medicine

Abstract: The role of thymosin, a hormone of the
thymus gland, as well as the hormones of other
endocrine organs, in host immunological competence is based on the effects of these hormones
on lymphoid tissue structure and function.
These effects may be either to enhance or to
inhibit the proliferation of lymphoid cells,
thus influencing the number of cells available
for participation in immunological phenomena, or
to alter the rate of maturation and degree of
responsivity of pre-existing precursor cells
that are in a more primitive stage of development. The role of hormones in the regulation
of host immunological competence also encompasses a variety of non-hormonal agents and
stimuli, which may exert marked effects on the
rates of synthesis and secretion of one or more
hormones that have lymphoid cells as a target
tissue. Of the lymphoid organs, the thymus has
the highest rate of cell proliferation and
turnover and appears to be the most sensitive
to hormonal influence. In view of the prime
contributions of the thymus to host immunological competence, it is not surprising that these
functions, including secretion of hormonal products, are strikingly modulated in their
expression by the blood concentrations of other
hormones, particularly those under the regulatory control of the hypothalamic-adenohypophysial axis.

INTRODUCTION

This presentation will consider the effects of thymosin, the secretory product of a new endocrine gland, the thymus, and other hormones in the regulation of host immunological competence. This topic can be discussed by considering three questions:

1. What are the primary cells contributing to host immunological competence?

2. What are the hormonal and related factors influencing the structure and functions of these cells?

3. What are the interrelationships that obtain among the regulatory actions of these hormones and other stimuli affecting host immunological competence?

PRIMARY CELLS CONTRIBUTING TO HOST IMMUNOLOGICAL COMPETENCE

The production of antibody in lymphoid structures was first implied by the studies of McMaster and Hudack (1) in 1935 and further emphasized by Ehrich and Harris (2) in 1942. Two years later, in collaboration with Dr. Thomas F. Dougherty, we reported the presence in lymphoid cells of a protein with the electrophoretic mobility of serum γ-globulin (3,4). The subsequent demonstration in our laboratory of antibody globulin in lymphocytes of immunized animals (5) focused attention on the role of the lymphocyte in immunological phenomena. These observations, followed by evidence for the role of lymphoid cells in the induction of delayed hypersensitivity (6,7), provided the initial basis for the subsequent prominence of the lymphocyte in host immunological competence.

In the light of both experimental and clinical investigations of the past decade, the fundamental roles of lymphoid cells in host immunological competence, both humoral and cell-mediated, have assumed major biological significance. Aspects of these roles have been presented by previous speakers in this Symposium and have been adequately reviewed in the literature (8-15). In brief, the established roles of the lymphocyte in humoral and cell-mediated immunity can be summarized as follows:

1. To participate in cooperative reactions with other cells of the lymphomyeloid complex to promote antibody synthesis.

2. To function in cell-mediated immunological phenomena.

3. To function selectively in host delineation of the recognition of self and non-self.

HORMONAL AND RELATED FACTORS INFLUENCING LYMPHOID TISSUE STRUCTURE AND FUNCTION

The role of hormones in the regulation of host immunological competence also encompasses a variety of non-hormonal agents and stimuli, which exert marked effects on the rates of synthesis and secretion of one or more hormones that act upon lymphoid cells. Thus, physical, chemical and neural stimuli, nutritional status, aging phenomena, as well as agents either administered or arising within the organism, *e.g.*, epinephrine, alter hormonal balance primarily as a result of the integration of the nervous and endocrine systems at the level of the hypothalamus.

The factors regulating lymphoid tissue structure and function may exert their influence in either of two ways, or both. (a) To alter by a proliferative effect the numbers of lymphoid cells available for participation in humoral and cell-mediated immunological phenomena, and (b) to alter the rate of maturation and degree of responsivity of lymphoid cells already present in the host but of a more primitive precursor stage of development.

Of the diverse structures of the mammalian organism, lymphoid cells have one of the highest rates of turnover, exceeded only by that of the cells of the intestinal mucosa. The rate of this turnover and replacement of lymphoid cells, either by homopoietic or heteropoietic proliferative mechanisms, is markedly altered by hormones. Table 1 lists those endocrine glands, and their hormonal products, that have been established as exerting an influence on the rate of proliferation of lymphoid organs.

TABLE 1

Endocrine glands affecting lymphoid
tissue structure and function

Endocrine gland	Hormone	Direction of effect*
Thyroid	Thyroxine, triiodo- thyronine	↑
Ovary	Estradiol	↑
Adenohypophysis	Somatotropin	↑
Thymus	Thymosin	↑
Adrenal cortex	Cortisol	↓
Testis	Testosterone	↓
Corpus luteum	Progesterone	↓

*↑ = proliferation; enhancement
 ↓ = involution; inhibitory

Let us consider first the endocrine glands that exert a proliferative control of lymphoid tissue structure and function. The influence of the thyroid gland on lymphoid tissue has added significance in the common embryological origin of the thyroid and the thymus. Clinical co-existing thyrotoxicosis and myasthenia gravis has been recorded, accompanied occasionally by thymomas. It might be assumed that any hormone that alters rates of metabolism would also affect lymphoid cell proliferation, particularly when viewed in the light of the lymphocyte production pathway during its repeated divisions. Varying degrees of lymphocytosis have been reported in both experimental and clinical hyperthyroidism, while thyroidectomy in experimental animals results in thymic atrophy. In our own studies, the rate of regeneration of lymphoid tissue in mice following whole body X-irradiation was markedly delayed if the animals were previously thyroidectomized.

The proliferative action of thyroxine on lymphoid tissue is seen in either adrenalectomized, gonadectomized, adrenalectomized-gonadectomized or hypophysectomized animals (16). Thus, this action of thyroxine is not dependent upon mediation by other endocrine glands.

Only brief reference is required to the established proliferative action of estradiol, the prime ovarian follicular hormone, on lymphoid tissue (12) Administration of the hormone leads to lymphoid tissue hypertrophy, characterized initially by active epithelial cell proliferation of the thymus. Prolonged exposure of mice of a specific strain to estrogens can lead to lymphoid tumors. In connection with the present discussion it may be noted that the total amount of lymph nodes and splenic lymphatic tissue is generally greater in female than in male experimental animals. This is probably of significance for the greater capacity for antibody synthesis during immunization exhibited by female animals in comparison to males (12). The possible contributions of sex differences to the expression of cell-mediated immunological phenomena remain to be explored. Data from studies of the incidence of malignancy and a possible causal relationship between decline in immunological competence and aging indicate that sex hormones may have a definite role as one of the factors modulating other immunological parameters in addition to the capacity for antibody synthesis.

The role of somatotropin (growth hormone) in the regulation of lymphoid tissue structure and function has assumed increasing importance. Somatotropin is of particular interest because its action on lymphatic tissue appears to be directed more specifically to the thymus (17,18). The administration of somatotropin increased the size of the thymus of intact and hypophysectomized animals. Prolonged injection of growth-hormone-containing extracts into rats produced generalized lymphoid tissue hyperplasia and, in some animals, lymphosarcomas in the lung tissue (19). This latter localization was probably due to stimulation by growth hormone of areas of peribronchial lymphoid tissue. Other lymphoid organs, *e.g.*, spleen and lymph nodes, also proliferate under the influence of growth hormone (20-22). Moreover, somatotropin administration to hypophysectomized rats elevated their depressed immune response (22).

Similar lymphoid cell hyperproliferative effects due to somatotropin occurred (23) in mice treated with mineral oil as a tumorigenic agent, as well as with the hormone alone. Accelerated plasma cell development was followed by production of lymphosarcomas. Tumor masses were present in the thymus, lung, peritoneal cavity, spleen and liver, with infiltration of lymphocytes into the spleen and significant enlargement of spleen and lymphoid tissue surrounding the thymus.

In contrast, administration to mice (18,24) of rabbit immune globulins isolated from an antiserum to purified somatotropin led to atrophied thymus glands, involuted splenic lymphoid tissue and the appearance of a wasting syndrome reminiscent of that seen in neonatally thymectomized mice (8,14). However, if somatotropin was administered simultaneously with the immune globulins, the effects of the latter were completely prevented.

The role of somatotropin in host immunological competence is reflected in the failure of development of the thymus-lymphatic tissue in the Snell-Bagg (dw) mouse with hereditary hypopituitary dwarfism (25,26). The hypophysis of this animal lacks somatotropic- and thyrotropic hormone-producing cells and these deficiencies are accompanied by hypoplasia of central and peripheral lymphoid tissues. Treatment with somatotropin and thyroxine prevented the thymus involution and the cellular depletion in the peripheral lymphoid tissue (27). The prophylactic influence of these hormones on lymphoid tissue structure and function of the Snell-Bagg mouse was reflected in a reconstitution of 19 S antibody production (18,27,28).

One of the longest studied and most recently accepted members of the list of endocrine glands implicated in influencing lymphoid tissue structure and function is the thymus (*c.f.*, 9,10,12,13,29). Of the diverse lymphoid structures, the thymus has three unique aspects. These are 1) a rate of replacement or turnover of lymphoid cell populations that is approximately three to five times that of the lymph nodes and spleen; 2) secretory reticuloepithelial cells that produce and release one or more hormones; and 3) the provision of an *in situ* microenvironment essential for completing the maturation of specific classes of lymphoid cells.

The high rate of replacement and turnover of lymphoid cell populations of the thymus ranks this gland as the most important of the lymphocytopoietic organs. This is reflected in the early production and export by the thymus to the peripheral lymph nodes and spleen of lymphoid cells that seed these structures and provide the basis for endowment of the host with immunological responsivity.

The second unique aspect of the thymus, namely the presence of secretory reticuloepithelial cells that produce and release one or more hormones, has long been explored but its significance only recently experimentally established. Our earlier observation (30) that cell-free extracts of calf and rat thymic tissue specifically produced a lymphocytosis and lymphoid tissue hypertrophy when administered to normal rats was confirmed by Gregoire and Duchateau (31) and by Metcalf (32). Subsequently, in collaboration with Dr. Allan Goldstein and Dr. Arabinda Guha, and utilizing calf thymus as the starting material, we achieved the purification and characterization of the first thymic polypeptide hormone (33). We had previously named this principle, thymosin (34). Earlier in this Symposium, Dr. Goldstein has described a subsequent modification of the preparative procedure for thymosin (15,35) and presented certain of its properties.

Histochemical and electron microscopic evidence supports the conclusion that the thymic epithelial cells are the site of hormone synthesis and secretion (36,37). Recently, Pyke and Gelfand (38) reported the presence of thymosin-like activity in the medium in which human thymic epithelial cells had been cultured.

Thymosin has a marked proliferative action on lymphoid tissue *in vivo*. This has been demonstrated following administration of thymosin fractions to normal or adrenalectomized adult mice, neonatally thymectomized mice, adult lethally X-irradiated mice, germ-free mice, congenitally athymic nude mice, normal adult guinea pigs, and dogs. This proliferative action of thymosin has been studied in some detail in mice, and is reflected both in an increase in lymphoid tissue weight, a stimulation of mitotic activity of lymphoid cells and an increased degree of incorporation of radioactive labeled precursors into the total DNA, RNA and protein of peripheral lymphoid structures. Histological and radioautographic studies (38) suggest that thymosin has a stimulatory effect particularly on the more primitive immature cells of proliferating lymph nodes. This latter action is significant for the role of thymosin in the development and maturation of lymphoid cells, a role that has been demonstrated in a wide variety of *in vitro* and *in vivo* model systems. These are summarized in Tables 2 and 3.

TABLE 2

Biological activities of thymosin
in *in vitro* models

Conversion of precursor cells to immunologically competent lymphocytes in the following:

- -Rosette assay
- -Cytotoxicity assay: expression of θ and TL antigens
- -Responsivity to mitogens
- -Mixed lymphocyte interaction
- -Secondary antibody response
- -Conversion of bone marrow cells *in vitro* into cells reactive in the graft vs host reaction *in vivo*
- -T and B cell cooperation (*in vitro* → *in vivo*)

TABLE 3

Biological activities of thymosin in *in vivo* models

Normal mice:

  -Lymphocytopoiesis
  -Enhanced rate of allograft rejection
  -Enhanced resistance to progressive growth of
   Moloney virus induced sarcoma
  -Enhanced mixed lymphocyte reaction (*in vivo* →
   in vitro)
  -Enhanced lymphoid cell response to mitogens (*in
   vivo* → *in vitro*)

Germ free mice:

  -Lymphocytopoiesis

Adrenalectomized mice:

  -Enhanced lymphocytopoiesis

Neonatally thymectomized mice:

  -Increased survival and rate of growth
  -Lymphocytopoiesis
  -Restoration of ability to reject skin allograft
  -Enhancement of mixed lymphocyte interaction

Athymic "nude" mice:

  -Lymphocytopoiesis
  -Restoration of response of lymphoid cells to
   mitogen
  -Reduction of allogeneic and xenogeneic tumor
   growth rate

Immunosuppressed mice:

  -Enhancement of ability to reject skin allograft

NZB mice:

  -Delay of appearance of abnormal thymocyte differentiation, with loss of suppressor function

---

The data available indicate that thymosin functions by accelerating the development and maturation of stem cells that are predetermined, under a thymic influence, to function as mature, immunologically competent lymphocytes. Thymosin can exert its influence both in the thymus and in extra-thymic loci. The action of the hormone on stem cells (predetermined T-cells or T_0 cells) promotes their maturation to T_1 cells and accelerates the progress of the latter to T_2 cells. The T_1 cells that mature under the influence of thymosin may function in at least three ways : 1) In cell-mediated immunological phenomena; 2) in cooperative reactions with B-cells to promote antibody synthesis; and 3) as cells with specialized functions, $e.g.$, as suppressor T-cells (40). These functions of thymosin, a hormone of the thymus, together with the role of this organ as a source of production and export of lymphoid cells to the peripheral tissues, notably to the spleen and lymph nodes, as well as the provision by the thymus of an intra-thymic micro-environment that contributes to the expression of specific parameters of host immunological competence, place the thymus, the newest member of the endocrine family, in a position of prime importance in assessing normal and aberrant immunological states.

Let us now indicate briefly the roles of the several hormones that decrease lymphoid tissue size and have an inhibitory influence on the expression by lymphoid cells of immunological responses. In general, it might be expected that the utility of hormones as a basis for immunotherapy in a variety of immunological deficient states, including cancer, would be directed toward augmenting host immunological competence by increasing numbers of lymphoid cells for participation in phenomena described previously. However, lymphoid tissue involution and inhibition of expression of specific lymphoid cell functions can be of significance in specific circumstances, $e.g.$, unrestrained lymphoid tissue proliferation and achievement of an immunosuppressed state prior and subsequent to tissue or organ transplantation. In addition, lymphoid tissue involution can serve as a stimulus for production of new lymphoid cells, under regulatory influences designed to maintain homeostasis.

Our demonstration in collaboration with Dr. T. F. Dougherty that lymphoid cells are a prime target of hypophysial (adrenocorticotropin)-adrenal cortical (11-hydroxy steroids, *e.g.*, cortisol) secretion, with a resultant marked, acute lympho-cytokaryhorrexsis and a concomitant lymphopenia, focused attention on the hormonal regulation of lymphoid tissue structure and function, including the relationship of this regulatory mechanism to antibody production (4). The dissolution of lymphoid tissue by adrenal steroids, with destruc-tion of the site of antibody synthesis, laid the basis for the demonstration by Heilman and Kendall (41) of the effectiveness of cortisol in restrain-ing the growth of a transplantable sarcoma in the mouse and for the subsequent use of lymphocytolytic steroids as immunosuppressive agents (42).

Of the lymphoid structures studied, the thymus gland is the most sensitive to the involutionary effects of the hypophysial-adrenal cortical axis. Of significance for more recent studies of the endocrine role of the thymus was the observation that due to hormonal treatment, "the disappearance of the numerous lymphocytes ordinarily present in the medulla of the thymus left the endodermal reticular cells more exposed, thus giving the im-pression that an increase in these cells had occurred" (43). These and subsequent studies (17, 44) have indicated that these cells, the probable site of thymic hormone synthesis (36-38), are relatively hydrocortisone-resistant.

Although the steroids of the adrenal cortex are probably the most potent of the hormonal agents that suppress lymphoid tissue proliferation and function, including these reflected in immune phenomena, two additional endocrine products have similar actions. Either testosterone or proges-terone, administered in a variety of animal models, diminishes lymphoid tissue size (17) and immunologi-cal responsivity (12,45). A dramatic example of this action of androgens was described by Szenberg and Warner (46). Injection of androgenic steroids into chick embryos caused marked involution of bursal lymphoid cells, as well as a decrease in the epithelial cells of the bursa. The decreased response of male animals to antigen, in comparison to the female, can be maintained at higher levels by prior castration (47). Evidence that orchidectomy in mice causes enlargement of lymphoid tissue and delays the normal rate of thymic involution has recently been reported (48), together with the demonstration that, in the operated animals, cell-mediated immunological competence is enhanced (49).

Although progesterone was initially described as lacking significant immunosuppressive activity (50), this was subsequently attributed to the dose of steroid used (51). Evidence now available supports the conclusion that progestins, including naturally occurring progesterone and certain of the synthetic steroids, *e.g.*, medroxy-progesterone, given in non-physiological large doses, are immunosuppressive agents (52). Whether or not the variable degree of host immunological responsiveness that has been reported in human pregnancy (53) bears a causal relationship to the elevated blood levels of progesterone remains to be established.

INTEGRATION OF HORMONAL REGULATION OF HOST IMMUNOLOGICAL COMPETENCE

The influence of individual hormones on the structure and function of lymphoid tissue can be dissected experimentally. However, it is obvious that in both normal and diseased states the interrelationships among the endocrine glands may markedly modify the nature of the final expression of host immunity. These interrelationships among hormones affecting lymphoid tissue structure and function are of particular significance since, among the lymphoid organs, the thymus and its hormonal secretions, including thymosin, have a central role in host immunological competence.

The striking proliferative effects of somatotropin on the thymus has raised the question of whether the hypothalamic-adenohypophysial axis exerts a trophic influence on the secretory activity of the thymus. Comsa and co-workers have recently reported (54) that the deficient antibody production in hypophysectomized-thymectomized rats could not be restored by repeated injections of somatotropin or a thymic hormone preparation. However, administration of both hormonal preparations fully restored to normal the response to antigen.

The influence of other endocrine glands on the thymus may be the basis of the role of this gland in lymphocytopoiesis and could determine the extrathymic classes of lymphocytes available to function in specific immunological responses. Thus, the lymphocytopoietic actions of thymosin are synergistic with somatotropin and antagonistic to the secretions of the adrenal cortex. Indeed, thymectomy does not result in a lymphophenia if the animal is previously adrenalectomized (55). Thus, *in vivo*, the influence of the thymus on lymphoid tissue may be mediated, at least in part, by the hypophysial-adrenal cortical axis.

The previously described lymphocytopoietic action of thyroxine is not manifested in the thymectomized guinea pig, indicating a possible thymotropic action of the thyroid gland. This recalls earlier observations (*c.f.*, 56) that the development of leukemia in mice is inhibited by either thymectomy or thyroidectomy, lending further emphasis to the interrelationship of these two endocrine glands.

The opposing actions of the adrenal cortex and the thymus on lymphocytopoiesis could influence the nature of the populations of T-cells available for immunological functioning. In view of the selective lymphocytolytic action of adrenal steroids on more immature T-cells, namely T_0 and T_1, and since thymosin action appears to be localized at an early stage of T-cell maturation (12,13,15), it is apparent that the numbers of <u>potential</u> immunologically competent cells available to the host may be determined by the relative blood concentrations of adrenal steroids, somatotropin, and thymosin. Thus, the effectiveness of thymosin in enhancing host immunological competence is integrated *in vivo* with the rates of secretion of other endocrine glands, notably, that of the adenohypophysis. The latter regulates the secretory rates of somatotropin, adrenal steroids, and thyroxine, and thus may exert a trophic influence on the secretion of thymosin. Figure 1 depicts some of the endocrine effects and interrelationships that have been discussed.

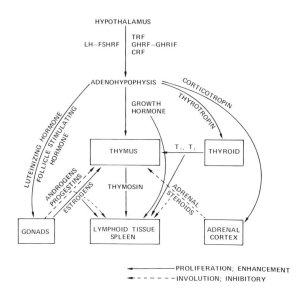

Fig. 1: Interrelationships of the thymus and other endocrine glands in the regulation of lymphoid tissue structure and function. LH-FSHRF, luteinizing hormone-follicle stimulating hormone regulatory factor; TRF, thyrotropin regulatory factor; GHRF-GHRIF, growth hormone releasing-growth hormone inhibitory factors; CRF, adrenocorticotropin regulatory factor; T₃, triiodothyronine; T₄, thyroxine

The possible thymotropic influence of somatotropin should be viewed in the light of the role of this hypophysial hormone in regulating blood levels of other proliferative factors, namely, the somatomedins (57). It is possible that thymosin, and perhaps other described thymic factors, may be members of a somatomedin-like family in that their production and/or secretion by the thymus gland may be influenced by one or more adenohypophysial hormones.

REFERENCES

(1)   P.D. McMaster and S. Hudack. J. Exp. Med.
       61 (1935) 783.

(2)   W.E. Ehrich and T.N. Harris. J. Exp. Med.
       76 (1942) 335.

(3)   A. White and T.F. Dougherty. Ann. N.Y. Acad.
       Sci. 46 (1946) 859.

(4)   A. White. Harvey Lectures. 43 (1947-48) 43.

(5)   T.F. Dougherty, J.H. Chase and A. White.
       Proc. Soc. Exp. Biol. Med. 57 (1944) 295.

(6)   E. Macher and M.W. Chase. J. Exp. Med.
       129 (1969) 81.

(7)   E. Macher and M.W. Chase. J. Exp. Med.
       129 (1969) 103.

(8)   J.F.A.P. Miller and D. Osoba. Physiol. Revs.
       47 (1967) 137.

(9)   A. White and A.L. Goldstein, in: Control
       Processes in Multicellular Organisms, Ciba
       Foundation Symposium, eds. G.E.W. Wolstenholme
       and J. Knight (Churchill, London, 1970)
       p. 210.

(10)   A. White and A.L. Goldstein, in: Hormones
       and the Immune Response, Ciba Foundation
       Study Group No. 36, eds. G.E.W. Wolstenholme
       and J. Knight (Churchill, London, 1970) p.3.

(11)   J.M. Yoffey and F.C. Courtice. Lymphatics,
       Lymph and the Lymphomyeloid Complex
       (Academic Press, New York, 1970).

(12)   A. White and A.L. Goldstein, in: Immuno-
       genicity. Physico-chemical and Biological
       Aspects, ed. F. Borek (North-Holland Pub-
       lishing Co., Amsterdam, 1972) p. 334.

(13)   A.L. Goldstein and A. White. Contemporary
        Topics in Immunobiol. 2 (1973) 239.

(14)   N. Trainin. Physiol. Revs. 54 (1974) 272.

(15)   A. White and A.L. Goldstein. Adv. in Metabo-
        lic Disorders. 8, Nobel Symposium #28 (1975),
        In press.

(16)   U. Ernström. Acta Pathol. et Microbiol.
        Scand. 63 (1965) Suppl. 178.

(17)   T.F. Dougherty. Physiol. Revs. 32 (1952) 379.

(18)   W. Pierpaoli and E. Sorkin, in: The Immune
        Response and Its Suppression, ed. E. Sorkin
        (Karger, New York, 1969) p. 122.

(19)   H.D. Moon, M.E. Simpson, C.H. Li and H.M.
        Evans. Cancer Res. 10 (1950) 297.

(20)   H.D. Moon, M.E. Simpson, C.H. Li and H.M.
        Evans. Cancer Res. 12 (1952) 448.

(21)   T.F. Dougherty, in: The Hypophyseal Growth
        Hormone, Nature and Actions, eds. R.W. Smith,
        Jr., O.H. Gaebler and C.N.H. Long (Blakiston,
        New York, 1955) p. 148.

(22)   M.R. Pandian and G. P. Talwar, J. Exp. Med.
        134 (1971) 1095.

(23)   K. Takakura, H. Yamada and V.P. Hollander.
        Cancer Res. 27 (1967) 2034.

(24)   W. Pierpaoli and E. Sorkin. J. Immunol. 101
        (1968) 1036.

(25)   C. Baroni. Acta Anatomica 68 (1967) 361.

(26)   C. Baroni. Experientia 23 (1967) 282.

(27)   C.D. Baroni, N. Fabris and G. Bertoli.
        Immunol. 17 (1969) 303.

(28)   W. Pierpaoli, C. Baroni, N. Fabris and E.
        Sorkin. Immunol. 16 (1969) 217.

(29)   A. White and A.L. Goldstein. Perspectives
       Biol. & Med. 11 (1968) 475.

(30)   S. Roberts and A. White. J. Biol. Chem. 178
       (1949) 159.

(31)   C. Gregoire and G. Duchateau. Arch. Biol.
       (Liège). 67 (1956) 269.

(32)   D. Metcalf. Brit. J. Cancer 10 (1956) 442.

(33)   A.L. Goldstein, A. Guha, M.M. Zatz, M.A.
       Hardy and A. White. Proc. Natl. Acad. Sci.
       U.S. 69(1972) 1800.

(34)   A.L. Goldstein, F.D. Slater and A. White.
       Proc. Natl. Acad. Sci. U.S. 56 (1966) 1010.

(35)   J.A. Hooper, M.C. McDaniel, G.B. Thurman,
       G.H. Cohen, R.S. Schulof and A.L. Goldstein,
       Ann. N.Y. Acad. Sci. (1975) In press.

(36)   A.L. Goldstein and A. White. Current Topics
       in Exp. Endocrinol. 1 (1971) 121.

(37)   J.M. Vetters and R.F. Macadam. J. Clin. Path.
       26 (1973) 194.

(38)   K.W. Pyke and E.W. Gelfand. Nature 251 (1974)
       423.

(39)   A.L. Goldstein, S. Banerjee, G.L. Schneebeli,
       T.F. Dougherty and A. White. Radiation Res.
       41 (1970) 579.

(40)   M.J. Dauphinee, N. Talal, A.L. Goldstein and
       A. White. Proc. Natl. Acad. Sci. U.S. 71
       (1974) 2637.

(41)   F.R. Heilman and F.C. Kendall. Endocrinology
       34 (1944) 416.

(42)   R.S. Schwartz, in: Immunobiology, eds. R.A.
       Good and D.W. Fisher (Sinauer Associates,
       Stamford, Conn. 1971) p. 240.

(43)   T.F. Dougherty and A. White. Am. J. Anat.
       77 (1945) 81.

(44)   D. Metcalf, in: The Thymus in Immunobiology.
       Structure, Function and Role in Disease, eds.
       R.A. Good and A.E. Gabrielsen (Hoeber Medi-
       cal Division, Harper & Row, Publishers, New
       York, 1964) p. 150.

(45)   R.B. Markham, A. White and A.L. Goldstein.
       Proc. Soc. Exp. Biol. Med. 148 (1975) 190.

(46)   A. Szenberg and N.L. Warner. Brit. Med. Bull.
       23 (1967) 30.

(47)   J.R. Batchelor, in: Hormonal Control of Anti-
       body Production, ed. B. Cinader (Thomas,
       Springfield, Ill., 1968) p. 276.

(48)   J.E. Castro. Proc. Roy. Soc. London B. 185
       (1974) 425.

(49)   J.E. Castro. Proc. Roy. Soc. London B. 185
       (1974) 437.

(50)   J.F. Hulka, K. Mohr and M.W. Lieberman.
       Endocrinology 77 (1965) 897.

(51)   L. Felner and M.G. Rhoades. J. Amer. Geriat.
       Soc. 13 (1965) 765.

(52)   J.S. Munroe. Res. J. Reticuloendothel. Soc.
       9 (1971) 361.

(53)   M.B. Thong, R.W. Steele, M.M. Vincent, S.A.
       Hensen and J.A. Bellanti. New Engl. J. Med.
       289 (1973) 604.

(54)   J. Comsa, J.A. Schwarz and H. Neu. Immunol.
       Communications 3 (1974) 11.

(55)   D. Metcalf and R.F. Buffett. Proc. Soc. Exp.
       Biol. Med. 95 (1957) 576.

(56)   J. Comsa, in: Thymic Hormones, ed. T.D.
       Luckey (University Park Press, Baltimore,
       1973) p. 59.

(57)   R. Luft and K. Hall, eds. Adv. in Metabolic
        Disorders, 8, Nobel Symposium #28 (1975),
        In press.

DISCUSSION

I. Schenkein, New York University: Dr. White, is there a sexual dimorphism for thymosine, like, for example, for the nerve growth factor, NGF, isolated from the mouse submandibular gland? The levels of NGF in glands from a male can be some ten times higher than those in the female gland. Is there any measurable difference in the levels of thymosin between male and female?

A. White, Syntex Research: I don't think that data are available as yet to answer that question. In preliminary radioimmunological assays that Dr. Goldstein referred to in his lecture, developed by Dr. Richard Schulof, the number of human subjects studied was too few to permit that conclusion. The studies were directed more toward thymosin blood levels in various age groups, and in selected diseases, rather than toward possible sex differences. Perhaps Dr. Goldstein would like to comment on whether sex differences obtain in blood levels of thymosin.

A.L. Goldstein, University of Texas: We have not looked at the question yet.

J. Schultz, Papanicolaou Cancer Research Institute: You recall that we both came from the same laboratory about 30 years ago, or 35, haven't we? And on the basis of that, I think you have little problem answering these questions. I think that fundamentally in a lot of what's going on here, is the assumption that cancer or tumor-bearing animals could respond equally as well to hormones and other factors as a normal, and that most experiments of controlled animals are under the same diet as the experimental animals and we all assume that demands and needs for certain factors are going to be the same with both. But what I think is missing here is that we do not have a figure for the half-life of the lymphocyte. What is the daily productive capacity, or needs, for the production of lymphocytes as a total requirement by the animal and I know that even tumor-bearing rats cannot respond to a sterile abscess, the same as a normal rat so, I wonder what consideration has been given to these

292

factors, as the ability of tumor-bearing animals to respond without the additional need for other nutritional factors, because there is a greater demand than in a normal control? I think that the best example, of course, is pernicious anemia in cells of Whipple's experiments which gave rise eventually, to the B-12 vitamins.

A. White: Could you focus that into a single question? As I understand, are you referring to the rate of production of lymphoid cells under various conditions?

J. Schultz: Well, in a normal animal you have a figure of lymphocyte production. Can the tumor bearing rat respond to the same stress to produce that many lymphocytes if necessary, regardless of the quality and the kind of lympho-cytes that are necessary. You fed sodium benzoate to rats and made them glycine dependent for growth. The presence of the tumor could well limit availability of factors for lymphocyte production.

A. White: There are data for lymphocyte production by the thymus of the normal guinea pig, derived from studies of Dr. Ernster in Stockholm. In addition, experiments of the type conducted by Professor Gowans and his colleagues have yielded data on lymphocyte numbers in rat thoracic-duct lymph under a variety of conditions. Measurements of numbers of peripheral blood lymphocytes give little information of lymphocyte production because addition to and removal from the blood of lymphocytes are going on simultaneously. I do not have a quantitative number to give you. However, a tumor-bearing animal is probably in a degree of adrenal stress. Depending upon the degree of the latter, lymphoid cell populations in the tumor-bearing animal would be fewer in number. Thus, lymphoid cells available to participate in immunological phenomena could be significantly reduced. This is true in undernourished animals because of non-specific pituitary adrenal-cortical stimulation resulting from caloric deprivation.

J. Schultz: Thank you.

M. M. Sigel, University of Miami School of Medicine: There appears to be a dichotomy in the effect of estrogens on the intact thymus and on the peripheral T cells. As you indicated, __in vivo__ estrogens cause proliferation and increas-ing function of the thymus but __in vitro__ estrogen causes a decrease in lymphocytes response to mitogens. This was found in several laboratories including ours (studies by Dr. Rippe and Mrs. Meltz). This has also been found the sera of pregnant women and block cellular responses. Thus what may work in the intact thymus may not hold for T cells.

A. White: In your in vitro studies, were physiological concentrations of estradiol used? In vivo, and in the pregnant woman, estrogens are not only present in elevated concentrations, but also progesterone levels are higher than normal. Progresterone may be immunosuppressive.

M.M. Sigel: Well, actually the concentrations that were effective in vitro were as low as one microgram. We have not tested the effect of progesterone.

L. Muschal, American Cancer Society: Is it fair to say Dr. White, that thymosin can account for the entire activity of the thymus gland?

A. White: As of today, the answer is no. As many of you are aware, several laboratories have described purified or partially purified cell-free products extracted from calf thymus tissue. Each of these has been reported to function in one or more of the several models in which thymosin is also active. The molecules from calf thymus have been described with molecular weights ranging from 3,200 to 70,000. In addition, Dr. J.F. Bach has purified from pig serum a polypeptide of molecular weight approximately 1200, which has thymosin-like activity. These data are the basis for my suggesting, in my presentation, that a family of thymic hormones may exist. Perhaps more than a single thymic product may be required to mimic completely all of the immunological functions assigned to the thymus and to thymus-derived T-cells.

P. Alexander, Chester Beatty Research Institute: Dr. White, is the thymus stimulating hormone growth hormones or a related pituitary hormone which is trophic for the thymus?

A. White: The data with growth hormone preparations of varying degrees of purity indicate that both in vitro and in vivo growth hormone stimulates lymphoid cell proliferation. Dr. Talwar and his colleagues in New Delhi have demonstrated a stimulatory effect of growth hormone on thymocyte metabolism. Also, in vivo, the administration of growth hormone to hypophysectomized animals with a lower than normal capacity to make antibody stimulates the synthesis of antibody in these animals. There may be a compensatory action of other endocrine systems in vivo, i.e., in the dwarf due to thyroid insufficiency and in the acromegalic.

P. Alexander: I know that the growth hormone preparations worked in your systems, but such preparations are not pure and they could contain in addition a thymus-trophic hormone.

A. White: You are correct. Until the postulated thymotropic action has been demonstrated with a growth hormone preparation of unequivocal purity, the assignment of this property to growth hormone is premature. However, more recent studies, for example those from Dr. Talwar's laboratory, have utilized a highly purified growth hormone preparation. It may be of interest to study this problem with the product obtained by partial proteolysis of growth hormine, described by Dr. Martin Sonnenberg and confirmed recently by Dr. C.H. Li.

TRANSFER FACTOR AND CANCER

H. SHERWOOD LAWRENCE
Infectious Disease and Immunology Division
Department of Medicine
New York University School of Medicine

Abstract: Transfer Factor (TF_D) is a dialysable ($<10,000$ M.W.) non-antigenic, non-toxic moiety prepared from lymphocytes of immune donors that selectively restores and/or augments both specific and non-specific DTH and CMI responses in recipients without concomitant Ig production. Application of TF_D as immunotherapy for a broad category of disease syndromes characterized by deficient cellular immunity (congenital immunodeficiency diseases; intracellular microbial and viral infections; "autoimmune" states and metastatic cancer) has resulted in immunologic improvement in 2/3 and clinical improvement in 1/2 of this group of patients. There is little question about the causal relationship of TF_D administration to the restoration of cellular immunity documented in such patients, nevertheless the early promise of clinical improvement remains to be substantiated by the results of properly controlled clinical trials.

INTRODUCTION:

In the preceding chapters various facets of the immunological plight of the tumor bearing patient have been delineated and the promise offered by a diversity of immunotherapeutic approaches has been summarized. Certainly there is something for everyone, particularly immunologists, in this catalogue either relating to the pathogenesis or to the treatment of cancer. This may be a good thing since at the very least it has brought a great deal of additional interest, activity and new viewpoints to focus on a complicated and evasive problem, even though the achievements to date have been either modest or disappointing. Still it is a beginning and even categorical basic science has a way of converging in the end on the in vivo realities to which we give a name and call disease. In this atmosphere of restrained optimism we plan to summarize briefly the recent application of Transfer Factor to the immunotherapy of cancer.

BACKGROUND -- BIOLOGICAL PROPERTIES OF TF

Transfer Factor (TF) is a convenient descriptive designation of the material or materials present in the circulating leukocytes of immune human donors that will confer cellular immunity upon non-immune individuals. This activity is present in viable cell-populations (1) as well as in leukocyte extracts (2). Although the precise identity of the cell population which possesses TF activity is unknown (e.g.T-cell, B-cell, macrophages), crude approaches have revealed that the activity resides in mononuclear cells that do not adhere to glass (3) nor to nylon (4). This conclusion has been supported by most recent work on this problem which has employed Ficoll-Hypaque purified mononuclear cell suspensions (95% Lymphocytes - 5% Monocytes) for the preparation of TF for in vivo use.

TF can be separated from the macromolecules of the disrupted mononuclear cells that bear it by dialysis through a cellophane sac and the dialysate can be concentrated by lyophilization (5). Further purification of the active moiety in raw leukocyte dialysates can be achieved by Sephadex (G-25) fractionation with the isolation of a peak that contains the biological activity (5-7). The most recent application of Sephadex chromatography has demonstrated the immunologic specificity of TF isolated as a single narrow peak that is more potent in vivo than the raw dialysate which may contain inhibitors of this activity (8). Thus TF has emerged as a non-antigenic, non-immunoglobulin moiety of $<$10,000 M.W. which is comprised of a peptide-nucleotide complex and is possessed of immunologic specificity (9, 10). Moreover, administration of TF to patients with deficient or absent cellular immunity has revealed that certain non-specific consequences ensue (e.g. augmented PHA, E-rosette, and MLC responses) indicating that a general augmentation of cell-mediated immunity (CMI) occurs (11-13). This result accrues in addition to the transfer of antigen-specific cutaneous DTH and CMI in vivo with concurrent lymphocyte transformation and lymphokine production (e.g. MIF, lymphotoxin, interferon) upon exposure of recipient lymphocytes to specific antigens in vitro (14-16).

Of further interest is the observation that TF has only resulted in the transfer of DTH and CMI and has not been found capable of transferring antibody production to the same antigenic determinants (e.g. diphtheria toxoid) to which DTH has been transferred (17). Nevertheless, in view of the overall augmentation of CMI that is induced by TF it is probable that facilitation of T-B cell cooperation does ensue indirectly, and this event may affect host antibody production to environmental antigens in general.

The extensive experience with TF as a potent, non-toxic immune reagent that selectively initiates, restores and/or augments CMI in humans has encouraged its recent application to the immunotherapy of a variety of disease syndromes that result as a consequence of or are associated with depressed DTH and CMI (18).

IMMUNOTHERAPY WITH DIALYSABLE TRANSFER FACTOR (TF$_D$)

The clinical experience with TF$_D$ immunotherapy is still largely fragmentary and anecdotal in nature and the current approaches are of necessity empirical. The variables encountered in the regimens employed from clinic to clinic, from country to country and from disease to disease are, of course, considerable (19). Moreover, the patients that have been selected for this new experimental therapeutic agent are either gravely or terminally ill and have been subject to all conventional therapeutic modalities without effect on the relentless course of their disease. In this bleak setting it is surprising that TF$_D$ is effective in restoring immunological competence in two-thirds of the patients treated, let alone resulting in clinical improvement in one-half (10).

Nevertheless, a general principle is beginning to emerge from such diverse, yet cumulative experience which would suggest that the administration of TF$_D$ may be expected to benefit those patients suffering from disease syndromes that either result directly from or indirectly cause depressed or absent CMI responses (19).

The diseases that have responded favorably and for which the administration of TF$_D$ shows promise for further exploitation are the congenital immunodeficiency syndromes, disseminated intracellular infections, certain diseases with intimations of autoimmunity and certain metastatic malignancies.

Congenital Immunodeficiency Disease

The congenital immunodeficiency syndromes that have been reconstituted for CMI responses by TF$_D$ include the Wiskott-Aldrich Syndrome (14, 20); Swiss type Agammaglobulinemia (21), Ataxia Telangiectasia (11); and Severe Combined Immuno-deficiency Disease (22, 23).

These patients generally acquire antigen-specific cutaneous DTH responses and CMI in vivo, as well as MIF production and/or lymphocyte transformation in vitro concordant with immune reactivity of the TF$_D$ donor. In addition, such patients have experienced a general non-specific augmentation of CMI as evidenced by the restoration of lymphocyte respon-siveness to PHA, to sheep RBC and to Mixed Leukocyte Culture reactivity in vitro and acquisition of the capacity to recognize and respond to environmental antigens (e.g. DNCB sensitization) in vivo. Concomitant with the restoration of CMI responses such patients have also experienced general clinical improvement, mainly related to the eradication of the indigent infections that beset them (14, 24, 25).

Intracellular Infectious Disease

The disseminated intracellular infections that have responded to TF$_D$ administration are those of viral, fungal and mycobacterial origin. The Viral infections include giant cell measles pneumonia, and congenital herpes simplex (26); herpes zoster in immunosupressed Hodgkins Disease (27), chronic active hepatitis (28, 29) and chicken pox pneumonia (30). The fungal infections include chronic mucocutaneous candidiasis (31-35), disseminated coccidioidomycosis (15, 36-37); and histoplasmosis (38). The mycobacterial infections include lepromatous leprosy (39), and systemic tuberculosis (40, 41).

In this category of disease the patients are usually anergic to the antigens of the replicating infectious agent and exhibit a general depression of CMI responses in the face of brisk and sustained humoral antibody production. Following administration of TF$_D$ there ensues the restoration of cutaneous DTH in vivo, as well as lymphocyte transforma-tion and/or lymphokine production in vitro to the antigens of the infectious agent. A variable degree of general clinical improvement and either suppression or eradication of the infectious agent is associated with or occurs subsequent to this augmentation and/or restoration of CMI responses.

The immune adaptation of patients faced with such massive antigen-overload consequent to dissemination of replicating microbes may be viewed as a state analagous to "high-zone" tolerance and it is possible that TF_D administration in augmenting CMI selectively results in a concomitant decrease in the microbial population may break such tolerance. There may be some analogy between this type of host-parasite relationship and that encountered in the tumor-bearing host similarly confronted with a replicating antigen (42).

"Autoimmune" Disease Syndromes

There is a group of disease syndromes where TF_D immunotherapy has been attempted and variable degrees of clinical improvement observed. These syndromes share in common certain clinical and laboratory stigmata of autoimmunity thought to be a consequence of chronic indolent infection perhaps of viral origin. This group includes: Subacute Sclerosing Panencephalitis (SSPE) associated with measles virus (26, 43, 44); chronic active hepatitis (28, 29); multiple sclerosis (45-47); Juvenile Rheumatoid Arthritis (48); and Behçet's Syndrome (49).

Rationale for TF_D Immunotherapy of Cancer

In addition to its demonstrable lack of toxicity (50,51), the paucity of untoward reactions (20, 52) and the potency of TF_D in restoring and/or augmenting CMI responses one should consider what, if any, rationale should guide the choice of TF_D for immunotherapy of malignancy.

As for any other type of immunotherapy, the effectiveness of this approach also depends greatly upon the interpretation of the immunological relationship of the tumor to the host and the nature and significance of the host's immune response to the tumor. Two questions are critical in this regard: 1) is the tumor really an allograft that exhibits tumor specific transplantation antigens that differ, however weakly, from the HLA antigens of the host? and 2) if such is the case, is the host making a sustained yet ineffective immune response to the tumor as suggested by the work of the Hellström's (53) whereby circulating tumor

301

antigen-antibody complexes (and antigen) that blindfold reactive lymphocytes and camouflage tumor target cells to
thwart recognition and rejection of the tumor?

If the tumor really functions as an allograft in vivo
then the fact that TF has been shown in humans to confer the
capacity for accelerated allograft rejection from immune to
non-immune normal individuals (54) becomes germane to the
rationale of its exploration in tumor immunotherapy. Briefly,
these studies indicated that in nature one individual does
not normally possess a TF vs. another individual's allograft
antigens. However, immunization of the prospective TF donor
with skin allografts from another individual (A) resulted in
the de novo appearance of leukocytes bearing a TF specific
for the tissues of A. The injection of such allograft-
specific anti-A TF of immune leukocyte extracts into non-
immune individuals resulted only in the accelerated rejection
of skin allografts obtained from A, but not allografts from
other individuals that were resident in the same individual.

Additionally, in individuals where allograft-specific
TF was effective in causing accelerated rejection of the
related target graft; non-specific TF was not effective and
immune serum was not effective. These results do provide
clues to a strategy for tumor immunotherapy, but they cannot
be extrapolated in toto since, unlike an allograft, the tumor
is an invasive, replicating, autonomous colony of cells and
the foreign histocompatibility mosaics expressed by the tumor,
when present, are weak antigens that are subject to constant
modulation by the host.

Hence, if the replicating colony of cells that comprise
the tumor possess surface antigens that are foreign to the
host, and if the main immunologic deficiency arises from
exuberant antibody production and depressed CMI, then TF_D
may be expected to restore and augment CMI to tumor specific
antigens selectively without concomitant transfer of antibody production.

Background Studies on the Transfer of Microbial DTH to Cancer Patients:

A. Using Viable Cells Muftuoglu and Balkuv (55)
demonstrated successful transfer of cutaneous DTH to tuberculin to 3 of 4 patients with acute leukemia; 2 of 2

patients with chronic myeloid leukemia; 3 of 4 patients with lymphosarcoma and 2 of 2 patients with carcinoma. In this series 21 of 22 patients with Hodgkins disease failed to respond to transfer of tuberculin DTH. Good et al (56) had reported earlier on the failure to transfer DTH to 13 of 13 patients with Hodgkins disease, as did Fazio and Calciati (57) in 7 of 7 patients.

It should be noted that these failures to transfer cutaneous DTH to patients with Hodgkin's disease were probably the result of giving an inadequate dose of TF in viable cells on only one occasion. Subsequent studies by Drew et al (27) employed a single injection of TF_D prepared from 7.5×10^8 cells of a donor immune to Herpes Zoster and reported on the recovery from disseminated Zoster infection in an immunosuppressed patient with Hodgkin's disease. In addition to the initial inflammatory response exhibited by the herpetic lesions in response to TF_D administration, the latter began to heal and the viral cultures became negative coincident with the onset of reactivity to Zoster antigen and PHA in the patient's lymphocytes.

Hattler and Amos (4) studied the response of 18 patients with advanced malignancy employing the technique of "local transfer" and using nylon column purified 90 - 98% lymphocytes. They achieved successful transfer in 17 of 18 patients to a variety of antigens (mumps, trichophytin, candida, tuberculin and histoplasmin). The recipients responded only to those antigens to which the donor reacted and not to antigens to which the donor did not react.

B. Using Dialysable Transfer Factor (TF_D): Our laboratory (58) conducted an early prospective study on the incidence of anergy and its meaning in 150 cancer patients and 80 control patients who were skin tested with a battery of antigens (SK-SK, PPD, Diphtheria Toxoid, Histoplasmin, coccidioidin and mumps).

Of passing interest, it was observed that 110 of 150 cancer patients were anergic to all skin test antigens used whereas 66 of 80 control subjects reacted to at least one of the battery of antigens used. When correlated with the presence or absence of metastases, 94 of the 110 anergic cancer patients (85%) had evidence of metastases at subsequent operation, whereas 29 of 40 cancer patients who had expressed a DTH response to one or more antigens had no evidence of metastasis.

The effect of dialysable Transfer Factor (TF_D) administered to 10 cancer patients anergic to all antigens was studied, using donors sensitive to SK-SD and the technique of local transfer. In 10 of 10 such anergic cancer patients each responded with vigorous cutaneous DTH following injection of SK-SD atop the local site of TF_D deposition. However, the intensity of systemic transfer was feeble (1+ reaction to SK-SD challenge at remote skin site) and, unlike the response of normal individuals, was not enduring.

These early studies provided background information suggesting that patients with a wide variety of metastatic malignancies possess the cell populations and the immunologic capacity to respond to transfer of cutaneous DTH either when viable leukocytes were used as vehicles of TF or when the partially purified product of such cells, dialysable Transfer Factor (TF_D) is administered. Implicit in such findings was the promise that should a tumor-specific TF_D be administered to cancer patients, the transfer of tumor immunity may be anticipated.

Immunotherapy of Metastatic Malignancy with TF_D

The application of TF_D to the immunotherapy of metastatic malignancy is just about getting underway and this is not the place to go into extensive clinical detail. Suffice it to say, that TF_D administration does augment the CMI responses of the patient toward his tumor antigens. In some instances such immunological improvement is associated with regression of the metastases and general improvement of the patients clinical state for variable periods of time. The patients in this mixed group that have been treated with TF_D share in common the clinical designation of advanced metastatic malignancy that has not responded to the gamut of conventional therapeutic modalities and for whom no other therapy is available. With these limitations in mind we list below the different types of cancer in which evaluation of TF_D immunotherapy is currently under assessment.

Breast Cancer - Effects of Pooled "non-specific" TF_D

With colleagues at the Sloan-Kettering Institute we undertook a collaborative study to assess the therapeutic potential and safety of TF_D administration to patients with cancer (50, 51). For this study 5 patients with advanced metastatic breast cancer of the "inflammatory" type were given pooled TF_D obtained from blood leukocytes of 177 normal women over 45 years of age. It was assumed that some of the healthy donors in this category may have met and responded to mutant neoplastic breast cells via immune surveillance from puberty onwards and thereby possess tumor-specific TF_D in memory of that event.

For this purpose TF_D was administered in doses of 1-4 ml. dialysate subcutaneous daily or three times weekly for periods ranging from 21 to 310 days. The total dose of TF_D given to individual patients was equivalent 20 to 257 ml. of packed WBC (20 ml. = 17 Billion Cells). Either tuberculin (PPD) or SK-SD cutaneous reactivity in the donors were used as markers and the respective DTH was transferred to 3 of 5 patients. Only 1 of the 5 patients was observed to have a temporary remission of the breast lesions which lasted for 6 months before relapse.

TF_D given repeatedly in such large doses did not cause any inflammatory or hypersensitivity reactions, nor were any hematological, biochemical or enzymatic abnormalities detected, or other harmful side effects observed. There were no changes detected in immunoglobulin levels (IgM, IgA, IgG) nor were antibodies detected to 24 human leukocyte antigens for which tests were performed and neither AU antigen nor AU antibodies were detected in these recipients of pooled TF_D.

From this limited study no conclusions can be drawn concerning the efficacy or potential usefulness of "pooled" non-specific TF_D as immunotherapy for breast cancer. Nevertheless, the data do allow the conclusion that TF_D itself is a non-toxic preparation that can be administered to patients with safety in large doses (257 ml. TF_D equivalent to 217 Billion Cells) repeatedly (125 injections) and over prolonged periods of time (310 days). The therapeutic margin of safety is therefore wide, in view of the fact that the average dose of TF_D currently used to treat infectious or immunodeficiency diseases effectively is prepared from 1×10^9 lymphocytes.

Malignant Melanoma - Effects of Tumor Specific TF

Brandes et al (59) sensitized melanoma patient A with melanoma tissue from patient B to serve as a source of tumor-specific TF. Following the subcutaneous injection of TF from frozen and thawed leukocyte extracts, patient B responded vigorously to his metastatic tumor nodules both locally and systemically. The local response consisted of inflammation and rejection of the tumor nodules in the skin and was of greater intensity in sites where leukocyte extract had been injected locally. The patient also experienced a systemic febrile response and the appearance of lymphobasts in his circulation. He died subsequently of brain hemorrhage.

Spitler et al (60) made the interesting observation that family contacts of melanoma patients possessed lymphocyte reactivity (transformation, MIF production) to the patients melanoma antigens. They prepare dialysable melanoma - specific transfer factor (TF_D) from such family contacts and administered it to 9 corresponding patients with malignant melanoma. Only 2 of the 9 patients responded immunologically with acquisition of lymphocyte transformation to their re-spective tumor antigens and clinically with regression of tumor lesions. One patient remained free of metastatic lesions for 7 months but developed new metastatic lesions 1-1/2 years later coincident with loss of lymphocyte trans-formation and MIF production to tumor antigens despite con-tinued administration of TF_D.

Morse et al (61) have also reported on regression of lesions and reactions of tumor rejection in 4 of 10 melanoma patients treated with melanoma-specific TF_D. Their source of TF_D was the leukocytes of cancer patients that had been sensitized to the prospective transfer factor recipient's killed tumor tissue.

Osteogenic Sarcoma - Effects of Tumor Specific TF_D

Levin et al (62, 25) have compared the effects of administration of tumor-specific TF_D with those of non-specific TF_D in the immunotherapy of 12 patients with osteogenic sarcoma. They observed immunologic improvement (i.e. lymphocyte mediated cytotoxicity vs. osteogenic sarcoma cultures,increased numbers of E-Rosettes, lymphocytic infil-trates and inflammatory reactions induced around metastatic lesions) to occur in such patients only after the administration of osteogenic sarcoma specific TF_D. When these effects of one dose of TF_D had waned with the passage of time, the same patient was given an equivalent dose of non-specific TF_D which produced no immunological improvement. However, upon repeat administration of osteogenic sarcoma specific TF_D to the same patient, the immunologic improvement noted above was restored. The authors conclude that administration of tumor-specific TF_D resulted in an increase of tumor-specific lymphocyte-mediated cytotoxicity and administration of non-specific TF_D was associated with a decrease in cytotoxic activity of the patient's lymphocytes. TF_D specific for osteogenic sarcoma was prepared from the lymphocytes of domiciliary relatives of the respective index case who had demonstrable lymphocyte-mediated cytotoxicity when tested vs. osteogenic sarcoma cell lines.

The clinical response in 8 of 12 patients has been favorable as assessed by regression of metastases and no new metastatic disease. Although 4 of the 8 patients in this group have been followed from 10 - 20 months and 4 have been followed 3 - 8 months, it is still early to reach definite conclusions. Of the remaining 4 patients: 1 patient exhibited no response; 1 patient experienced a remission and died 7 months after TF_D administration had ceased and 2 patients died with extensive pulmonary metastases.

Neidhart and Lo Buglio (63) have reported tumor-specific TF_D administration to a patient with osteogenic sarcoma whose pulmonary metastases disappeared after 4 months of adriamycin and diimidazolecarboxamide therapy. Osteogenic-sarcoma specific TF_D was prepared from the patient's father. Chemotherapy was discontinued and tumor-specific TF_D administered to the patient in doses of 15 units (1 unit = 10^8 lymphocytes) every 2 weeks. This regimen resulted in the initial transfer of KLH sensitivity in vivo and in vitro which had been used as a marker and subsequent development of MIF production by the patient's lymphocytes versus her own tumor antigens. The patient remains free of disease 17 months following initiation of TF_D therapy.

Earlier, Lo Buglio's (64) group had treated a patient with alveolar sarcoma resistant to chemotherapy with tumor-specific TF_D obtained from an identical twin and demonstrated the transfer of tumor-specific immunity to the patient (MIF production in the presence of patient's tumor antigens) after two injections of 15 units of TF_D. The MIF production was

307

transient and after a third injection of TF_D remained positive for 3 weeks. The patient gained weight, became asymptomatic and refused further therapy. The pulmonary lesions
remained stable for a year thereafter, but at 14 months the
disease flared and he died.

Acute Lymphocytic Leukemia
Effects of Leukemia-Specific TF_D

Neidhart and Lo Buglio (63) have treated 5 patients with
acute lymphocytic leukemia with tumor-specific TF_D obtained
from domiciliary family members that exhibit a positive MIF
test to the respective patients leukemia antigens. Two of
the 5 patients developed transiently positive MIF tests to
their own leukemia antigens, yet none of the patients have
responded clinically. The authors suggest the failure to
respond to TF_D may be related to the known immunosuppresive
effects of the chemotherapy on which the patients were maintained.

Nasopharyngeal Carcinoma
Effects of E-B virus specific TF_D

Goldenberg and Brandes (65) prepared TF_D from E-B virus
positive adults who had recovered from Infectious mononucleosis and administered it to 2 patients with refractory
Nasopharyngeal carcinoma. Following TF_D administration
tumor regression was observed in both patients. In one
patient the clinical improvement was associated with lymphocytic infiltration in the tumor biopsy, conversion of
cutaneous DTH to tuberculin and to T. Rubrum and a fall in
antibody titer to viral capsid antigen of the E-B virus. In
the second patient the tumor regression was temporary.

Under the auspices of the Canadian National Research
Council, Goldenberg and Brandes are conducting a double-
blind field trial of TF_D immunotherapy of Nasopharyngeal
carcinoma in Hong Kong where this disease is endemic.

GENERAL COMMENT

As may be seen from this mere recital of anecdotes the
application of TF_D to the immunotherapy of cancer has just
about begun and no conclusions can be reached. The augmentation of immunological responses following administration of

TF_D ensues with regularity yet clinical improvement, when it occurs, is transient and unpredictable. This should come as no surprise, since the whole enterprise is at a crude, empirical level and the patients selected are at the end-stage of a disease that has proved refractory to conventional therapy.

The promise afforded by TF_D administration rests solely on its established capacity to selectively augment cell-mediated immunity to the tumor-specific antigens of the host without concomitant antibody production and with relative safety over a wide range of dosage schedules. In addition to the transfer of tumor-specific immunity, the fact that TF_D also results in a non-specific boost of cell-mediated immune responses in general, could be construed as an added benefit.

Only time and carefully controlled clinical trials may provide the firm data upon which the role of TF_D in the immunotherapy of cancer can be decided (66-68). Although an appreciation of the potential of TF took two decades to reach the present stage of awareness, the momentum derived from the current pace of basic investigations (69, 70) as well as clinical applications (66-68) makes it likely that future progress will proceed at an accelerated rate.

The author's work has been supported by: The National Institute of Allergy and Infectious Diseases Research Grant AI-01254-19, Training Grant AI-00005-16 and the National Cancer Institute Program Project 1 P01-CA-16247-01.

BIBLIOGRAPHY

1. Lawrence, H.S. Proc. Soc. Exp. Biol. and Med.
    71 (1949) 516.

2. Lawrence, H.S. J. Clin. Invest. 34 (1955) 219.

3. Slavin, R.G. and J.E. Garvin. Science 145 (1964) 52.

4. Hattler, B.G. and D.B. Amos. J. Nat. Cancer Inst.
    35 (1964) 927.

5. Lawrence, H.S., S. Al-Askari, J. David, E.C. Franklin,
    and B. Zweiman. Trans. Assoc. Amer. Physicians
    76 (1963) 84.

6. Neidhart, J.A., R.S. Schwartz, P.E. Hurtubise,
    S.G. Murphy, E.N. Metz, S.P. Balcerzak, and
    A.F. Lo Buglio. Cell. Immunol. 9 (1973) 319.

7. Gottlieb, A.A., L.G. Foster, S.R. Waldman, and
    M. Lopez. Lancet 2 (1973) 822.

8. Zuckerman, K.S., J.S. Neidhart, S.P. Balcerzak and
    A.F. Lo Buglio. J. Clin. Invest. 54 (1974) 997.

9. Lawrence, H.S. Advan. Immunol. 11 (1969) 195.

10. Lawrence, H.S. Harvey Lect. Series 68,
    (Academic Press, New York 1974) p. 239.

11. Griscelli, C., J.P. Revillard, H. Beutel, C. Herzog,
    and J.L. Touraine. Biomedicine 18 (1973) 220.

12. Wybran, J., A.S. Levin, L.E. Spitler and H.H. Fudenberg.
    N. Engl. J. Med. 228 (1973) 710.

13. DuPont, B., M. Ballow, J.A. Hansen, C. Quick, E.J. Yunis
    and R.A. Good. Proc. Natl. Acad. Sci. (USA)
    71 (1974) 867.

14. Spitler, L.E., A.S. Levin, D.P. Stites, H.H. Fudenberg,
    B. Pirofsky, C.S. August, E.R. Stiehm, W.H. Hitzig
    and R.A. Gatti. J. Clin. Invest. 51 (1972) 3216.

15. Cloninger, P., L.D. Thrupp, G.A. Granger, and H.S. Novey. West. J. Med. 120 (1974) 322.

16. Emodi, G., M. Just and P. Grob. Lancet 2 (1973) 1382.

17. Lawrence, H.S. and A.M. Pappenheimer, Jr. J. Exp. Med. 104 (1956) 321.

18. Lawrence, H.S. New Engl. J. Med. 283 (1970) 411.

19. Lawrence, H.S., In: Clinical Immunobiology, Vol. 2, ed. F.H. Bach and R.A. Good. (Academic Press, New York, 1974) p. 115.

20. Ballow, M., B. Dupont and R.A. Good. J. Pediat. 83 (1973) 772.

21. Hitzig, W.H., H.P. Fontanellaz, U. Muntener, S. Paul, L.E. Spitler and H.H. Fudenberg. Schweiz. Med. Wochenschr. 102 (1972) 1237.

22. Mogerman, S.N., A.S. Levin, L.E. Spitler, D P. Stites, H.H. Fudenberg and H.R. Shinefeld. Clin. Res. 21 (1973) 310.

23. Montgomery, J.R., M.A. South, R. Wilson, E. Richie, L.R. Heim, S. Criswell and J.J. Trentin. Clin. Res. 21 (1973) 118.

24. Levin, A.S., L.E. Spitler and H.H. Fudenberg. Annu. Rev. Med. 24 (1973) 175.

25. Fudenberg, H.H., A.S. Levin, L.E. Spitler, J. Wybran and V. Byers. Hosp. Pract. 9 (1974) 95.

26. Moulias, R., J.M. Goust, P. Reinert, J.J. Fournel, A. Deville-Chabrolle, N. Duong, C.N. Muller-Berat and P. Berthaux. Nouv. Presse Med. 2 (1973) 1341.

27. Drew, W.L., M.R. Blume, R. Miner, I. Silverberg and E.H. Rosenbaum. Ann. Int. Med. 79 (1973) 747.

28. Kohler, P.F., J. Trembath, D.A. Merrill, J.W. Singleton and R.S. DuBois. Clin. Immunol. and Immunopath. 2 (1974) 465.

29. Shulman, S., M. Schulkind and E. Ayoub. Lancet
    2 (1974) 650.

30. Nitschke, R., S. Oleinick, G.B. Humphrey, J. Lankford
    and R. Orr. Clin. Res. 23 (1975) 68A.

31. Schulkind, M.L., W.H. Adler, W.A. Altemeir and
    E.M. Ayoub. Cell. Immunol. 3 (1972) 606.

32. Pabst, H.F. and R. Swanson. Brit. Med. J. 2 (1972) 442.

33. Kirkpatrick, C.H., R.R. Rich and T.K. Smith.
    J. Clin. Invest. 51 (1972) 2948.

34. Valdimarsson, H., C.B.S. Wood, J.R. Hobbs and
    P.J.L. Holt. Clin. Exp. Immunol. 11 (1972) 151.

35. Bläker, F., P.J. Grob, H.H. Hellwege and
    K.H. Schulz. Dtsch. Med. Wschr. 98 (1973) 415.

36. Graybill, J.R., J. Silva, R.H. Alford and D.E. Thor.
    Cell. Immunol. 8 (1973) 120.

37. Cantanzaro, A., L. Spitler and K.M. Moser.
    J. Clin. Invest. 54 (1974) 690.

38. Smith, C.R., D. Griffith, K. Baughman and J.R. Graybill.
    Clin. Res. 22 (1974) 708A.

39. Bullock, W.E., J.P. Fields and M.W. Brandriss.
    N. Engl. J. Med. 287 (1972) 1053.

40. Whitcomb, M.E. and R.E. Rocklin. Ann. Int. Med.
    79 (1973) 161.

41. Thestrup-Pedersen, K., H. Thulin and H. Zachariae.
    Acta Allergol. 29 (1974) 101.

42. Lawrence, H.S. in: Clinical Immunobiology, Vol. 1,
    ed. F.H. Bach and R.A. Good. (Academic Press,
    New York, 1973) p. 48.

43. Vandvik, B., S.S. Froland, H.M. Hoyeraal, R. Stien and
    M. Degre. Scand. J. Immunol. 2 (1973) 367.

44. Valdimarsson, H., G. Agnarsdottir and P.J. Lachman.
    Proc. Roy. Soc. Med. 67 (1974) 1125.

45. Jersild, C., P. Platz, M. Thomsen, G.S. Hansen,
    A. Svejgaard, B. DuPont, T. Fog, A.K. Ciongoli and
    P. Grob. Lancet 2 (1973) 1382.

46. Utermohlen, V. and J. Zabriskie. J. Exp. Med.
    138 (1973) 159.

47. Platz, P., B. DuPont, T. Fog, L. Ryder, M. Thomsen,
    A. Svejgaard and C. Jersild. Proc. Roy. Soc. Med.
    67 (1974) 1133.

48. Kass, E., S.S. Froland, J.B. Natvig, P. Blichfeldt,
    H.M. Hoyeraal and E. Munthe. Scand. J. Rheumat.
    3 (1974) 113.

49. Denman, A.M. in: Infectious Agents in Rheumatic
    Diseases ed. D.C. Dumonde (Blackwell, Oxford 1975)
    in press.

50. Oettgen, H.F., L.J. Old, J.H. Farrow, F.T. Valentine,
    H.S. Lawrence and L. Thomas. J. Clin. Invest.
    50 (1971) 71A.

51. Oettgen, H.F., L.J. Old, J.H. Farrow, F.T. Valentine,
    H.S. Lawrence and L. Thomas. Proc. Natl. Acad. Sci.
    (USA) 71 (1974) 2319.

52. Gelfand, E.W., R. Baumal, J. Huber, M.C. Crookston and
    K.H. Shumak. New Engl. J. Med. 289 (1973) 1385.

53. Hellström, K.E. and I. Hellström. Annu. Rev. Microbiol.
    24 (1970) 373.

54. Lawrence, H.S., F.T. Rapaport, J.M. Converse and
    W.S. Tillett. J. Clin. Invest. 39 (1960) 185.

55. Muftuoglu, A.U. and S. Balkuv. N. Engl. J. Med.
    277 (1967) 126.

56. Good, R.A., W.D. Kelly, J. Rotstein and R.L. Varco.
    Progr. Allergy 6 (1962) 187.

57. Fazio, M. and A. Calciati. Panminerva Med. 4 (1962) 164.

58. Solowey, A.C., F.T. Rapaport and H.S. Lawrence in:
    Histocompatibility Testing (S. Karger, Basel, 1967)
    p. 75.

59. Brandes, L., D.A.G. Galton and E. Wiltshaw. Lancet
    2 (1971) 293.

60. Spitler, L.E., J. Wybran, H.H. Fudenberg, A.S. Levin and
    M. Lewis. Clin. Res. 21 (1973) 221.

61. Morse, P.A., G.D. Deraps, G.V. Smith, S. Raju and
    J.D. Hardy. Clin. Res. 21 (1973) 71.

62. Levin, A.S., V.S. Byers, H.H. Fudenberg, J. Wybran,
    A.J. Hackett and J.O. Johnston. J. Clin. Invest.
    1975 in press.

63. Neidhart, J.A. and A.F. Lo Buglio. in: Seminars in
    Oncology, Vol. 1 ed. J. Yarbro (Grune and Stratton,
    New York, 1974) p. 379.

64. Lo Buglio, A.F., J.F. Neidhart, R.W. Hilberg, E.N. Metz
    and S.P. Balcerzak. Cell. Immunol. 7 (1973) 159.

65. Goldenberg, G. and L. Brandes. Clin. Res. 20 (1972) 947.

66. Editorial. Transfer Factor. Lancet 2 (1973) 79

67. Editorial. Transfer Factor. Brit. Med. J. II
    (1974) 397.

68. Valdimarsson, H. Workshop on Transfer Factor:
    Clinical Application in: Progress in Immunology II
    Vol. 5 ed. L. Brent and J. Holbrow (American-
    Elsevier, New York, 1974) p. 377.

69. Kirkpatrick, C.H. and D. Rifkind. Meeting Report on
    Basic Properties and Clinical Applications of
    Transfer Factor. Cell. Immunol. 10 (1974) 165.

70. Gottlieb, A.A. Workshop on Transfer Factor: Biological
    Properties in: Progress in Immunology II Vol. 5 ed.
    L. Brent and J. Holbrow (American-Elsevier, New York,
    1974) p. 371.

DISCUSSION

M. Cohn, Salk Institute: The experiment that is critical to understanding "transfer factor" is the one which you transfer the specificity to an HLA determinant assayed by an accelerated rejection of a skin graft; however, in that experiment the cycle is not completed because the source of transfer factor is an extract of peritoneal leukocytes made by freezing and thawing, but it is not one that has been purified further by separation through the dialysis tubing. So the question that I have to ask you is: do you have two low molecular weight substances below 10,000 molecular weight which will distinguish specifically two HLA types.

H.S. Lawrence, New York University School of Medicine: The answer is no. We did, however, elucidate additional information on this point in subsequent studies in humans where ultracentrifugal fractions of leukocyte extracts (mitochondria, microsomes, endoplasmic reticulum) were observed to actively immunize naive individuals to skin allografts obtained from the leukocyte donor. (Rapaport, F.T., Dausset, J., Converse, J.M. and Lawrence, H.S., Transplantation 3 (1965) 490). This HL-A antigenic activity of leukocyte extracts was found to be non-dialysable and repeated injection of materials in the dialysate failed to immunize individuals to the skin allograft of the leukocyte donor. In the allograft system then we were able to separate the HL-A antigens from the dialysable constituents of leukocytes-of which TF_D is one.

M. Cohn: Yes, that I would expect; that's all right. Now, let me ask you this question, in the case where transfer factor of low molecular weight has been used, that is dialyzable, do you have any examples, where an autoimmune response is provoked in that individual? I would expect a generally heightened cell mediated responsiveness which should lead to autoimmunity in some cases.

H.S. Lawrence: An example of this may be found in the observations of Griscelli et al. (Biomedicine 18 (1973) 220) made in children with congenital immunodeficiency who could not respond to DNCB sensitization before TF administration yet did respond after TF$_D$, despite the fact that the TF$_D$ donors were unreactive to DNCB. This result has been interpreted to document the non-specificity of TF$_D$. However, transfer of DNCB sensitivity from negative donors seems unlikely since TF$_D$ obtained from donors with marked sensitivity to both DNCB and tuberculin has been found to transfer cutaneous DTH only to tuberculin but not to DNCB when given to the same recipient (Brandriss, M.W., J. Clin. Invest. 47 (1968) 2152). Eisen has reported identical results using leukocyte extracts to transfer tuberculin but not DNCB sensitivity despite the donor's exquisite sensitivity to both PPD and DNCB (Eisen, H.N. IN: 3EDIATORS OF CELLULAR IMMUNITY, Ed. H.S. Lawrence and M. Landy (Academic Press, N.Y., 1969) p. 206.

Griscelli has more recently reported similar results in immunodeficient children who have failed to reject skin allografts before TF$_D$ administration and who then develop inflammatory reactions around the graft after each systemic injection of TF$_D$ which then subsides and the grafts are not rejected (cf Gottlieb, A.A., Transfer Factor: Biological Properties Workshop, IN: Progress in Immunology II (Academic Press, N.Y. 1974). These effects could be viewed to result from acquisition of the capacity to recognize environmental antigens following reconstitution of CMI by TF$_D$.

However, I think that Fudenberg, and his colleagues, may have done the experiment you request using TF$_D$ in transferring tumor specific CMI, a form of allograft immunity, to patients with osteogenic sarcoma. (Fudenberg, et al. Hosp. Pract. 9 (1974) 95). In these observations only osteogenic sarcoma specific TF$_D$ was effective in conferring on such patients in vivo and in vitro CMI to osteogenic sarcoma antigens, whereas TF$_D$ with specificities for another tumor (e.g., hypernephroma) was not effective in this regard.

There are, however, documented non-specific consequences of TF$_D$ administration to patients (e.g. acquisition and/or augmentation of lymphocyte responses to PHA; to sheep RBC for E rosettes; and to other lymphocytes in the mixed leukocyte culture test). Nevertheless, the immunologic specificity of TF$_D$ has been confirmed on repeated occasions and the most recent work employed a single peak isolated from TF$_D$ after

passage through Sephadex G-25 (Zuckerman et al. J. Clin.
Invest 54 (1974) 997). Using a single peak fraction of TF$_D$
these authors transferred specific cutaneous DTH _in vivo_ to
KLH to 10/10 individuals only when the material was obtained
from KLH immune donors. Identical Sephadex purified peaks
of TF$_D$ prepared from tuberculin positive donors who were not
immune to KLH, failed to transfer delayed reactivity to KLH
while transferring tuberculin reactivity to 11 additional
individuals.

N. Felberg, Wills Eye Hospital and Research Institute:
Does the fact that transfer factor is found in unaffected
family members of melanoma and sarcoma patients suggest to
you that there may be a viral etiology in these two malignancies, and is it possible that in premalignant cancers, or
cancer such as adenocarcinoma of the colon, which seems to
be familial, that unaffected members may have transfer
factor that would be useful in treating the affected member.

H.S. Lawrence: Yes. Much of this data has come from
Fudenberg's and from LoBuglio's laboratories. For example,
one patient of Spitler's with melanoma was treated with a
melanoma-positive transfer factor taken by leukophoresis
from an uncle, and responded immunologically as well as
clinically with regression of metastases for a year. At the
end of a year the metastases recurred despite continued
administration of TF$_D$. Upon re-testing the uncle at this
time he had lost CMI to the melanoma antigen. Following a
2-3 week respite from leukophoresis, the uncle re-acquired
CMI to melanoma antigens.

N. Felberg: Does a patient in remission, after receiving transfer factor, then have transfer factor in his
white cells?

H.S. Lawrence: I don't know. There is just one type
of experiment that answers that. I refer to our experiments
that showed serial passage of cutaneous DTH to tuberculin or
to streptococcal antigens from individual A to B to C.
Since that time there has been repeated demonstration that
all recipients of transfer factors, sick or well, acquire a
population of circulating lymphocytes that will proliferate
in the presence of antigen and produce lymphokines (MIF, LT,
Interferon). My guess is that if you prepared TF$_D$ from such
antigen-reactive circulating lymphocytes and injected it
into a secondary recipient that you would transfer DTH
reactivity, just as we did in the original experiments cited

317

(Lawrence J. Clin. Invest. 34 (1955) 219).

P. Alexander, Chester Beatty Research Institute: Dr. Fudenberg, do you want to comment on your experiences?

H.H. Fudenberg, University of California School of Medicine: First of all, I would like to say that we never used "recovered" patients, as a source of donors of white cells to make transfer factors. First of all the vast majority of these five years after removal of their primary have lost cellular immunity to the neoplasm; secondly, we think that it is unethical, not justified, because if the patient develops metastasis, six months, one or two years later, one can never be sure whether it resulted from partial removal of his protective mechanism. What we used is, as Jerry (Dr. Lawrence) pointed out, household contacts not necessarily family members, just household contacts; parents, sibs, guardians, servants, who had not "transfer factor" because everyone has transfer factors, but whose lymphocytes, (T cells) possess the specific ability, to kill, for example, osteosarcoma cells in long term in vitro culture and the data observed in these studies is by far the most convining arguments for specificity. For if transfer factor is prepared for in family members who lack that specificity, for (osteosarcoma) there is no rise in the patient's T cell mediated cytotoxicity, which would be expected to act as a hinderence to the expected development of metastasis. If one uses tumor-specific dializable transfer factors one obtains a rise of cytotoxicity in the thymocytes of the patient.

R. Bollinger, Duke University: The matter of transferring accelerated homograft rejection and the fact that you can now do it in primates, raises an interesting question that's important, also for the mechanism of maintenance of self-tolerance. If you did your experiment, for example, in monkeys, transferring skin from monkey "A" to monkey "B", thus raising a transfer factor in "B", what would be the effect of putting that transfer factor back in monkey "A"? Exactly, this might happen at some time in the future during clinical trials, were we to inadvertently obtain transfer factor from a donor previously sensitized to histocompatibility antigens of the recipient.

H.S. Lawrence: Goran Möller asked me that identical question in relation to humans some years ago and I would shudder to think of possible autoimmune tissue damage that might be launched. Those of you who've worked with this molecule, however small, are convinced of its great potency. Additionally, Peter Behan of Glasgow, has produced either allergic encephalitis, or allergic neuritis in monkeys, and transferred that lesion from monkey to monkey with dialyzable transfer factor. He finds the specificity of the cutaneous DTH transferred by TF$_D$ was determined by the species of origin of the encephalitogenic material (e.g., turtle vs. mammalian myelin protein) used to raise TF$_D$ in the donor.

E.W. Lamon, University of Alabama: There seems to be several paradoxes here that puzzle me, but I'd like to ask about one in particular, and that is that some of the diseases that you treated successfully have a definite...

H.S. Lawrence: Actually, I was citing the clinical experiences of others.

E.W. Lamon: ...have a definite component of delayed type hypersensitivity which contributes to the lesion, or contributes to the disease; on the other hand, other cases require an increase in cellular mediated immunity to be overcome. Do you have any hypothesis which would explain this? Perhaps activating suppressor T cells in one instance, and not in the other? How would you explain this phenomenon?

H.S. Lawrence: Well, it is not so much a paradox. It suggests that cell mediated immunity is the mechanism that is responsible for eradication of intracellular parasites and that when TF$_D$ confers cell-mediated immunity on the anergic patient in the face a replicating antigen flung throughout his tissues, then the DTH response is apt to cause inflammation. These patients do get an inflammatory response and care must be taken to keep it minimal (e.g. smaller doses of TF$_D$ or administration of prednisone as Bullock showed to dampen the expression of DTH yet not interfere with the underlying transfer).

R.E. Parks, Jr., Brown University: I wonder whether you could offer further clarification on two points. The first has to do with the chemistry of transfer factor. Did I understand correctly that at present you believe it to be a relatively low molecular weight polypeptide associated with a nucleic acid?

H.S. Lawrence: Nucleotides?

R.E. Parks, Jr.: Do you have any idea which nucleotides

319

are involved? What have been the problems of identifying the chemical structures?

H.S. Lawrence: Well, Arthur Gottlieb, who's done most of the recent work on this, suggests that they are nucleotides of RNA and probably the single stranded variety.

R.E. Parks, Jr.: Do you know whether these are individual nucleotides bound to the polypeptide or whether there are internucleotide linkages?

H.S. Lawrence: The biochemistry hasn't got to that degree of precission.

R.E. Parks, Jr.: However, I believe that you stated that transfer factor is not destroyed by pancreatic ribonuclease.

H.S. Lawrence: It's not destroyed by pancreatic ribonuclease. Indeed, it was this property that led us to suggest that <u>should</u> it turn out to be a polynucleotide, then it would probably be one of double, rather than single, stranded RNA, but at the same time emphasizing the presence and possible role of peptides in the dialysate. There are a number of small peptides that do have specificity.

R.E. Parks, Jr.: Is the activity of transfer factor destroyed by exposure to various proteinases?

H.S. Lawrence: In some experiments that Dr. Lynne Spitler has done, she has inactivated the capacity of TF_D to transfer cutaneous DTH <u>in vivo</u> in humans with pronase.

R.E. Parks, Jr.: The other point relates to the extent of species-to-species transfer of immunity. In other words, could you immunize a horse with someone's tumor cells and then isolate an effective transfer factor from the white cells of the horse?

H.S. Lawrence: I don't know about a horse, but you can immunize a monkey.

R.E. Parks, Jr.: Well, the monkey is very close to man. How about other species more distantly related?

H.S. Lawrence: The only evidence of that possibility has been reported by Nornong et al. who immunized chimpanzees with a human melanoma, prepared chimp transfer factor and gave it back to the patient (Clin. Res. 32 (1973) 1035).

Does Human Carcinogenesis Involve Derepressive Gene
Activation?: Oncocolon Antigens, A Model System.

Allyn H. Rule, Graduate Department of Biology, Boston College
(02167) and Tufts University, School of Medicine, Boston, MA.
(02111).

Earlier work by Gold and Freedman (1) suggested that the
carcinoembryonic antigen (CEA) was the product of derepressive dedifferentiating oncogenic mechanisms.

Newer data obtained using CEA-radioimmunoassay with
isoelectric focusing profiles of individual as well as tumor
pools of adenocarcinomas of the colon suggest that this antigen
belongs to a family of phase specific oncocolon antigens. Most
of the data are in accordance with the idea that partially overlapping gene sets are expressed in mammallian embryogenesis
and carcinogenesis (2). Some, none or all oncocolon antigens
may be found in various colon samples. These include: fetal
colon sources, normal colon and individual tumors.

Gene sets for colon antigens expressed early in embryo-
logic development which proceed through adulthood include
those found with pK_i at pH 2, 2.5, 4.5, 5.0, 6.0, 6.5 and
8.0. The carcinoembryonic type (pH 4.0) is expressed pre-
dominately in the first and second trimester which oncofoetal
type (pH 3.0) is found in the second and third trimester in
utero. These latter two antigens are not normally expressed
in adult colon but may precede and include neoplastic colon
changes.

Some of these data also suggest that in a few cases, oncogenesis may proceed from the multiplication of primitive
colon cells and need not reflect dedifferentiating mechanisms.

REFERENCES

1. Gold, P. and Freedman, S.O., J. Experimental Med. 121
   (1965) 439.

2. Rule, A.H. and Goleski-Reilly, C., Cancer Research 34
   (1974) 2083.

GENETIC CONTROL OF LYMPHOCYTE TRANSFORMATION BY PHA

H.J. Heiniger and B.A. Taylor, The Jackson Laboratory, Bar Harbor, Maine

By use of our easily reproducible micromethod[1] for the culture of peripheral mouse lymphocytes we could test their response to PHA in single animals without sacrificing them; thus, genetic studies of the blastogenic transformation of lymphocytes have become feasible. We analyzed the PHA-response of circulating peripheral lymphocytes from 59 inbred strains, substrains, and hybrid lines of mice. The DBA and C3H families of mice were low responders; the A strains exhibited an intermediate response, and the C57 group responded best to PHA. Of all strains, DBA/2J responded least, whereas PL/J exhibited the highest incorporation of tritiated thymidine (^{3}H-TdR).

There is a correlation between the PHA response and the spontaneous incidence of leukemia among the inbred strains of mice: the strains (C58/J, AKR/J, HRS/J, and PL/J) which exhibit a high incidence of leukemia were good responders to PHA and no leukemia strain was found among the low responder group. Leukemic lymphoid cells themselves were not, or only to a small extent, responsive to PHA.

The fact that the overall strain-distribution of response was continuous suggested that several genes must determine blastogenic transformation of lymphocytes. Our findings suggest that 2 to 4 loci are involved; the major histocompatibility locus, H-2, does not appear to affect the response as revealed by the analysis of 11 congenic resistant strains. Using an analysis of variance, the heritability (H^2) of responsiveness was found to be very high (75-80%) and the reproducibility of our results between several experiments was better than 80%.

REFERENCE

(1) H.J. Heiniger, J.M. Wolf, H.W. Chen, and H. Meier, Proc. Soc. Exp. Biol. Med. 143 (1973) 6.

Supported by Research Contract N01 CP 33255 of the National Cancer Institute.

Carcinoembryonic Antigen Levels in Normal Blood Bank Donors

E. B. Rosenberg, P.M. Smith, and R.D. Safian, Division of Nuclear Medicine, University of Miami School of Medicine and Mount Sinai Medical Center, Miami, Florida.

Sera from 475 normal blood donors were assayed for carcinoembryonic antigen (CEA) using a double antibody triple isotope radioimmunoassay. This assay, developed at the City of Hope Hospital, Duarte, California, utilizes ^{125}I-CEA, ^{131}I goat IgG, and ^{22}Na. ^{131}I is used as an internal control to assure that all samples are processed appropriately and ^{22}Na serves as a volume marker allowing rapid sample processing. All results are generated on punch tapes and are processed on a NOVA 1200 data processor.

Using this radioimmunoassay, higher CEA levels were found in smokers than in nonsmokers. Highest CEA levels were found in individuals who smoked more than one pack per day or who had been smoking for at least 10 years. Individuals with anti-A antibodies in their blood were found to have elevated CEA titers when compared to other blood donors. Donors with Rh+ blood had higher CEA levels than those with Rh- blood. The mean CEA level of individuals over the age of 30 was nearly 1.4 times that of individuals below the age of 20. Mean CEA levels were not found to differ in blacks and caucasians, or in males and females.

The double antibody triple isotope radioimmunoassay for quantitating CEA has provided valuable information which emphasizes that any other studies associating CEA levels with various diseases should include consideration of smoking history, blood group, and age, because certain CEA elevations might be attributable to these factors.

REFERENCES:

(1) M.L. Egan, J.T. Lautenschleger, J.E. Coligan, and C. W. Todd, Immunochem. 9 (1972) 289.
(2) W.D. Terry, P.A. Henkart, J. E. Coligan, and C.W. Todd, Transplant. Rev. 20 (1974) 100.

CEA FAMILY SYNDROME: ABNORMAL CARCINOEMBRYONIC ANTIGEN (CEA) LEVELS IN FAMILIES WITH RETINOBLASTOMA.

N.T. Felberg, J.B. Michelson, and J.A. Shields, Wills Eye Hospital & Research Institute, Philadelphia, Pennsylvania.

Retinoblastoma is the most common ocular malignancy of childhood. It is either transmitted as an autosomal dominant trait (hereditary), or is a somatic cell mutation (sporadic). Pathologically proven retinoblastoma patients and their family members were examined for plasma CEA levels. We have defined those families where a closely related family member, other than the propositus, presents with an abnormally elevated plasma CEA level in the absence of demonstrable disease, as belonging to the CEA FAMILY SYNDROME.

Of the 17 sporadic retinoblastoma families studied, 9 (52.9%) were found to have the CEA FAMILY SYNDROME. In 6 of these 9 families, the relative involved was the mother of the index case. In total, 19 of the 65 family members (29.2%) had elevated plasma CEA ($P < 4 \times 10^{-8}$, when compared to the 3% elevated in the normal population). Two families in this study were exceptional. In Family No. 8, the mother in all 5 siblings were elevated. In Family No. 17, the mother, father and all 3 siblings were elevated. Of even greater interest in this family, is the history of both maternal grandparents dying of cancer. The maternal grandmother had adenocarcinoma of the colon, and 12 years later she succumbed to cancer of the stomach. The history of this family may classify it as a member of both the CEA FAMILY SYNDROME and the CANCER FAMILY SYNDROME (Lynch & Krush, Surg. Gynecol. Obstet 132 (1971) 247).

The CEA FAMILY SYNDROME has several similarities to the CANCER FAMILY SYNDROME. Both appear to be either autosomal dominant or selective maternal transmission. Both exhibit unaffected family members with elevated plasma CEA levels. However, whereas individuals with abnormal CEA values who belong to the CANCER FAMILY SYNDROME have a 50% possibility of getting adenocarcinoma of the colon, individuals with abnormal CEA values who belong to the CEA FAMILY SYNDROME, are very unlikely to get retinoblastoma. Perhaps, the so-called "spontaneous" retinoblastoma seen here, actually follows a selective maternal or cytoplasmic inheritance as does the elevated CEA level.

NORMAL HUMAN SERA DETECTING HUMAN LEUKEMIA ASSOCIATED ANTIGENS

B. Schacter, K. Hopkins and W.B. Bias,   The Johns Hopkins
University, Baltimore, Maryland   21205

There is growing evidence for the appearance of new antigenic determinants on the surface of human leukemia cells (1).
The nature and significance of these leukemia associated antigens however remains obscure. We have under study 11 sera
from normal, healthy individuals which demonstrate highly
specific complement dependent cytotoxic antibody against cells
of some patients with diseases affecting the proliferation
and maturation of leukocytes. Cells are prepared from fresh
peripheral blood by passage thru a column of packed nylon
followed by density gradient centrifugation over a layer of
Ficoll-Hypaque (2). Complement dependent cytotoxicity is
tested by slight modification of the Amos method (3). The
highest frequency of reactivity with these sera (designated
HUNAT) is seen with cells of patients with acute lymphoblastic leukemia. Less frequently, reactivity with HUNAT
sera is seen with cells of patients with acute myelocytic
leukemia, acute monocytic leukemia, leukolymphosarcoma and
chronic myelogenous and lymphocytic leukemia. HUNAT sera
were unreactive with all remission cells tested, including
cells of six patients whose admission cells were previously
reactive with one or more HUNAT sera. Cells of seven
patients with infectious mononucleosis were unreactive with
the HUNAT sera. Normal cells, representing 27 first and
second locus HL-A antigens, were unreactive with the HUNAT
sera, suggesting that the HUNAT sera are not detecting normal
human transplantation antigens. Several lymphoblastoid cell
lines are reactive with the HUNAT sera, and cross absorption
tests with one serum suggests that the HUNAT antigen present
on a reactive leukemic cell is also present on several cell
lines. Analysis of the pattern of reactivity with five
HUNAT sera suggest that at least two partially overlapping
specificities are detected on the leukemia cells. These results suggest the existence of a set of human leukemia associated antigens which are immunogenic in man.

References:

1. R. Harris Nature 241 (1973) 95.
2. E. Thorsby and A. Bratlie Histocompatibility Testing
    (1970) p. 655-656. Munksgaard, Copenhagen.
3. D.B. Amos, et al. Transp. 7 (1969) 220.

IMMUNODIAGNOSTIC TEST FOR OSTEOSARCOMA IN PATIENTS WITH A HIGH BODY BURDEN OF RADIUM*

E. L. Lloyd, M. Menon and J. L. Mitchen, Argonne National Laboratory, Argonne, Illinois

Persons carrying high body burdens of ^{226}Ra are predisposed to the development of osteosarcomas. Attempts have therefore been made to develop early immunological diagnostic tests for osteosarcomas in this high risk group. The present study describes the test in these patients for lymphocyte cytotoxicity to human osteosarcoma cells in culture. Fifteen patients with residual body burdens greater than 0.3 μCi ^{226}Ra, three of whom had previous amputations for osteosarcoma, were tested. These were matched by fifteen normal controls, whose lymphocytes were treated simultaneously.

With one exception, no cytotoxicity was observed in any of the patients studied. This is in agreement with the fact that no fresh osteosarcomas were diagnosed. The patient, in which cytotoxicity was observed, was suffering from an inflammatory lesion involving bone due to a foreign body reaction at the time of the first test. When the test was repeated 10 months later, no cytotoxicity was observed. No significant nonspecific cytotoxicity was observed using lymphocytes taken from normal control subjects with any of the target cell lines used.

* Work performed under the auspices of the U. S. Atomic Energy Commission.

IMMUNOCHEMICAL DEMONSTRATION OF α-LACTALBUMIN SYNTHESIS IN A HUMAN MAMMARY CARCINOMA CELL LINE

H. N. Rose and C. M. McGrath, Michigan Cancer Foundation, Detroit, Michigan 48201

A stable cell line (MCF-7) has been cultured from a pleural effusion of a patient with metastatic breast carcinoma[1]. Although MCF-7 exhibits the structural characteristics of mammary epithelial cells, definitive biochemical evidence is necessary to verify that the cells, after long-term culture, are indeed human and mammary[1,2].

The protein α-lactalbumin (α-LA) is a specific product of functional differentiation of mammary epithelial tissue under hormonal regulation[3]. α-LA was isolated from human milk. Rabbits were immunized and a radioimmunoassay (RIA) developed capable of detecting 12×10^{-15} moles (170 pg) of α-LA. The anti-α-LA was highly specific, demonstrating no cross-reactivity with rodent, ruminant and porcine α-LA or human lysozyme.

Three human tumor cell lines, breast (MCF-7), throat (D-562) and cervical (HeLa) were grown in Hank's Medium 199 with 10% calf serum and insulin (10 µg/ml). Supernatants (100,000 X g) were prepared from harvested cells and assayed for human α-LA by RIA. Only MCF-7 was found to contain α-LA (155 ng/mg protein). Each cell line was exposed to prolactin (10 µg/ml) for periods up to 10 days and again assayed for α-LA. MCF-7 contained α-LA (172 ng/mg protein). D-562 and HeLa were negative.

These results give strong evidence that MCF-7 are mammary epithelial cells of human origin. The apparent loss of hormonal control of α-LA synthesis may be related to the tumorigenic nature of the cells.

REFERENCES

(1) H. D. Soule, J. Vazquez, A. Long, et al., J. Nat. Cancer Inst. 51 (1973) 1409.
(2) G. C. Buehring and A. J. Hackett, J. Nat. Cancer Inst. 53 (1974) 651.
(3) R. L. Hill, K. Brew, T. C. Vanamen, et al., Brookhaven Symp. Biol. 21 (1968) 139.

IMMUNOGENICITY OF HUMAN BREAST CANCER; ANTIGENIC SIMILARITY TO MURINE MAMMARY TUMOR VIRUS (MuMTV)

M.M. Black, R.E. Zachrau, B. Shore, D.H. Moore[*], and H.P. Leis, Jr., New York Medical College, New York, New York, and Institute for Medical Research[*], Camden, New Jersey.

Prognostically significant immunogenicity of human breast cancer tissue is recognizable microscopically in the form of lymphoreticuloendothelial (L-RE)[1] responses in the primary lesion and regional lymph nodes. As judged by L-RE responses, skin tests and in vitro leukocyte migration procedures immunogenicity is maximal during the developmental (in situ) stage and decreases with the progression of the disease.[2,3] In vitro measurements also indicate that 1. there is a high level of antigenic similarity among L-RE positive breast cancer tissues. 2. Leukocyte preparations having hypersensitivity responses to L-RE positive breast cancer tissues commonly cross react with MuMTV.[4] 3. Leukocyte responsiveness to MuMTV is commonly associated with cross reactivity against immunogenic breast cancer tissues. The findings are consistent with viral participation in the developmental phase of human breast cancer and with the potential for immunoprophylaxis.[5]

Since the biological behavior of breast cancer reflects dynamic interactions between the intrinsic aggressive potential of the cancer cells, the immunogenicity of the cancer cells and the specific cellular hypersensitivity of the host there can be no single treatment which is equally "best" for all patients. Therapy, be it surgical, radiation, chemical or immunological or combinations, should be matched to the needs of individual patients.

REFERENCES

(1) M.M. Black, Natl Cancer Inst Monograph 35 (1972) 73.
(2) M.M. Black and H.P. Leis, Jr., Cancer 32 (1973) 384.
(3) M.M. Black, H.P. Leis, Jr., B. Shore, and R.E. Zachrau, Cancer 33 (1974) 952.
(4) M.M. Black, D.H. Moore, B. Shore, R.E. Zachrau, and H.P. Leis, Jr., Cancer Research 34 (1974) 1054.
(5) M.M. Black, S.J. Cutler, and T.H.C. Barclay, Cancer 29 (1972) 61.

ATTEMPT TO DISTINGUISH SURFACE ANTIGENS OF WILMS' TUMOR DERIVED CELLS

Pavel Koldovsky, Ursula Koldovsky and Klaus Hummler, Childrens' Hospital of Philadelphia, Philadelphia, Pennsylvania.

Substantial evidence has accumulated in recent years that a patient can react immunologically against his own cancer. Such reaction can be detected in vitro by cell mediated and/or serum mediated cytotoxicity. This reaction is usually detectable not only against autologous tumor cells but also against allogeneic tumor cells of the same histological type. This is in sharp contrast from the pattern of the reactivity observed in animal experiments: the specificity of the animal tumors is determined by the inducing agent - in the case of the viral induced tumors by the virus.

Many antigens are or may be associated with the cell membrane of a malignant cell. The most important groups seems to be: H-LA, organ (tissue) associated and tumor associated antigens. In previous experiments we have been able to show that patients with mailgnant brain tumors and Wilms' tumors can develope an immunological reaction against respective tissue associated antigens. In the presented paper will be discussed the possibility to distinguish the reactivity against antikidney associated antigens and against antitumor associated antigens in the serum and immunocytes from Wilms' tumor patient. For differentiation of these reactions blocking techniques were employed. Significance of these findings is discussed from the view of immunopathology as well as from the view of the research for candidates for oncogeneic viruses.

LIPID COMPOSITION OF PLASMA MEMBRANES OF SPONTANEOUS MAMMARY CARCINOMAS IN MICE

T.L. Rednour and A.S. Bennett, Ball State University, Muncie, Indiana

Interferences with molecular interactions among membrane lipids and proteins could cause a reduction in membrane fluidity[1] and alterations in the distribution of surface antigens[2,3], producing membrane characteristics associated with abnormal cells.

Plasma membranes were isolated by differential centrifugation from mammary tumors produced in Strong A mice. Lipids were extracted with chloroform-methanol (2:1), separated by TLC and saponified. The resulting fatty acids were methylated, then identified and quantified by GLC. Significant alterations in the fatty acid composition of triglycerides (TG), free fatty acids (FFA), cholesterol esters (CE), and phospholipids (PL) were found. Carcinoma samples had up to 40 percent less short chain fatty acids and two times the amount of 16:0, 16:1, 18:0, and 18:1 acids. Normal cell membranes had up to 29 percent 21:0 but fractions from carcinoma membranes contained no more than 10 percent. As much as 10 percent of the fatty acids in CE, TG and PL fractions of tumors was 17:2, an acid rarely found in normal cells. A shift from a de novo to a chain elongation pathway as the principal route for the synthesis of fatty acids is suggested.

REFERENCES
(1) R.Barnett, L.Furcht and R.Scott, Proc. Nat'l. Acad. Sci.,U.S. 71 (1974) 1992.
(2) S.Singer and G.Nicholson, Science 175 (1972) 720.
(3) M.C.Raff and S.DePetris, Fed. Proc. 32 (1973) 48.

THE SPECIFIC IMMUNE-PRECIPITATION OF INTRACELLULAR PRE-CURSOR-LIKE POLYPEPTIDES OF RAUSCHER LEUKEMIA VIRUS

R. B. Naso, L. J. Arcement, and R. B. Arlinghaus, The University of Texas System Cancer Center, M. D. Anderson Hospital and Tumor Institute, Houston, Texas

Antisera to disrupted Rauscher leukemia virus (RLV) or to the purified Rauscher viral 30,000 mol. wt. polypeptide were used to specifically precipitate newly synthesized intracellular viral polypeptides from extracts of infected NIH Swiss mouse cells (JLS-V16). Analysis by SDS-polyacrylamide gel electrophoresis (SDS-PAGE) of extracts from cells pulse-labeled for 10-20 min with ^{35}S-methionine showed that immune precipitates contained none of the non-glycosylated internal structural polypeptides of mature viruses. The major viral-specific polypeptides labeled in 10 min included polypeptides of 180,000, 140,000, 110,000, 80,000, and 60,000 daltons with minor polypeptides of 65,000, 50,000, and 40,000 daltons. Labeling the intracellular viral-specific polypeptides with ^{14}C-glucosamine indicated that the 180,000, 110,000, 80,000, and 60,000 dalton polypeptides were glycosylated and all but the 110,000 dalton polypeptides are contained in the mature virions. Based on pulse-chase experiments, it appears that at least 3 of the large polypeptides (140,000, 65,000, and 50,000 daltons) are precursors to the three major internal structural polypeptides of the mature virions.

REFERENCES

(1) R.B. Naso, L.J. Arcement, and R.B. Arlinghaus, Cell, In Press.
(2) R.B. Arlinghaus, R.B. Naso, and L.J. Arcement, XI International Cancer Congress, In Press.

PARTIAL ISOLATION, SPECIFICITY AND IMMUNOGENICITY OF ANTIGENS ASSOCIATED WITH THE B16 MELANOMA

I. Schenkein and J.-C. Bystryn, New York University Medical Center, New York, New York

B16 melanoma cells were incubated with ^{3}H-leucine, and radioactive proteins secreted or shed by the cells into the medium were concentrated and fractionated using $(NH)_2SO_4$, G-200 Sephadex and DEAE cellulose. A rabbit antiserum raised against injected radiated melanoma cells and exhaustively absorbed with normal syngeneic mouse tissue can be used successfully in conjunction with a goat anti-rabbit serum in a "sandwich" technique to assay for antigens associated with the B16 melanoma. The antigens studied so far appear to be glycoproteins whose precipitability is greatly enhanced by treatment with neuraminidase. Specificity of the partially purified melanoma associated antigens (MAA) was studied by absorption and radioimmunoassay. They appear to be quantitatively or qualitatively different from normal syngeneic adult and fetal antigens, from antigens derived from unrelated syngeneic tumors and allogenic melanomas and from murine type C viral proteins. Mice immunized with the partially purified MAA developed antibodies to this material. Detection was done by a sensitive double antibody-antigen binding assay. The protective effect of immunization to lethal doses of injected viable melanoma cells is being studied.

CELLULAR LOCALIZATION OF HSV-2 ASSOCIATED ANTIGENS IN TRANSFORMED MOUSE CELLS

T.W. Orme, B.A. McCaw, C.W. Boone and A.L. Boyd,
NCI Frederick Cancer Research Center, Frederick, Maryland

UV-irradiated HSV-2 (Savage strain) was used to transform BALB/c mouse embryo cells[1]. The transformed cells induce tumors in normal immunocompetent BALB/c mice (TD_{50} ~ 5 X 10^3). X-irradiated transformed cells immunize normal mice against a challenge with 1 X 10^6 tumor cells. The in vitro cultured transformed cells and a number of cultures explanted from tumors display cytoplasmic and nuclear antigens associated with the continued presence of the HSV-2 genome. Indirect immunofluorescence tests revealed that antisera directed against virion antigens produce only a weak reaction with cytoplasmic antigens in the transformed cells. Tumor-bearer serum reacts more strongly with these antigens. At early stages in tumor development the fluorescence is primarily cytoplasmic, but as the tumor progresses the pattern becomes distinctly nuclear and reminiscent of classical T antigens. A correlation between nuclear fluorescence and HSV-2 neutralizing activity by tumor-bearer serum was established. Mice bearing small tumors have a delayed hypersensitivity response to tumor cells. Mice bearing large tumors and having antibody against nuclear antigens have lost this response.

REFERENCES

(1) A.L. Boyd, T.W. Orme and C.W. Boone, 2nd International Symposium on Herpesvirus and Oncogenesis, Nuremberg, Germany (1974).

Research sponsored by the National Cancer Institute under Contract No. NO1-CO-25423 with Litton Bionetics, Inc.

IMMUNOCHEMICAL STUDIES IN EXPERIMENTAL GLIOMA

J.S. Lo and J.A. Kellen (Dept. of Clinical Biochemistry,
Sunnybrook Hospital, University of Toronto, Toronto, Canada).

To our knowledge, the systemic immune response of the host
to experimental transplanted brain tumours has not been investigated. In our studies, Zimmerman's transplantable ependy-
moblastoma (induced by methylcholanthrene) has been used and
maintained in inbred C57Bl/6J female mice[1]. The tumours were
excised at the end of the third week after transplantation
and homogenized; a cytoplasmic protein fraction was extracted
and separated by centrifugation at 105.000xg. This fraction,
together with Freund's adjuvant, was used to immunize rabbits.
The antiserum obtained was examined for antibodies against
tumour-associated proteins in the soluble protein fraction by
immunodiffusion and immunoelectrophoresis; further isolation
and purification were carried out with column chromatography
and isoelectric focusing.

In parallel studies, antisera against intact tumour cells
have been produced. From both antisera, the gamma globulin
fractions were isolated and conjugated with Fluorescein
isothiocyanate. Differential binding of the labelled antibodies in histological sections from tumours and normal
organs has been observed (methodology as sub 2).

Spleen cells of normal and tumour-bearing mice were separated by velocity sedimentation[3]; a sandwich technique was
applied to detect binding of the fluorescent antisera to
various cell populations by UV microscopy. Preferential
binding to the T and B cell populations with anticellular
and anti-cytoplasmatic conjugates respectively has been
recorded, proving a cellular immune response of the host.

REFERENCES

(1) H.M. Zimmerman and H. Arnold, Cancer Res. 1:919-938,1970.
(2) J.A. Kellen and A.C.-H.Lo, Oncology 27:315-323,1973.
(3) G. Miller and R.A. Phillips, J. Cellular Physiol.
    73:191,1969.

SCANNING AND TRANSMISSION ELECTRON MICROSCOPY OF HUMAN T CELL MEDIATED CYTOLYSIS

E. L. Springer, A. J. Hackett, and V. S. Byers, School of
Public Health, Cell Culture Laboratory, University of Cali-
fornia, Berkeley, California and U.S. Public Health Service
Hospital, San Francisco, California

Thymus derived lymphocytes with tumor specific cytotoxic activity, verified by the 51-chromium release assay
(1) were shown by SEM to attach to cultured mammary carcinoma (ALAB) cells (2,3). Lymphocytes from household contacts
of mammary carcinoma patients made multipoint attachments to
the tumor cell and destroyed it by stripping the membrane
away from the cytoplasm. No other type of cell was involved
in the process. Non-cytotoxic lymphocytes from individuals
with no known contact with a cancer patient also formed multipoint attachments to the tumor cells but did not destroy
the membrane. Monocytes also isolated by the Ficoll-hypaque
separation technique (4) interacted with both tumor cells and
lymphocytes via cytoplasmic bridges. Spherical bodies, 1
micron in diameter, were also found associated with the
lymphocytes. Platelets and erythrocytes were also observed.
The aspecimens were double fixed, critical point dried (5)
and rotary coated with carbon and gold, then examined in the
Stereoscan S4-10 scanning electron microscope operating at
10KV.

In situ fixed and embedded cytotoxic lymphocytes and
ALAB cells showed a fusion or merging of the plasma membrane
at the point of contact.

REFERENCES

(1) R. B. Faanes, Y. S. Choi and R. A. Good, J. of Exper.
     Medicine, 137 (1973) 171.
(2) M. V. Reed and G. O. Gey, Lab. Invest. 11 (1962) 638.
(3) G. C. Buehring and A. J. Hackett, J. Nat. Cancer Inst.
     53 (1974) 621.
(4) M. Wioland, O. Sabolovic, and D. Berg, Nature 237 (1972)
     274.
(5) T. E. Anderson, N. Y. Acad. of Sci., Trans. Ser. to 13
     (1951) 130.

Supported by:
Contract # E 73-2001-N01-CP-3-3237
Byers Contract# NIH Postdoctoral Fellowship 5-FO-2AI-53320

Tumor Cell Destruction by Lymphocytes Induced With Tumor
Specific IgM.

E.W. Lamon[1], H. Whitten[1], H.M. Skurzak[2], B. Andersson[2] and
E. Klein[2]

1 - Department of Surgery and Microbiology, University of
Alabama in Birmingham School of Medicine, Birmingham, Alabama, and, 2 - Department of Tumor Biology, Karolinska Institute, Stockholm, Sweden.

Antisera with specificity for Moloney leukemia virus (MLV)
determined antigen(s) were studied for their ability to induce MLV antigen target cell destruction by lymphocytes in
microcytotoxicity assays. Sera from animals which had re-
gressed Moloney Sarcoma virus(MSV) tumors as well as sera
from animals with progressively growing MSV tumors were
found to induce normal spleen lymphocytes to be active a-
gainst the targets. Regressor serum was found also to potentiate the activity of immune spleen cells from tumor bearing
(15 days after MSV) or regressor (50 days after MSV) animals.
Both 19S and 7S Sephadex G 200 fractions of the antisera
were found to induce cytotoxicity by normal spleen lymphocytes and to potentiate the activity of MSV immune spleen
lymphocytes. These activities were shown to be IgM and IgG
respectively by the use of sepharose coupled anti-mouse IgM
and anti-mouse IgG columns. All activity was removed by
passing sera over both columns. Recent experiments have
shown that IgM not only induces cytotoxicity by spleen
cells but will induce normal thymus cells to be cytotoxic
as well.

LEUKOCYTE AGGREGATION TEST: IN VITRO ASSESSMENT FOR TRANSPLANTATION AND TUMOR IMMUNITY

B.H. Tom, N.R. Pellis, and B.D. Kahan, Laboratory of Surgical Immunology, Northwestern University Medical School, Chicago, Illinois 60611

Cell-mediated transplantation immunity may be detected in vitro by assays reflecting: 1) lymphocyte contact and recognition of target antigens; 2) lymphocyte activation following contact; and 3) lymphocyte performance leading to alteration of function or destruction of target cells. The recognition phase represents the clearest expression of immunological specificity and, furthermore, is less prone to obfuscation by secondary cellular and humoral factors characteristic of the other stages. The leukocyte aggregation test (LAT) [1-3] based upon the formation of aggregates by immune leukocytes on corresponding target cells, measures an early event following recognition. This system displays specificity for the donor as opposed to third-party targets, and can be modulated by host serum. In the present studies its success in evaluating the immune status of clinical renal transplant patients was extended to the murine system. The LAT was capable of detecting specific immune aggregation of leukocytes to target cells, both in the case of skin allotransplants between DBA/2J (H2^d) and C3H/HeJ (H2^k) mice, and in syngeneic tumor grafts of 3-methylcholanthrene-induced sarcomas in C3H/HeJ mice. [4] These results suggested that there was: 1) a shift in the reactive lymphocyte population from the lymph nodes in first-set rejection to the spleen during second-set rejection; 2) a cyclic activity of immune cells during the rejection course; and 3) a differential reactivity of immune cells on skin or kidney targets, depending upon the immunizing graft.

REFERENCES

(1) B.D. Kahan, B.H. Tom, K.K. Mittal, and J.J. Bergan, The Lancet i (1974) 37.

(2) B.H. Tom, M.M. Jakstys, and B.D. Kahan, J. Immunology 113 (1974) 1288.

(3) B.H. Tom and B.D. Kahan, Clinical Immunobiology, Vol. 3, Academic Press, 1974, in press.

(4) N.R. Pellis, B.H. Tom, and B.D. Kahan, J. Immunology 113 (1974) 708.

SPECIFIC RECOGNITION OF MOUSE H-2

ALLOANTIGENS BY HUMAN LYMPHOCYTES

Kirsten F. Lindahl & Fritz H. Bach

Cytotoxic lymphocytes generated in transplantation reactions in vivo or in vitro are mainly directed against antigens of H-2, the major histocompatibility complex in mouse,
although the H-2 antigens only constitute a minor part of the
surface proteins of the lymphocyte. One possible reason for
this may be that the differences for non-H-2 antigens between
individuals of the same species are too small to induce a
cytotoxic response. Cytotoxic cells from another species
would be expected to differ strongly at many loci because of
the phylogenetic distance and would thus be expected to recognize more antigens as foreign. We have immunized human
lymphocytes against mouse spleen cells in vitro and tested
their cytotoxic potential on target cells of various strains
to assay whether the H-2 antigens also serve as the major
targets in such a cross-species combination. In mouse different strains are available which allow one to ask whether
H-2 antigens are of major import or whether antigens determined by other genetic loci (referred to as the "background")
can also serve as targets. The results, using a large number
of different strains to which human lymphocytes were sensitized, indicate that human lymphocytes after sensitization

340

in vitro (1) primarily recognize the antigens of H-2 as the cytotoxic targets (2) differentiate between different antigens of the H-2 complex (i.e. kill target cells carrying the H-2 antigens to which they were sensitized more effectively than target cells carrying different H-2 antigens), (3) cannot differentiate between non-H-2, or background, antigens of different strains although some low level cytotoxicity is associated with the non-H-2 targets. The evidence is consistent with the concept that the cytotoxicity associated with non-H-2 targets is non-specific. These findings suggest to us that the narrow specificity of allogeneic effector cells is the result of the nature of cell surface molecules, only a few of them being able to efficiently induce effector cells and to serve as targets. The reason could be their chemical nature, their density on the surface, their rate of turnover or other factors.

A MATHEMATICAL MODEL AND COMPUTER SIMULATION OF THE GROWTH AND REJECTION OF A MURINE ASCITES TUMOR ALLOGRAFT

Bagwell, C.B., Hudson, J.L. and Irvin III, G.L., Veterans Administration Hospital, Miami, Florida, 33125

An important process in the cellular immune rejection of an ascites tumor allograft involves the activation of host T-lymphocytes and macrophages. This process can be divided into at least eight phases: 1. tumor proliferation, 2. T-cell sensitization, 3. cytotoxic lymphocyte proliferation and/or recruitment, 4. lymphocyte cytotoxic activity, 5. macrophage sensitization, 6. macrophage accumulation, 7. macrophage cytotoxic activity, and 8. clearance of dead tumor cells. A differential equation was written to approximate each phase of the system. Using difference approximations to the differential equations, a digital computer simulation of the primary cellular immune response was obtained.

EL4 leukosis cells can be differentiated from a population of an allogeneic host's peritoneal exudate cells by their size (volume) characteristics. An accurate estimation of tumor cell numbers in the peritoneal cavity can be obtained by cell volume distribution analysis of the peritoneal exudate (Coulter electronic particle counter - Channelyzer system).

A least squares analysis (NONLIN program) of the differential equations in conjunction with cell volume distribution data resulted in estimations of parameters that describe the cellular immune response in this biological model.

IMMUNIZATION OF MICE AGAINST SYNGENEIC EL4 TUMOR CHALLENGE
BY INOCULATIONS OF RADIATION-BLOCKED EL4 CELLS

Johnson, T.S., Hudson, J.L., Feldman, M.E., Fuentes, M.P.
and Irvin III, G.L., Veterans Administration Hospital,
Miami, Florida, 33125

Six to eight week old female C57BL/6J (H-2^b) mice were
inoculated with multiple ip injections of syngeneic,
radiation-blocked EL4 leukosis cells (10^7 cells per
injection). Significant immunoprophylaxis was noted in
these sensitized animals upon ip challenge with 5 x 10^3
viable EL4 tumor cells while animals which received
inoculations of radiation-blocked allogeneic L1210 leukemia
cells, syngeneic C1498 myeloma cells or C57BL/6J normal
spleen cells were not protected and died at approximately
the same rate as nonsensitized controls (i.e. within 23 days
post challenge). Survival of the syngeneic host may be
associated with cell-mediated immunity since inoculations
of radiation-blocked EL4 cells stimulated the in vivo
development of lymphoid cells cytotoxic for EL4 as measured
by in vitro ^{51}Cr - release cytotoxicity assays. The
measured cytotoxic response elicited by radiation-blocked
EL4 cells was low yet significant ($p < 0.01$). In correlation
with the survival data, other experiments suggested that
such in vitro cell-mediated immunity was tumor specific.
These results indicate that a latent capacity for immune
recognition and rejection of the syngeneic EL4 tumor exists
in the C57BL/6J host and that this immune response can be
elicited without exogenous amplifiers such as immunoadjuvants, chemical modifiers and/or allogeneic information
transfer.

DETERMINATION OF COMPLEMENT-DEPENDENT ANTIBODY CYTOTOXICITY
FOR EL4 LEUKEMIA CELLS BY CELL VOLUME DISTRIBUTION ANALYSIS

Prudhomme, D.L., Hudson, J.L. and Irvin III, G.L., Veterans
Administration Hospital, Miami, Florida, 33125

Cell volume changes have been reported in many systems
following plasma membrane damage.[1] An electronic particle
counter has been used previously to count undamaged cells
remaining after treatment with serially diluted antibody
and complement.[2]

In the current study, an electronic particle counter and
multichannel analyzer system (Coulter Channelizer) was used
to determine the cell volume distribution of EL4 murine
leukemia cells damaged by anti-EL4 antiserum and complement.

Two distinct cell volume distributions were observed
for viable and damaged cells. The Channelizer displays
these two cell volumes as peaks on an oscilloscope screen
by size and number. By integrating data from these two
peaks, a ratio was obtained which could be expressed
directly as cell viability when the system was calibrated
with known concentrations of viable and damaged cells mixed
in appropriate ratios.

Viability data determined both by alcian blue and trypan
blue dye exclusion methods compared favorably with ratio
data determined by cell volume distribution analysis(CVDA).
Glutaraldehyde fixation of cell samples preserves the viable
and damaged cell volume relationships. This permits larger
scale assays than routinely possible with other methods
since test results can be monitored at a later, more
convenient time.

Data from CVDA is statistically preferable over that obtained by dye exclusion methods since several thousand
cells can be assayed for viability in a short period of time.
For laboratories having the instrumental capabilities, the
replacement of dye exclusion methods for measuring cytotoxic
activity by CVDA is recommended for its capacity, rapidity
and accuracy.

REFERENCES

(1) Laiho, K.V., Shelburne, J.D., Trump,B.F.,Am. J. Pathol.
     65 (1971) 203.
(2) Terasaki, P.I. and Rich, N.E., J. Immunol. 92 (1964)
     128.

IMMUNE DYSFUNCTION AND PULMONARY NEOPLASIA INDUCED BY CHRONIC PULMONARY IRRADIATION

S. A. Benjamin, F. F. Hahn, R. K. Jones and R. O. McClellan, Inhalation Toxicology Research Institute, Lovelace Foundation for Medical Education and Research, Albuquerque, NM 87108

Beagle dogs were exposed by inhalation to relatively insoluble fused clay particles containing beta- or beta-gamma emitting radionuclides for long-term toxicity testing. The specific radionuclides were chosen so that the effective half-life in the lung (^{90}Y, 2.6 days; ^{144}Ce, 180 days; ^{90}Sr, 370 days) would result in a variety of radiation dose patterns to pulmonary tissue. Early effects have included the development of radiation pneumonitis and progressive pulmonary fibrosis. Exposed dogs also developed peripheral lymphopenia, the course of which is dose-rate dependent. In dogs exposed to ^{144}Ce or ^{90}Sr fused clay, progressive lymphopenia developed and peripheral lymphocytes remained depressed through 2 to 3 years after exposure. The remaining peripheral lymphocytes from lymphopenic dogs exposed to ^{144}Ce or ^{90}Sr fused clay showed depressed function as measured by plant mitogen stimulation in vitro. These dogs also showed depressed humoral immune responses to heterologous erythrocytes. Dogs exposed to ^{90}Y fused clay developed an early lymphopenia which returned to normal by 6 months after exposure. Lymphocyte dysfunction was not found in these animals. The dogs exposed to ^{144}Ce and ^{90}Sr fused clay have developed a high incidence of primary lung neoplasms, mostly hemangiosarcomas, as early as 2 years post-exposure at times when lymphopenia is still manifest. Dogs exposed to ^{90}Y fused clay, which do not show the persistent lymphopenia, have developed few pulmonary tumors at comparable times, none of which have been hemangiosarcomas. Thus, pulmonary irradiation from internally deposited radionuclides can induce some degree of immunologic suppression which, when combined with the direct carcinogenic effect of the radiation, might be related to early development of pulmonary neoplasms.

Research performed under AEC Contract AT(29-2)-1013.

EVIDENCE INDICATING MALFUNCTION OF COMPLEMENT AS A VITAL FACTOR IN THE EVOLUTION OF ACUTE LYMPHOCYTIC LEUKEMIA

R. Spitzer, D. Kalwinsky, J. Urmson, and A. Stitzel, SUNY Upstate Medical Center, Syracuse, New York.

In acute lymphocytic leukemia (ALL), data has been obtained to indicate that (1) at the time of diagnosis, there is a demonstrable defect in the ability of both the classical and alternative pathways of complement to be activated; (2) this defect disappears after induction of a remission and during maintenance but returns during a relapse; (3) as a reflection of this failure to be able to activate complement, serum levels of C4 (classical pathway) and properdin factor B (alternative pathway) are elevated at diagnosis or in relapse; (4) as a manifestation of the disappearance of this defect, there is a marked fall in serum C4 and factor B to levels far below the normal range at the end of induction and a trend toward normal during maintenance therapy. These findings are consistant with the concept that the complement system may play a role in the immune elimination of tumor cells in ALL and suggests that failure of this biologic system to function may be a determining factor in the evolution of this disease.

Seven children with ALL were studied serially and 7 patients were evaluated at the time of diagnosis or in relapse only. Ability of the classical pathway to be activated was determined by assaying consumption of C4 when an immune precipitate (IMP) was added to the patient's serum. Ability of the alternative pathway to be utilized was determined by consumption of C3-C9 on the addition of zymosan (Z) or cobra venom factor (CoF) to the patient's serum. Serum levels of C4 and C3-C9 were determined by hemolytic assays; serum levels of C3 and factor B (B) were quantitated by radial immunodiffusion. At diagnosis or in relapse: (1) 80% of sera failed to consume C4 with an IMP and 13 of 14 failed to consume C3-C9 with Z or CoF; (2) 65% of sera had levels of C4, C3 and B significantly greater than normal and only 1 serum (for B) was below normal. After induction: (1) all sera but 1 were able to react normally with Z or CoF and an IMP; (2) serum levels were significantly reduced in 4 of 7 patients for C4 and B and in 3 of 7 for C3. During maintenance: (1) all sera were normal on the addition of an IMP or Z; (2) in all sera, levels of C3 returned to normal; in all but 1, levels of B were normal; however, in 3 of 7 patients, C4 levels remained depressed.

THE EFFECT OF PLASMACYTOMAS ON IMMUNOGLOBULIN LEVELS
AND ON THE PRIMARY IMMUNE RESPONSE OF BALB/C MICE

H. Francis Havas and Marilyn Fenton, Department of Microbiology and Immunology, Temple University School of Medicine,
Philadelphia, Pennsylvania 19140, U.S.A.

Patients with multiple myeloma often suffer from severe
recurrent infections, accompanied by reduced normal immunoglobulin levels and an impaired immune response. A study
was therefore undertaken to elucidate the immunological
defect of the myeloma-bearing host using plasmacytoma-bearing
mice as a model. For this purpose the effect of tumor
growth on serum immunoglobulin levels and on the primary immune response (IR) was investigated in Balb/c mice bearing
MOPC-173 (Ig2a), MOPC-104E (IgM), MOPC-315 and MOPC-460
(IgA). Levels of IgG2, IgA, and IgM were measured by radial
immunodiffusion and compared with controls. The IR to sheep
red blood cells (SRBC) of tumor-bearing mice was measured by
the localized hemolysin in gel (LHG) technique and by passive
hemagglutination (HA).
The initial increase of the myeloma protein coincided
with the first appearance of the tumor and increased with its
progression. However the level of myeloma, protein did not
appear to correspond to the tumor size at death. The level
of other immunoglobulins decreased with time. The depression
effects on the immunoglobulin levels were unrelated to the
tumor type: an increase in IgM during the first week after
tumor injection in mice bearing IgA and IgG2 plasmacytomas
was followed by a decrease in IgM levels in all tumor-bearing
mice. IgG2 levels were decreased 6-fold in mice bearing
MOPC-315 (i.p.) and 3-fold in those with MOPC-104E. The
decreases in immunoglobulin levels were not due to tumor
growth per se because all levels of immunoglobulin were increased in the presence of Sarcoma 37, a pleomorphic neoplasm.
The primary IR was not suppressed in the myelomatous
mice following a high immunizing dosage of SRBC, as measured
by the LHG and HA tests; however, lower dosages had an effect
on the number of antibody secreting cells and on reducing
serum antibody levels. The implications of these findings
will be discussed.

PERSISTENT CELL MEDIATED IMMUNE DEFICIENCY FOLLOWING INFANTILE DIARRHEA.

W. Dutz, E. Rossipal, H. Ghavami and K. Vessal, Pahlavi University, Shiraz, Iran.

The growth and intercurrent diseases of 50 institution-alized orphans during the first year of life was recorded. Cell mediated immunity in the same infants at age 3 - 5 years was determined with 2,4 DNCB skin testing. 10% of the children were nonreactive, 40% showed only minimal reactivity. All of the nonreactive children suffered from severe infectious diarrhoea with marasmus and radiologically verified thymic atrophy before the age of 6 months. Other infants showed graded deficiencies related to infections in the first six months of life. Infections after this time do not seem to interfere with the development of the cell mediated immune response. The high suceptibility of people in developing nations to tuberculosis and other diseases related to cell mediated immune response, the high frequency and early onset of lymphoma and rapid ageing are probably at least partially related to persistent cell mediated immune deficiency.

IMMUNOSTIMULANT PROPERTIES OF AMPHOTERICIN B

T. Blanke, R. Little, R. Lynch, H. Lin and G. Medoff,
Washington University School of Medicine, St. Louis, Mo.

Immunological adjuvants have a potential role in the therapy of neoplastic and infectious diseases. We have ascribed immunostimulant properties to the polyene antibiotic Amphotericin B (AmB) because 1) it acts synergistically with 1,3, bis(2-chloroethyl)-1-nitrosourea (BCNU) in the cure of a transplantable AKR leukemia[1]; 2) it delays the development of spontaneous leukemia in AKR mice; and 3) it enhances resistance of mice to L. monocytogenes infection, and macrophages from recipient animals show enhanced phagocytosis and microbicidal activity[2]. We now report the stimulatory effects of AmB on murine humoral immune responses following immunization with trinitrophenylated human albumin (TNP-HSA) or sheep erythrocytes (SRBC), and on some of the biological effects of AmB on murine lymphocytes and lymphoid organs. AmB produces a concentration dependent cytotoxic effect which is most marked with thymocyte suspensions, lymph node and spleen cells exhibiting less susceptibility. Intraperitoneal (IP) administration of AmB also produces a reversible thymic involution with microscopic cortical depletion (2-5 days), and subsequently splenic weight and "red pulp" cellularity (8-11 days) increase significantly. Two to threefold increases in antibody titers result from a single IP administration of AmB accompanying immunization of mice with TNP-HSA or SRBC. Similarly AmB induces a two to threefold increase in IgM antibody-forming spleen cells in immunized mice. Other experiments indicate that AmB also affects T cell immune responses.

Since AmB is a chemically defined compound that binds to membrane sterols, these studies should provide insight into the cellular and molecular mechanisms of action of adjuvants.

REFERENCES

(1) G. Medoff, F. Valeriote, R. Lynch, D. Schlessinger and G. Kobayashi, Cancer Research 34 (1974) 974.

(2) M. Thomas, G. Medoff and G. Kobayashi, Journal of Infectious Diseases 127 (1973) 373.

THE IMMUNOTHERAPEUTIC AND ANTITUMOR PROPERTIES OF AMPHO-TERICIN B.

G. Medoff, F. Valeriote, R. Lynch and G.S. Kobayashi,
Washington University School of Medicine, St. Louis, Missouri

The use of the macrolide polyene antibiotic amphotericin B (AmB) in combination with 1,3-bis (2-chloroethyl)-1-nitrosourea (BCNU) to treat a transplanted AKR leukemia has cured a significant percentage of the animals of their leukemia (30%). Neither agent alone resulted in any cures (1). We think that the basis for the synergistic effect of the drug combination is an increased uptake of BCNU into the leukemic cells induced by the membrane effects of AmB, and a stimulation of host resistance to the tumor caused by the adjuvant properties of AmB.

Additional experiments with this system have shown that the cure rate of the leukemic mice can be increased by giving multiple injections of AmB and one injection of BCNU. Our present regimen of AmB 0.2 mgm intraperitoneally (I.P.), 1,2,3 and 4 days after injection of 10^6 leukemic cells; and BCNU 0.2 mgm on day 4 cures 60-80% of the mice. Similar to the single dose regimen, the combination results in an initial enhancement of the killing of leukemic cells over BCNU alone, followed by a period of stabilization of cell number, and then a complete disappearance of leukemic colony forming units from the femoral marrow (LCFU) (2).

The long term survivors have a high incidence of central nervous system (CNS) leukemia (25%). The pathology of the various treatment groups generally confirms the LCFU data, and also suggests that the CNS acts as a source for systemic dissemination in those long term survivors which develop late exacerbations of the leukemia.

We have also shown that AmB prophylaxis (0.5 mgm I.P. every 2 weeks) beginning at 8 weeks of age significantly delays the onset of spontaneous lymphoma in AKR mice. More-over some of the survivors of the AmB treated group died at 1 to 1-1/3 years of age of adenocarcinoma of the breast and had no evidence of lymphoma.

The significance of these findings in relation to human leukemia and the use of AmB in the treatment of malignancy will be discussed.

References:
1. Medoff, G. et al. Cancer Res. 34:974, 1974.
2. Bruce, W.R. and Van der Gaag, H. Nature 199:79, 1963.

ENHANCEMENT OF MYCOBACTERIA-INDUCED CELLULAR IMMUNE RESPONSES WITH ENDOTOXIN

H.B. Warner* and H.R. Strausser, Rutgers University, Newark, N.J. (*Presently at the New York State Institute for Basic Research in Mental Retardation, Staten Island, N.Y.)

Administration of systemic endotoxin at the appropriate time following a preparatory injection of complete adjuvant enhances a delayed hypersensitivity reaction in sensitized animals [1]. Endotoxin has been shown to stimulate both B cells and T cells[2]. The present study involves the effect of E. coli endotoxin systemically administered on local intracutaneous and renal fatpad lesions induced by Mycobacterium butyricum given 23-30 days earlier. The study was performed to determine if two different adjuvants could enhance a local tissue responsiveness. This would be important in the future treatment of neoplasma as well as providing a possible explanation for the mechanism of recurrent tissue destruction in certain autoimmune diseases.

One example of the enhancement of the local lesion is provided by the fact that when complete, Freund's adjuvant was administered intracutaneously to rabbits followed by E. coli endotoxin given intravenously 23 days later, hemorrhage and edema with surrounding necrosis occurred in most instances within 5-7 hours, whereas little or no evidence of this tissue destruction occurred with complete adjuvant alone. The lesions at this time contained a large number of macrophages and lymphocytes, typical of the classic delayed hypersensitivity response[3].

REFERENCES

1. J. Freund, J. Exp. Med. 60 (1934) 669.

2. A.C. Allison, P. Davis, and R.C. Page. J. Infect. Dis. S128 (1973) 128.

3. H.H. Gadebusch in "Macrophages and Cellular Immunity" (A. Laskin and H. Lechevalier, eds.) (1972) p. 7, CRC Press, Cleveland, Ohio.

MACROPHAGE MEDIATED ANTITUMOR ACTIVITY INDUCED BY A SYNTHETIC IMMUNOPOTENTIATOR (PYRAN)

P.S. Morahan, A.M. Kaplan, M.J. Snodgrass, and W. Regelson, Virginia Commonwealth University, Richmond, Virginia.

Treatment of mice with pyran (25mg/kg, i.p.), a synthetic polyanionic immunopotentiator, activates a population of macrophages which is capable of recognizing and destroying tumor cells, while being relatively nontoxic for normal mouse embryo fibroblasts. This tumor cell cytotoxicity, as shown by isotope release from ^{125}IUDR labelled cells, occurs primarily between 24 and 48 hr. Preliminary evidence indicates that pyran activated macrophages also exert a cytostatic effect on target cells.

Activated macrophages have also been recovered from the peritoneal cavity of pyran-treated mice bearing the Lewis lung carcinoma. These mice show a significant delay in tumor growth, and tumor metastasis, and prolongation of mean survival time (MST). The recovered macrophages are cytotoxic for other tumor cells in addition to the Lewis lung cells, but not for normal cells. Histopathological studies of tumors removed from the tumor-bearing mice protected with pyran have shown there is a greater histiocytic response in pyran-treated mice than in untreated tumor-bearing mice.

In addition to these lines of evidence for macrophage involvement in pyran activity against solid tumors, administration of pyran-activated macrophages to tumor bearing mice prolongs MST. Lewis lung carcinoma was implanted s.c., surgically excised on day 14 (when 100% of the mice show metastasis), and the mice injected 5 times with 10^7 activated peritoneal cells. Mice from whom the tumor was removed showed a MST of 34.0 ± 1.8 days, while macrophage treated mice showed a significantly prolonged MST of 41.6 ± 2.1 days. Thus, results from several different experimental approaches have implicated macrophages in the antitumor activity of pyran against solid tumors. (Supported in part by USPHS Grant CA1537 and Contract CB-43877).

ANTI-TUMOR EFFECT OF *C.PARVUM*: EFFECT ON THE IMMUNE RESPONSE
TO LIVE AND IRRADIATED TUMOUR. Abdul Ghaffar, University of
Edinburgh, Department of Surgery, University Medical School,
Teviot Place, Edinburgh, EH8 9AG, Scotland.

C. parvum given 3 days after live tumour inoculation retarded

the tumour growth in mice. Furthermore, immunization with

irradiated cell protected mice completely against a subse-

quent challenge with live cells. However, if *C. parvum* was

administered prior to immunization with irradiated cells it

partially abolished the protective effect of irradiated cells.

The mechanism of *C. parvum* action has been investigated and

will be discussed.

GRAFT VERSUS LEUKEMIA VI. ADOPTIVE IMMUNOTHERAPY IN COMBINATION WITH CHEMORADIOTHERAPY FOR AKR SPONTANEOUS LEUKEMIA-LYMPHOMA[1]

Mortimer M. Bortin, Alfred A. Rimm, William Rose, Robert L. Truitt and Edward C. Saltzstein, Mount Sinai Medical Center and The Medical College of Wisconsin, Milwaukee, WI 53233

Following clinical diagnosis of spontaneous leukemia-lymphoma, AKR ($H-2^k$) mice were randomized and entered into a test group, or one of three concurrent control groups. Test mice were treated with adoptive immunotherapy in combination with chemoradiotherapy. The chemoradiotherapeutic regimen caused tumor cytoreduction and was sufficiently immunosuppressive to assure engraftment of immunocompetent cells from allogeneic donors (adoptive immunotherapy). A total of 40 leukemic AKR mice were given bone marrow and lymph node cells from histoincompatible DBA/2 ($H-2^d$) mice. After 6 days the mice were "rescued" from graft-versus-host disease by killing the DBA/2 cells and restoring hematopoiesis using cells transplanted from histocompatible RF ($H-2^k$) donors. From the last day of treatment, the median survival time (MST) was 56 days, and 45% (18/40) survived more than 60 days.

The MST of 22 untreated mice was 17 days, and none of the mice survived 60 days. A total of 17 leukemic AKR mice received the full chemoradiotherapeutic regimen, but no transplant. From the last day of treatment, the MST was 16 days, and none survived 60 days. A final control group of 30 leukemic AKR mice received the full chemoradiotherapeutic regimen plus two transplants of bone marrow and lymph node cells from non-leukemic AKR donors (in place of cells from DBA/2 and RF donors). From the last day of treatment the MST was 18 days, and 17% (5/30) survived more than 60 days.

Thus, adoptive immunotherapy plus chemoradiotherapy resulted in significant prolongation of MST, and a significantly greater proportion of 60-day survivors when compared with untreated controls, chemoradiotherapy controls, or control mice that received cells from syngeneic donors ($P < 0.05$ to < 0.001).

[1]Research supported by NIH Contract N01-CB-33853 and the Trustees, Mount Sinai Medical Center

A MODEL FOR DETERMINING THE MINIMAL RESIDUAL TUMOR CELL NUMBERS

R.N. Hiramoto and V.K. Ghanta, Department of Microbiology, University of Alabama in Birmingham, Birmingham, Alabama

The general principles of cancer chemotherapy based on cell cycle nonspecific (CCNS) and cell cycle specific (CCS) agents and drug cell-kill kinetics, are fairly well understood. The development of therapeutic programs based on first order kill kinetics are theoretically sound. They require repeated use of near toxic levels of drugs over long periods of time, which inevitably leads to resistant cell lines.

Immunotherapy by virtue of its specificity could be a logical means to destroy the small foci of drug resistant mutants that might arise. An animal model that can simulate as in humans the entire course of tumor growth under partially effective chemotherapy is required. The necessary conditions that such an animal model must meet are, 1) all assessments must be made in a single animal; 2) the animal must be allowed to bear large numbers of tumor cells which can be numerically assessed accurately at any time interval during the tumor growth period; 3) the tumor cells must be disseminated to other parts of the body; 4) the tumor number must be experimentally reduced to a minimal number by a partially effective chemotherapy regimen; and 5) the absolute number of viable residual tumor cells at any instant of time must be assessed during the period of cell kill.

If all of the above conditions can be met, we could establish the minimum number of tumor cells that the original tumor mass must be reduced to before immunotherapy with either humoral antibody or a cell mediated response can be used effectively. Experiments are designed to see whether a model which can meet essentially all of the requirements outlined. 1) All assessments of tumor numbers were carried out in individual mice in which tumor was disseminated by i.v. injection of 1×10^6 cells at day 0. The tumor grew linearly from day 10 to 21 at which time the tumor cell numbers ranged from 0.26-2.9×10^9 cells/mouse. 2) Tumor cell numbers were experimentally reduced with cytoxan (200 mg/kg, i.p.) on day 21 and the number of viable cells were determined during the period of tumor cell kill. By day 39 the minimal number of tumor cells detectable were reduced to 1-2×10^6 cells/mouse. The model is useful to establish minimal number of residual tumor cells which could be successfully eliminated by immunotherapeutic modalities.

IMMUNOFLUORESCENT IDENTIFICATION OF DNA REPLICATION IN SINGLE CELLS WITH ANTI-BRDU ANTIBODIES

H.G. Gratzner, R.C. Leif, D.J. Ingram and A. Castro, Papanicolaou Cancer Research Institute, Miami, Fla. 33136.

Antibodies specific for 5-bromodeoxyuridine (BrdU) were produced in rabbits[1] with the antigen, Bromouridine-Bovine serum albumin (BSA-BrU)[2].

Studies of the antiserum by double-diffusion in agarose demonstrated that a single precipitin band was present with BSA-BrU and undiluted antiserum, with some slight cross reaction with BSA-Thymidine. Titers determined by microcomplement fixation were: 1/400 for BSA-BrU, 1/2400 for denatured BrdU-DNA, 1/50 denatured DNA, 1/50 for BSA.

Antibody specific for BrdU was produced by affinity chromotography[3] on sepharose 4B-Bromouridine columns.

Immunofluorescence studies with cultured cells demonstrated that fluorescent antibody (indirect) can be used to detect recently replicated BrdU-labeled DNA in single cells. The addition of BrdU to antiserum used to stain fixed cells eliminates fluorescence, whereas addition of thymidine does not. The technique has been applied to studies of cell kinetics by fluorescence methods. Cultured cells in S phase can be detected, and the labeling indices correspond to those found with the classical autoradiographic method utilizing (^{3}H) TdR.

Supported by NCI Grant CA 13441, NCI contracts NO1-CB-43962, and NO1-CB-33861.

REFERENCES

(1) B.F. Erlanger, S.M. Beiser, Proc. Nat'l. Acad. Sci. USA 52 (1964) 68.
(2) D.L. Sanicri, B.F. Erlanger, S.M. Beiser, Science 174 (1971) 70.
(3) D. Eichler and D.G. Glitz, Biochim. Biophys. Acta. 335 (1974) 303.

A 5
B 6
C 7
D 8
E 9
F 0
G 1
H 2
I 3
J 4